YO-BCF-906

HIV ESSENTIALS

Fourth Edition

Paul E. Sax, MD
Clinical Director
Division of Infectious Disease and HIV Program
Brigham and Women's Hospital
Associate Professor of Medicine
Harvard Medical School
Boston, MA

Co-Editors

Calvin J. Cohen, MD, MS
Director of Research
Community Research Initiative of New England
Instructor of Medicine
Harvard Medical School
Boston, MA

Daniel R. Kuritzkes, MD
Director of AIDS Research
Brigham and Women's Hospital
Associate Professor of Medicine
Harvard Medical School
Boston, MA

2011

JONES & BARTLETT
LEARNING

1404496
AUG 31 2011

World Headquarters

Jones & Bartlett Learning
40 Tall Pine Drive
Sudbury, MA 01776
978-443-5000
info@jblearning.com
www.jblearning.com

Jones & Bartlett
   Learning Canada
6339 Ormindale Way
Mississauga, ON L5V 1J2
Canada

Jones & Bartlett
   Learning International
Barb House, Barb Mews
London W6 7PA
United Kingdom

Jones & Bartlett Learning books and products are available through most bookstores and online booksellers.
To contact Jones & Bartlett Learning directly, call 800-832-0034, fax 978-443-8000, or visit our website at
www.jblearning.com.

Substantial discounts on bulk quantities of Jones & Bartlett Learning publications are available to corporations,
professional associations, and other qualified organizations. For details and specific discount information,
contact the special sales department at Jones & Bartlett Learning via the above contact information or send an
email to specialsales@jblearning.com.

Production Credits

Executive Publisher: Christopher Davis
Editorial Assistant: Sara Cameron
Production Director: Amy Rose
Senior Production Editor: Daniel Stone
Medicine Marketing Manager: Rebecca Rockel
V.P., Manufacturing and Inventory Control: Therese Connell

Composition: diacriTech, Chennai, India
Cover Design: Kristin E. Parker
Printing and Binding: Cenveo, Inc.
Cover Printing: Cenveo, Inc.

ISBN-13: 978-1-4496-1339-6

6048

Printed in the United States of America
14 13 12 11 10   10 9 8 7 6 5 4 3 2 1

EDITORIAL NOTE

Over the last several years, HIV treatment has improved substantially—so much so that virtually every patient who is able to take antiretroviral therapy can achieve virologic suppression, even those with extensive resistance from prior treatment eras. Clinicians continue to gain further experience with the newest of our antiretroviral agents (maraviroc, raltegravir, and etravirine), and are incorporating them (especially raltegravir) increasingly into earlier lines of therapy. With the extraordinary success of currently-available regimens, emphasis has shifted in many patients from the sole goal of suppressing viremia to the long term need to prevent and manage non-HIV related complications, in particular cardiovascular disease and malignancies.

The goal of this guide is to provide practitioners actively involved in HIV care with rapid access to practical information useful for patient management. When possible, we have cited US national guidelines from the Department of Health and Human Services and the International AIDS Society–USA; these are available at aidsinfo.nih.gov or www.iasusa.org respectively, and readers are advised to check these sites for the most recent updates. We have also provided recommendations based on our interpretation of clinical trials, cohort studies, case reports, and personal experience.

We continue to dedicate this volume to people living with HIV who have partnered with us to learn how to manage this condition, and to the doctors, nurses, social workers, pharmacists, and other healthcare professionals who focus on HIV as a specialty and continue to teach us how to get better at what we do.

Paul E. Sax, MD
Calvin J. Cohen, MD, MS
Daniel R. Kuritzkes, MD

TABLES AND FIGURES

TABLE OF CONTENTS

CONTRIBUTORS

Paul E. Sax, MD
Clinical Director, Division of
  Infectious Diseases and HIV Program
Brigham and Women's Hospital
Associate Professor of Medicine
Harvard Medical School
Boston, Massachusetts

Calvin J. Cohen, MD, MS
Director of Research, Community
  Research Initiative of New England
Instructor of Medicine
Harvard Medical School
Boston, Massachusetts

Daniel R. Kuritzkes, MD
Director of AIDS Research
Brigham and Women's Hospital
Associate Professor of Medicine
Harvard Medical School
Boston, Massachusetts

Burke A. Cunha, MD
Chief, Infectious Disease Division
Winthrop-University Hospital
Mineola, New York
Professor of Medicine
SUNY School of Medicine
Stony Brook, New York

David W. Kubiak, PharmD, BCPS
Infectious Disease Clinical Pharmacist
Brigham and Women's Hospital
Adjunct Clinical Assistant
Professor of Pharmacy
Bouvé College of Health Sciences
School of Pharmacy
Northeastern University
Boston, Massachusetts

Damary C. Torres, PharmD
Clinical Pharmacy Specialist
Winthrop-University Hospital
Mineola, New York
Associate Clinical Professor of Pharmacy
College of Pharmacy
St. John's University
Queens, New York

Athe Tsibris, MD
Instructor in Medicine
Harvard Medical School
Massachusetts General Hospital
Boston, Massachusetts

Ruth Tuomala, MD
Director of Ob/Gyn Infectious Diseases
Brigham and Women's Hospital
Assistant Professor of Obstetrics,
Gynecology, and Reproductive Biology
Harvard Medical School
Boston, Massachusetts

ACKNOWLEDGMENTS

To accomplish the task of presenting the data compiled in this reference, a small, dedicated team of professionals was assembled. This team focused their energy and discipline for many months into typing, revising, designing, illustrating, and formatting the many chapters that make up this text. We wish to acknowledge Monica Crowder Kaufman for her important contribution. We would also like to thank the many contributors who graciously contributed their time and energy.

Paul E. Sax, MD
Calvin J. Cohen, MD, MS
Daniel R. Kuritzkes, MD

NOTICE

ABBREVIATIONS FOR ANTIRETROVIRAL AGENTS

3TC	lamivudine	FTC	emtricitabine
ABC	abacavir	IDV	indinavir
ATV	atazanavir	LPV/r	lopinavir/ritonavir
d4T	stavudine	MVC	maraviroc
ddC	zalcitabine	NFV	nelfinavir
ddI	didanosine	NVP	nevirapine
DLV	delavirdine	RAL	raltegravir
DRV	darunavir	RTV	ritonavir
EFV	efavirenz	SQV	saquinavir
ENF	enfuvirtide	TDF	tenofovir disoproxil fumarate
ETR	etravirine	TPV	tipranavir
FPV	fosamprenavir	ZDV	zidovudine

OTHER ABBREVIATIONS

AFB	acid fast bacilli	Enterobacteriaceae:	Citrobacter,
ALT	alanine transferase		Edwardsiella, Enterobacter, E. coli,
ANC	absolute neutrophil count		Klebsiella, Proteus, Providencia,
ARC	AIDS-related complex		Salmonella, Serratia, Shigella
ARDS	adult respiratory distress syndrome	ESR	erythrocyte sedimentation rate
ART	antiretroviral therapy	ESRD	end-stage renal disease
AST	aspartamine transferase	ET	endotracheal
β-lactams	penicillins, cephalosporins,	FUO	fever of unknown origin
	cephamycins (not monobactams	GI	gastrointestinal
	or carbapenems)	gm	gram
BAL	bronchoalveolar lavage	GU	genitourinary
BID	twice daily	HSV	herpes simplex virus
ICU	intensive care unit	HU	hydroxyurea
CD4	CD4 T-cell lymphocyte	I & D	incision and drainage
CIE	counter-immunoelectrophoresis	IFA	immunofluorescent antibody
CMV	cytomegalovirus	IgA	immunoglobulin A
CNS	central nervous system	IgG	immunoglobulin G
CPK	creatine phosphokinase	IgM	immunoglobulin M
CrCl	creatinine clearance	IM	intramuscular
CSF	cerebrospinal fluid	INH	isoniazid
CT	computerized tomography	INSTI	integrase strand
DFA	direct fluorescent antibody		transfer inhibitor
DIC	disseminated intravascular coagulation	IRIS	immune reconstitution
DNA	deoxyribonucleic acid		inflammatory syndrome
DS	double strength	IV/PO	IV or PO
e.g.	for example	IV	intravenous
ELISA	enzyme-linked immunosorbent assay	kg	kilogram
EMB	ethambutol	L	liter
ENT	ear, nose, throat	LFT	liver function test

MAC	*Mycobacterium avium* complex	PZA	pyrazinamide
mcg	microgram	q__d	every__days
mcL	microliter	q__h	every__hours
mg	milligram	QD	once daily
mL	milliliter	qmonth	once a month
min	minute	qweek	once a week
MRI	magnetic resonance imaging	RBC	red blood cells
MRSA	methicillin-resistant *S. aureus*	RBV	ribavirin
MSSA	methicillin-sensitive *S. aureus*	RNA	ribonucleic acid
NNRTI	non-nucleoside reverse transcriptase inhibitor	RT-PCR	reverse-transcriptase polymerase chain reaction
NRTI	nucleoside reverse transcriptase inhibitor	SGOT/SGPT	serum transaminases
		SLE	systemic lupus erythematosus
NSAID	nonsteroidal anti-inflammatory drug	sp.	species
OI	opportunistic infection	SQ	subcutaneous
PBS	protected brush specimen	SS	single strength
PCP	*Pneumocystis jirovecii* (carinii) pneumonia	TB	tuberculosis
		TID	three times per day
PCR	polymerase chain reaction	TMP	trimethoprim
PI	protease inhibitor	TMP-SMX	trimethoprim-sulfamethoxazole
PMN	polymorphonuclear leucocytes	VCA	viral capsid antigen
PPD	purified protein derivative	VZV	varicella zoster virus
PO	oral	WBC	white blood cells

Chapter 1

Overview of HIV Infection

OVERVIEW OF HIV INFECTION

Infection with Human Immunodeficiency Virus (HIV-1) leads to a chronic and, without treatment usually fatal infection characterized by progressive immunodeficiency, a long clinical latency period, and opportunistic infections. The hallmark of HIV disease is infection and viral replication within T-lymphocytes expressing the CD4 antigen (helper-inducer lymphocytes), a critical component of normal cell-mediated immunity. Qualitative defects in CD4 responsiveness and progressive depletion in CD4 cell counts increase the risk for opportunistic infections such as *Pneumocystis jiroveci (carinii)* pneumonia, and neoplasms such as lymphoma and Kaposi's sarcoma. HIV infection can also disrupt blood monocyte, tissue macrophage, and B-lymphocyte (humoral immunity) function, predisposing to infection with encapsulated bacteria. Direct attack of CD4-positive cells in the central and peripheral nervous system can cause HIV meningitis, peripheral neuropathy, and dementia.

More than 1 million people in the United States and 30 million people worldwide are infected with HIV. Without treatment, the average time from acquisition of HIV to an AIDS-defining opportunistic infection is about 10 years; survival then averages 1–2 years. There is tremendous individual variability in these time intervals, with some patients progressing from acute HIV infection to death within 1–2 years, and others not manifesting HIV-related immunosuppression for > 20 years after HIV acquisition. Antiretroviral therapy and prophylaxis against opportunistic infections have markedly improved the overall prognosis of HIV disease. The approach to HIV infection is shown in Figure 1.1.

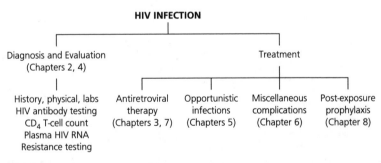

Figure 1.1. Approach to HIV Infection

STAGES OF HIV INFECTION

A. **Viral Transmission.** HIV infection is acquired primarily by sexual intercourse (anal, vaginal, infrequently oral), exposure to contaminated blood (through sharing of needles by injection drug users, less commonly transfusion of contaminated blood products), or maternal-fetal (perinatal) transmission. Sexual practices with the highest risk of transmission include unprotected receptive anal intercourse (especially with mucosal tearing), unprotected receptive vaginal intercourse (especially during menses), and unprotected rectal/vaginal intercourse in the presence of genital ulcers (e.g., primary syphilis, genital herpes, chancroid). Lower risk sexual practices include insertive anal/vaginal intercourse and oral-genital contact. The risk of transmission after a single encounter with an HIV source has been estimated to be 1 in 150 with needle sharing, 1 in 300 with occupational percutaneous exposure, 1 in 300–1000 with receptive anal intercourse, 1 in 500–1250 with receptive vaginal intercourse, 1 in 1000–3000 with insertive vaginal intercourse, and 1 in 3000 with insertive anal intercourse. Transmission risk increases with the number of encounters and when the source of infection has higher HIV RNA plasma levels (Lancet 2001;357:1149–53). The mode of transmission does not affect the natural history of HIV disease, though patients with active or past injection drug use may have shortened survival due to comorbid complications (AIDS 2007;21:1185–97).

B. **Acute (Primary) HIV Infection (pp. 4–5).** Acute HIV occurs 1–4 weeks after transmission and is accompanied by a burst of viral replication with a decline in CD4 cell count. Most patients manifest a symptomatic mononucleosis-like syndrome, which is often overlooked. Acute HIV infection is confirmed by demonstrating a high HIV RNA in the absence of HIV antibody.

C. **Seroconversion.** Development of a positive HIV antibody test usually occurs within 4 weeks of acute infection, and invariably (with few exceptions) by 6 months.

D. **Asymptomatic HIV Infection.** Asymptomatic HIV lasts a variable amount of time (average 8–10 years) and is accompanied by a gradual decline in CD4 cell counts and a relatively stable HIV RNA level (sometimes referred to as the viral "set point").

E. **Early Symptomatic HIV Infection.** Previously referred to as "AIDS Related Complex (ARC)," findings include thrush or vaginal candidiasis (persistent, frequent, or poorly responsive to treatment), herpes zoster (recurrent episodes or involving multiple dermatomes), oral hairy leukoplakia, peripheral neuropathy, diarrhea, or constitutional symptoms (e.g., low-grade fevers, weight loss).

F. **AIDS is defined** by a CD4 cell count < 200/mm³, a CD4 cell percentage of total lymphocytes < 14%, or one of several AIDS-related opportunistic infections. Common opportunistic infections include *Pneumocystis jiroveci (carinii)* pneumonia, cryptococcal meningitis, recurrent bacterial pneumonia, *Candida esophagitis*, CNS toxoplasmosis, tuberculosis, and non-Hodgkin's lymphoma. Other AIDS indicators in HIV-infected patients include candidiasis of the bronchi, trachea, or lungs; disseminated/extrapulmonary coccidiomycosis, cryptococcosis, or histoplasmosis; chronic (> 1 month) intestinal cryptosporidiosis or isosporiasis; Kaposi's sarcoma; lymphoid interstitial pneumonia/pulmonary lymphoid hyperplasia; disseminated/extrapulmonary mycobacterial (non-tuberculous) infection; progressive multifocal leukoencephalopathy (PML); recurrent *Salmonella septicemia*; or HIV wasting syndrome.

G. Advanced HIV Disease corresponds with a CD4 cell count < $50/mm^3$. Most AIDS-related deaths occur at this point. Common late stage opportunistic infections are caused by CMV disease (retinitis, colitis) or disseminated *Mycobacterium avium* complex (MAC).

ACUTE (PRIMARY) HIV INFECTION

A. Description. Acute clinical illness associated with primary acquisition of HIV, occurring 1–4 weeks after viral transmission (range: 6 days to 6 weeks). Symptoms develop in 50–90%, but are often mistaken for the flu, mononucleosis, or other nonspecific viral syndrome. More severe symptoms may correlate with a higher viral set point and more rapid HIV disease progression (J AIDS 2007;45:445–8). Even without therapy, most patients recover, reflecting development of a partially effective immune response and depletion of susceptible CD4 cells. Unfortunately, damage to the immune system through depletion of the gut-associated lymphoid tissue occurs rapidly (AIDS 2007;21:1–11) and may not be preventable even with effective ART.

B. Differential Diagnosis includes **EBV, CMV**, viral hepatitis, enteroviral infection, secondary syphilis, toxoplasmosis, HSV with erythema multiforme, drug reaction, Behçet's disease, acute lupus.

C. Signs and Symptoms usually reflect hematogenous dissemination of virus to lymphoreticular and neurologic sites (N Engl J Med 1998;339:33–9):
- Fever (97%).
- Pharyngitis (73%). Typically non-exudative (unlike EBV, which is usually exudative).
- Rash (77%). Maculopapular viral exanthem of the face and trunk is most common, but can involve the extremities, palms and soles.
- Arthralgia/myalgia (58%).
- Neurologic symptoms (12%). Headache is most common. Neuropathy, Bell's palsy, and meningoencephalitis are rare, but may predict worse outcome.
- Oral/genital ulcerations, thrush, nausea, vomiting, diarrhea, weight loss.

D. Laboratory Findings
  1. CBC. Lymphopenia followed by lymphocytosis (common). Atypical lymphocytosis is variable, but usually low level (unlike EBV, where atypical lymphocytosis may be 20–30% or higher). Thrombocytopenia occurs in some.

2. **Elevated Transaminases** in some but not all patients.

3. **Depressed CD4 Cell Count.** Can rarely be low enough to induce opportunistic infections, most commonly PCP or mucosal candidiasis.

4. **HIV Antibody.** Usually negative, although persons with prolonged symptoms of acute HIV may have positive antibody tests if diagnosed late during the course of illness.

E. **Confirming the Diagnosis of Acute HIV Infection**
   1. **Obtain HIV Antibody** to exclude prior disease.

   2. **Order Viral Load Test** (HIV RNA PCR), preferably RT-PCR. HIV RNA confirms acute HIV infection prior to seroconversion when the HIV antibody test is concurrently negative. Most individuals will have very high HIV RNA (> 100,000 copies/mL). Be suspicious of a false-positive test if the HIV RNA is low (< 10,000 copies/mL) (J Infect Dis 2004;190:598–604). For any positive test, it is important to repeat HIV RNA and HIV antibody testing. p24 antigen can also be used to establish the diagnosis, but is less sensitive than HIV RNA PCR.

   3. **Order Other Tests/Serologies if HIV RNA Test is Negative.** Order throat cultures for bacterial/viral respiratory pathogens, EBV VCA IgM/IgG, CMV IgM/IgG, HHV-6 IgM/IgG, and hepatitis serologies as appropriate to establish a diagnosis for patient's symptoms.

F. **Management of Acute HIV Infection**
   1. **Initiate Antiretroviral Therapy.** Patients with acute HIV infection should be referred to an HIV specialist, who ideally will enroll the patient into a clinical study. Some clinicians recommend antiretroviral therapy for patients who are highly symptomatic or have severe disease, although no long-term clinical studies comparing treatment vs. observation have been conducted. The optimal duration of therapy and role of intermittent treatment are under investigation. Regimens for treatment are similar to those outlined for chronic HIV infection (Table 3.3). Some clinicians elect to start with PI-based treatment given the higher risk of transmitted NNRTI than PI resistance.

   2. **Obtain HIV Resistance Genotype** (Chapter 4) because of the possibility of transmission of antiretroviral therapy-resistant virus. A genotype resistance test is preferred; therapy can be started pending results of the test. Again, because transmitted NNRTI resistance completely reduces the activity of initial NNRTI-based therapy, initial treatment with two NRTIs plus a boosted PI is preferred in this setting. If no NNRTI resistance is detected on genotype, therapy may be changed if indicated.

   3. **Rationale for Treatment of Acute HIV Infection.** No prospective clinical studies have conclusively documented the benefits of therapy for acute HIV infection. Possible benefits include hastening symptom resolution, reducing viral transmission, lowering virologic "set point," and preserving virus-specific CD4 responses. Eradication of HIV is not possible with currently available agents (Nat Med 2003;9:727–8).

Chapter 2

Diagnosis and Evaluation of HIV Infection

HIV ANTIBODY TESTING

A. Standard HIV Antibody Tests (see also Clin Infect Dis 2007;45:S221–S225). HIV antibody tests (ELISA, Western blot) and quantitative plasma HIV RNA (HIV viral load) assays are used to diagnose HIV infection (Figure 2.1). Most patients produce antibody to HIV within 6–8 weeks of exposure; 50% will have a positive antibody test by 3–4 weeks, and nearly 100% will have detectable antibody by 6 months.

   1. ELISA. Usual screening test. All positives are routinely confirmed with Western blot or other more specific tests.

   2. Western Blot. CDC criteria for interpretation:

   a. Positive. At least two of the following bands present: p24, gp41, gp160/120

   b. Negative. No bands present

   c. Indeterminate. HIV band present, but does not meet criteria for positivity

   3. Test Performance. Standard method is ELISA screen with Western blot confirmation.

   a. ELISA negative. Western blot is not required (ELISA sensitivity 99.7%, specificity 98.5%). Obtain HIV RNA if acute HIV infection is suspected.

   b. ELISA positive. Laboratories will confirm results with Western blot. Probability that ELISA and Western blot are both false-positives is extremely low (< 1 per 140,000). Absence of p31 band could be a clue to a false positive Western blot.

   c. Unexpected ELISA/Western blot. Repeat test to exclude clerical/computer error, the most common cause of incorrect results.

   4. Indeterminate Western Blot. This occurs in approximately 4–20% of reactive ELISAs, usually due to a single p24 band or weak other bands. HIV-related causes include seroconversion in progress, advanced HIV disease with loss of antibody response, or infection with HIV-2. Non-HIV-related causes include cross-reacting antibody from pregnancy, blood transfusions, organ transplantation, autoantibodies from collagen vascular disease, influenza vaccination, or recipient of HIV vaccine. In low-risk patients, an indeterminate result rarely represents true HIV infection. Since seroconversion-in-progress is generally associated with high HIV RNA levels, the recommended approach is to obtain an HIV RNA test. In addition, most patients with indeterminate Western blots due to seroconversion-in-progress will develop a fully positive HIV test within 1 month.

B. Other HIV Antibody Tests

   1. Home Test Kit (Home Access HIV-1 Test System). This system can be purchased over-the-counter at pharmacies, or ordered by phone or over the Internet (www.homeaccess.com). Users receive a kit that includes a stylet for obtaining a sample of blood from the fingertip, which is then placed on filter paper and mailed to the company for testing. The standard test will return a result within 7 days and costs $44; users can purchase overnight shipping for an additional cost and a more rapid turnaround time. By using a code provided with each kit, users can call and obtain their results anonymously. Phone counseling is available to explain the results, as well as a database of local HIV providers if the test result is positive. The Home Access test employs ELISA testing, which is done in duplicate. All individuals with reactive tests on the system must have results confirmed by standard testing. As of 2009, there is no true home test that returns results to the user without the involvement of a central laboratory or healthcare facility; such tests are technically feasible and are being reviewed by the FDA.

2. **OraSure.** This office-based test was approved in 1996 and uses a special swab that collects oral mucosal transudate (not saliva) when it is held between the cheek and the gum. This system obtains quantities of antibody that are comparable to or exceed those from serum samples. Once the specimen is collected, it is sent to a central laboratory for ELISA and Western blot testing, which can be performed on the same sample. As a result, the sensitivity and specificity of the test are comparable to standard blood HIV antibody testing (JAMA 1997;277:254).

3. **Rapid HIV Tests (OraQuick ADVANCE Rapid HIV Test; Uni-Gold Recombigen HIV).** The OraQuick was approved in 2004 and can be performed on whole blood, plasma, or oral mucosal transudate samples. The UniGold test is limited to blood samples. Results are returned in 10–20 minutes and are comparable in accuracy to a single ELISA test. As a result, *a reactive rapid test must be confirmed with standard ELISA/Western blot serology.* A major advantage of this rapid test includes the ability to give patients a negative result at the time of care; there also is some evidence that individuals given a positive rapid test result are more likely to return for their confirmative serology results. Since the test can be done at the point of care (no CLIA certification is required), it is particularly useful in the evaluation of source patients of needlestick injuries and for women in labor who did not receive HIV testing during prenatal care. There have been reports of high rates of false positive rapid tests when oral samples are used in low-prevalence settings (Ann Intern Med 2008 Aug 5;149[3]:153–60); as a result, some sites have switched to using blood rapid testing, either with the OraQuick or the Uni-Gold.

C. **Selected Other Licensed HIV Diagnostic Tests**

1. **p24 Antigen.** Approved for diagnosis of acute HIV infection. However, due to low sensitivity of this test, HIV RNA has replaced p24 antigen in clinical practice, and hence this test is rarely ordered.

2. **Nucleic Acid Based Tests.** In the United States, donated blood has been screened with nucleic acid based tests since the late 1990s, shortening the time between infection and detectability of infection to about 12 days. As a result, the rate of acquiring HIV from a blood transfusion is now estimated at one infection per 2 million units transfused (JAMA 2003;289:959). A related test, the Aptima HIV-1 RNA Qualitative Assay, was approved for HIV diagnosis in 2006. Like quantitative HIV RNA tests, this assay can be used to diagnose acute HIV infection before antibodies develop, but results are provided only as positive or negative. Additionally, it can confirm HIV infection in a person with a positive HIV ELISA or rapid test. It is not known whether the rate of false positivity with the Aptima test is lower than the rate with RT-PCR or bDNA.

3. **ARCHITECT HIV Antigen/Antibody Combination Assay (Abbott).** Licensed for use in the United States in 2010, this is the first test that can detect both HIV antibody and

p24 antigen. As such, it turns positive before standard ELISA testing, hence shortens the window period between HIV acquisition and detection of antibody. The test can be run on a similar laboratory platform as some HIV antibody tests from this company. The sensitivity of the test for acute HIV compared with HIV RNA testing is not known.

QUANTITATIVE PLASMA HIV RNA (HIV VIRAL LOAD ASSAYS)

HIV viral load assays measure the amount of HIV RNA in plasma. The high sensitivity of these assays allows detection of virus in most patients not on antiretroviral therapy. These tests are used to diagnose acute HIV infection, and more commonly to monitor the response to antiretroviral therapy.

A. **Uses of HIV RNA Assay**

1. **Confirms Diagnosis of Acute HIV Infection.** A high HIV RNA with a negative HIV antibody test confirms acute HIV infection prior to seroconversion.

2. **Helps in Initial Evaluation of HIV Infection.** Establishes baseline HIV RNA and helps (along with CD4 cell count) determine whether to initiate or defer therapy, as HIV RNA correlates with rate of CD4 decline (Ann Intern Med 1997 Jun 15;126[12]:946–54). Of note, baseline HIV RNA is not as strong a determinant of the indication for therapy as the CD4 cell count.

3. **Monitors Response to Antiviral Therapy.** HIV RNA changes rapidly decline 2–4 weeks after starting or changing effective antiretroviral therapy, with slower decline thereafter. Patients who achieve virologic suppression (less than 50 copies per mL) have the most durable response to antiviral therapy and the best clinical prognosis. No change in HIV RNA suggests that therapy will be ineffective or the patient is noncompliant.

4. **Estimates Risk for Opportunistic Infection.** For patients with similar CD4 cell counts, the risk of opportunistic infections is higher with higher HIV RNAs. HIV RNA is not formally incorporated into opportunistic infection prevention guidelines.

B. **Assays and Interpretation**

1. **Tests, Sensitivities, and Dynamic Range.** Several assays are used, each with advantages and disadvantages; most US sites use RT-PCR or bDNA. Any assay can be used to diagnose acute HIV infection and guide/monitor therapy, but the same test should be used to follow patients longitudinally.

    a. **RT-PCR Amplicor** (Roche): Sensitivity = 400 copies/mL; dynamic range = 400–750,000 copies/mL

    b. **RT-PCR Ultrasensitive 1.5** (Roche): Sensitivity = 50 copies/mL; dynamic range = 50–75,000 copies/mL

    c. **bDNA Versant 3.0** (Bayer): Sensitivity = 75 copies/mL; dynamic range = 75–500,000 copies/mL

    d. **Nucleic acid sequence-based amplification** (NASBA), NucliSens HIV-1 QT (bioMerieux). Sensitivity = 176 copies/mL; dynamic range = 176–3.5 million copies/mL (depends on volume)

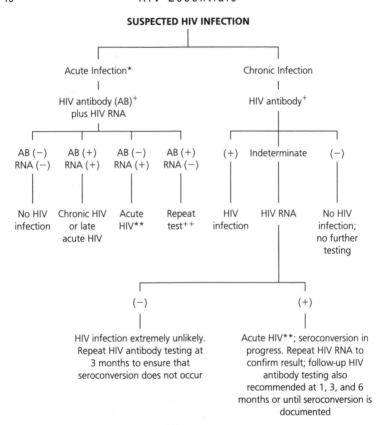

Figure 2.1. Approach to HIV Testing

(−) negative test; (+) positive test

*   Occurs 1–4 weeks after viral transmission. Most patients manifest a viral syndrome (fever, pharyngitis ± rash/arthralgias), which is often mistaken for mononucleosis or the flu and therefore overlooked

** HIV RNA in acute HIV infection should be very high (usually > 100,000 copies/mL)

+   All positive ELISA tests must be confirmed by Western blot; usually this is done automatically in clinical laboratories

++ May be long-term non-progressor or laboratory error

    e. Real Time HIV-1 assay (Abbott): PCR-based assay. Sensitivity = 40 copies/mL; dynamic range = 40–10 million copies/mL

    f. COBAS AmpliPrep/COBAS TagMan HIV-1 test (Roche): Sensitivity = 48 copies/mL; dynamic range = 48–10 million copies/mL

2. **Correlation Between HIV RNA and CD4 Cell Count.** HIV RNA assays correlate inversely with CD4 cell counts, but do so imperfectly (e.g., some patients with high CD4 counts have relatively high HIV RNA levels, and vice versa.) For any given CD4, higher HIV RNA levels correlate with more rapid CD4 decline. In response to antiretroviral therapy, changes in HIV RNA generally precede changes in CD4 cell count.

3. **Significant Change in HIV RNA Assay.** This is defined by at least a 2-fold (0.3 log) change in viral RNA (accounts for normal variation in clinically stable patients), or a 3-fold (0.5 log) change in response to new antiretroviral therapy (accounts for intralaboratory and patient variability). For example, if a HIV RNA result = 50,000 copies/mL, then the range of possible actual values = 25,000–100,000 copies/mL, and the value needed to demonstrate antiretroviral activity is ≤ 17,000 copies/mL.

C. Indications for HIV RNA Testing. This test is usually performed in conjunction with CD4 cell counts, and is indicated for the diagnosis of acute HIV infection and for initial evaluation of newly diagnosed HIV. It is also recommended 2–8 weeks after initiation of antiretroviral therapy and every 3–6 months in all HIV patients.

D. When to Avoid HIV RNA Testing

  1. **During Acute Illnesses and Immunizations.** Patients with acute infections (opportunistic infection, bacterial pneumonia, even HSV recurrences) may experience significant (> 5-fold) rises in HIV RNA, which return to baseline 1–2 months after recovery. Although data are conflicting, many studies show at least a transient increase in HIV RNA levels following influenza and other immunizations, which return to baseline after 1–2 months.

  2. **When Test Results Would Not Influence Therapy.** This is a frequent scenario in patients with advanced disease who have no antiretroviral options or cannot tolerate therapy.

  3. **As a Screening Test for HIV Infection,** except if acute (primary) HIV disease is suspected during the HIV antibody window (i.e., first 3–6 weeks after viral transmission). HIV RNA tests have an unacceptably high false-positive rate when used for this purpose (J Infect Dis 2004;190:598–604), and are much more costly than HIV antibody testing.

INITIAL ASSESSMENT OF HIV-INFECTED PATIENTS

A. Clinical Evaluation. The history and physical examination should focus on diagnoses associated with HIV infection. Compared to patients without HIV, the severity, frequency, and duration of these conditions are usually increased in HIV disease.

1. **Dermatologic:** Severe herpes simplex (oral/anogenital); herpes zoster (especially recurrent, cranial nerve, or disseminated); molluscum contagiosum; staphylococcal abscesses; tinea nail infections; Kaposi's sarcoma (from HHV-8 infection); petechiae (from ITP); seborrheic dermatitis; new or worsening psoriasis; eosinophilic pustular folliculitis; severe cutaneous drug eruptions (especially sulfonamides)

2. **Oropharyngeal:** Oral candidiasis; oral hairy leukoplakia (from EBV); Kaposi's sarcoma (most commonly on palate or gums); gingivitis/periodontitis; warts; aphthous ulcers (especially esophageal/perianal)

3. **Constitutional symptoms:** Fatigue, fevers, chronic diarrhea, weight loss

4. **Lymphatic:** Persistent, generalized lymphadenopathy

5. **Others:** Active TB (especially extrapulmonary); non-Hodgkin's lymphoma (especially CNS); unexplained leukopenia, anemia, thrombocytopenia (especially ITP); myopathy; miscellaneous neurologic conditions (cranial/peripheral neuropathies, Guillain-Barre syndrome, mononeuritis multiplex, aseptic meningitis, cognitive impairment)

B. Baseline Laboratory Testing (Table 2.1) (See also Clin Infect Disease 2009;49:651–681).

Table 2.1. Baseline Laboratory Testing for HIV-Infected Patients*

Test	Rationale
Repeat HIV serology (ELISA/ confirmatory Western blot)	Indicated for patients unable to document a prior positive test, and for "low risk" individuals with a positive test (to detect computer/clerical error). Repeat serology is now less important since HIV RNA testing provides an additional means of confirming HIV infection. Also useful in ruling out cases of suspected factitious HIV
CBC with differential, platelets	Detects cytopenias (e.g., ITP) seen in HIV. Needed to calculate CD4 cell count
Chemistry panel ("SMA 20")	Detects renal dysfunction and electrolyte/LFT/glucose abnormalities, which may accompany HIV and associated infections (e.g., HIV nephropathy, HCV)
Fasting lipid profile	Since HIV and many antiretroviral agents influence lipid levels, a lipid profile before treatment provides a useful baseline
CD4 cell count	Determines the need for antiretroviral therapy and opportunistic infection (OI) prophylaxis. Best test for defining risk of OI's and prognosis
HIV RNA assay ("viral load")	Provides a marker for the pace of HIV disease progression. Determines indication for and response to antiretroviral therapy
HIV resistance genotype	Identifies patients infected with a resistant virus (some resistance now detected in approximately 15% of newly diagnosed patients in the US)
Tuberculin skin test (standard 5 TU of PPD)	Detects latent TB infection and targets patients for preventive therapy. Anergy skin tests are not recommended due to poor predictive value. HIV is the most powerful co-factor for the development of active TB

Table 2.1. Baseline Laboratory Testing for HIV-Infected Patients* (cont'd)

Test	Rationale
PAP smear	Risk of cervical cancer is nearly twice as high in HIV-positive women vs. uninfected controls; some advocate anal pap smears for gay men
Toxoplasmosis serology (IgG)	Identifies patients at risk for subsequent cerebral/systemic toxoplasmosis and the need for prophylaxis. Those with negative tests should be counseled on how to avoid infection
Syphilis serology (VDRL or RPR)	Identifies co-infection with syphilis, which is epidemiologically-linked to HIV. Disease may have accelerated course in HIV patients
Hepatitis C serology (anti-HCV)	Identifies HCV infection and usually chronic carriage. If positive, follow with HCV genotype and HCV viral load assay. If patient is antibody-negative but at high-risk for hepatitis, order HCV RNA to exclude a false-negative result
Hepatitis B serologies (HBsAb, HBcAb, HBsAg)	Identifies patients who are immune to hepatitis B (HBsAb) or chronic carriers (HBsAg). If all three are negative, hepatitis B vaccine is indicated
Hepatitis A serology (anti-HAV)	Identifies candidates for hepatitis A vaccine; if anti-HAV positive, already immune
G6PD screen	Identifies patients at risk for dapsone or primaquine-associated hemolysis
CMV serology (IgG)	Identifies patients who should receive CMV-negative or leukocyte-depleted blood if transfused
VZV serology (IgG)	Identifies patients at risk for varicella (chickenpox), and those who should avoid contact with active varicella or herpes zoster patients. Serology-negative patients exposed to chickenpox should receive varicella-zoster immune globulin (VZIG); some advocate varicella vaccine if CD4 > 350/mm^3
Chest x-ray	Sometimes ordered as a baseline test for future comparisons. May detect healed granulomatous diseases/other processes. Indicated in all tuberculin skin test positive patients
HLA-B*5701	Needed if therapy with abacavir is planned. Patients negative for HLA-B*5701 have almost no risk of severe hypersensitivity reaction to abacavir

*   See also Clin Infect Dis 2009;49:651–681

Table 2.2. Use of CD4 Cell Count for Interpretation of Patient Signs and Symptoms in HIV Infection

CD4 (cells/mm³)	Associated Conditions
> 500	Most illnesses are similar to those in HIV-negative patients. Some increased risk of bacterial infections (pneumococcal pneumonia, sinusitis), herpes zoster, tuberculosis, skin conditions
200–500*	Bacterial infections (especially pneumococcal pneumonia, sinusitis), cutaneous Kaposi's sarcoma, vaginal candidiasis, ITP
50–200*	Thrush, oral hairy leukoplakia, classic HIV-associated opportunistic infections (e.g., *P. jiroveci [carinii]* pneumonia, cryptococcal meningitis, toxoplasmosis). For patients receiving prophylaxis, most opportunistic infection do not occur until CD4 cell counts < 100/mm³ (Ann Intern Med 1996;124:633–42)
< 50*	"Final common pathway" opportunistic infections (disseminated *M. avium* complex, CMV retinitis), HIV-associated wasting, neurologic disease (neuropathy, encephalopathy)

*   Patients remain at risk for all processes noted in earlier stages

C. CD4 Cell Count (Lymphocyte Subset Analysis)

1. Overview. Acute HIV infection is characterized by a decline in CD4 cell count, followed by a gradual rise associated with clinical recovery. Chronic HIV infection shows progressive declines (~ 50–80 cells/year, but with wide interpatient variability) in CD4 cell count without treatment, followed by more rapid decline 1–2 years prior to opportunistic infection (AIDS-defining diagnosis). Cell counts remain stable over 5–10 years in 5% of patients, while others may show rapid declines (> 300 cells/year). Since variability exists within individual patients and between laboratories, it is useful to *repeat any value before making management decisions*.

2. Uses of CD4 Cell Count

a. Gives context of degree of immunosuppression for interpretation of symptoms/signs (Table 2.2)

b. Used to guide therapy. Guidelines support CD4 cell counts < 350/mm³ as a threshold before which treatment should be initiated, regardless of HIV RNA or symptoms. For prophylaxis against PCP, toxoplasmosis, and MAC/CMV infection, CD4 cell counts of 200/mm³, < 100/mm³, and < 50/mm³ are used as threshold levels, respectively

c. Provides estimate of risk of opportunistic infection or death. CD4 cell counts < 50/mm³ are associated with a markedly increased risk of death (median survival 1 year without treatment), although some patients with low counts survive > 3 years even without antiretroviral therapy. Prognosis is heavily influenced by HIV RNA, presence/history of opportunistic infections or neoplasms, performance status, and the immunologic response to antiretroviral therapy

Chapter 3

Treatment of HIV Infection

INITIATION OF ANTIRETROVIRAL THERAPY (Figure 3.1 and Table 3.2)

Combination antiretroviral therapy has led to dramatic reductions in HIV-related morbidity and mortality for patients with severe immunosuppression (CD4 < 200 cells/mm³) or a prior AIDS-defining illness [N Engl J Med 1997 Sep 11;337(11):725–33]. Treatment of asymptomatic patients is also recommended for those with CD4 cell counts between 200–500 cells/mm³, as there is increasing evidence that such therapy is associated with a reduced risk of both HIV-related and non-HIV related complications. Potential benefits of starting antiretroviral therapy with relatively high CD4 cell counts include reduction in HIV RNA, prevention of immunodeficiency, delayed time to onset of AIDS, reduced non-AIDS morbidity (cardiovascular, hepatic, neoplastic), decreased risk of drug toxicity, viral transmission, and selecting resistant virus. A cohort study published in 2009 found that deferral of ART until after the CD4 cell count fell to < 500 cells/mm³ was associated with nearly a two-fold increased risk of death [Kitihata N Engl J Med 2009]; a second study suggested that improved outcome was seen when treatment was started before the CD4 reached 350, but not at higher levels [Lancet 2009; DOI: 10.1016/S0140–6736(09)60612–7]. Potential risks of early antiretroviral therapy include reduced quality of life (from side effects/inconvenience), earlier development of drug resistance (with consequent transmission of resistant virus), limitation in future antiretroviral choices, unknown long-term toxicity of antiretroviral drugs, and unknown duration of effectiveness.

The primary goals of therapy are prolonged suppression of viral replication to undetectable levels (HIV RNA < 50–75 copies/mL), restoration/preservation of immune function, and improved clinical outcome. Once initiated, antiretroviral therapy should be continued indefinitely, as intermittent treatment has been associated with increased risk of HIV-related and non-HIV-related complications (N Engl J Med 2006 Nov 30;355[22]:2283–96). One possible exception is when treatment is started in pregnant women with CD4 cell counts > 500 solely to reduce the risk of maternal-child transmission. Such women may have treatment stopped after delivery, based on patient and clinician preference. The safety of this strategy (versus continuous therapy) is currently under study.

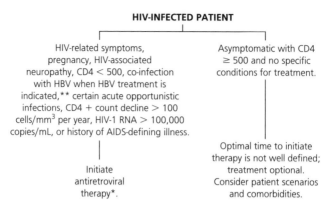

HIV-INFECTED PATIENT

HIV-related symptoms, pregnancy, HIV-associated neuropathy, CD4 < 500, co-infection with HBV when HBV treatment is indicated,** certain acute opportunistic infections, CD4 + count decline > 100 cells/mm^3 per year, HIV-1 RNA > 100,000 copies/mL, or history of AIDS-defining illness.

Asymptomatic with CD4 ≥ 500 and no specific conditions for treatment.

Optimal time to initiate therapy is not well defined; treatment optional. Consider patient scenarios and comorbidities.

Initiate antiretroviral therapy*.

Figure 3.1. Indications for Initiating Antiretroviral Therapy

* See Table 3.4.

** Treat with fully suppressive antiviral drugs active against both HIV and hepatitis B virus (HBV).

Adapted from: Guidelines for the Use of Antiretroviral Agents for HIV-1-infected Adults and Adolescents: Recommendations of the Panel on Clinical Practices for Treatment of HIV Infection; aidsinfo.nih.gov, December 1, 2009

Table 3.1. 2010 IAS-USA Guidelines: Recommendations for Initiating Antiretroviral Therapy (ART) in Treatment-Naïve Adults with HIV-1 Infection Who Are Ready To Begin Therapy

Measure	Recommendation
Specific conditions	ART is recommended regardless of CD4 cell count
Symptomatic HIV disease	
Pregnant women 2010 IAS-USA Guidelines:	
HIV-1 RNA >100,000 copies/mL	
Rapid decline in CD4 cell count, >100/μL per year	
Active hepatitis B or C virus coinfection	
Active or high risk for cardiovascular disease	
HIV-associated nephropathy	

Table 3.1. Recommendations for Initiating Antiretroviral Therapy (ART) in Treatment-Naïve Adults with HIV-1 Infection Who Are Ready To Begin Therapy (cont'd)

Measure	Recommendation
Symptomatic primary HIV infection	
Risk for secondary HIV transmission is high, eg, serodiscordant couples	
Asymptomatic, CD4 cell count ≤500/μL	ART is recommended
CD4 cell count <350/μL	
CD4 cell count 350–500/μL	
Asymptomatic, CD4 cell count >500/μL	ART should be considered, unless patient is an elite controller (HIV-1 RNA <50 copies/mL) or has stable CD4 cell count and low-level viremia in the absence of ART

Abbreviation: HIV, human immunodeficiency virus.

Adapted from Thompson, MA, Aberg, JA, Cahn, P., et al. Antiretroviral Treatment of Adult HIV Infection: 2010 Recommendations of the International AIDS Society USA Panel. *JAMA*. 2010;304(3):321–333 (doi:10.1001/jama.2010.1004)

Table 3.2. Antiretroviral Agents Used for HIV Infection

Drug (abbreviation; trade name, manufacturer)	Formulations	Usual Adult Dosing§
NUCLEOSIDE (AND NUCLEOTIDE) REVERSE TRANSCRIPTASE INHIBITORS (NRTIs)		
Abacavir sulfate (ABC; Ziagen, GlaxoSmithKline)	300-mg tablets; 20-mg/mL oral solution	300 mg BID or 600 mg QD
Abacavir sulfate/lamivudine (Epzicom, GlaxoSmithKline)	600/300-mg tablet	One 600/300-mg tablet QD
Abacavir sulfate/lamivudine/ zidovudine (Trizivir, GlaxoSmithKline)	300/150/300-mg tablet	One 300/150/300-mg tablet BID
Didanosine (ddI; Videx/Videx EC, Bristol-Myers Squibb; Oncology/Immunology; also available generically)	125-, 200-, 250-, 400-mg delayed-release enteric-coated capsules; 100-, 167-, 250-mg powder	Capsule: < 60 kg: 250 mg QD ≥ 60 kg: 400 mg QD 250 mg QD with tenofovir (best avoided) Powder: < 60 kg: 167 mg BID ≥ 60 kg: 250 mg BID probably

Table 3.2. Antiretroviral Agents Used for HIV Infection (cont'd)

Drug (abbreviation; trade name, manufacturer)	Formulations	Usual Adult Dosing§
NUCLEOSIDE (AND NUCLEOTIDE) REVERSE TRANSCRIPTASE INHIBITORS (NRTIs) (cont'd)		
		Administration: Take on empty stomach at least 30 minutes before or 2 hours after meal
Emtricitabine (FTC; Emtriva, Gilead Sciences)	200-mg capsule	200 mg QD
Lamivudine (3TC; Epivir, GlaxoSmithKline)	150-, 300-mg tablets; 10-mg/mL oral solution	150 mg BID or 300 mg QD
Lamivudine/zidovudine (Combivir, GlaxoSmithKline)	150/300-mg tablet	One 150/300-mg tablet BID
Stavudine (d4T; Zerit, Bristol-Myers Squibb Virology)	15-, 20-, 30-, 40-mg capsules; 1-mg/mL oral solution	< 60 kg: 30 mg BID ≥ 60 kg: 40 mg BID
Tenofovir disoproxil fumarate (TDF; Viread, Gilead Sciences)	300-mg tablet	One 300-mg tablet QD
Tenofovir disoproxil fumarate/emtricitabine (Truvada, Gilead Sciences)	300/200-mg tablet	One 300/200-mg tablet QD
Zidovudine (ZDV; Retrovir, GlaxoSmithKline; also available generically)	100-mg capsule; 300-mg tablet; 10-mg/5 mL oral solution; 10-mg/mL IV solution	200 mg TID or 300 mg BID (or with 3TC as Combivir or with abacavir and 3TC as Trizivir) 5–6 mg/kg daily
NON-NUCLEOSIDE REVERSE TRANSCRIPTASE INHIBITORS (NNRTIs)*		
Delavirdine mesylate (DLV; Rescriptor, Agouron)‡	100-, 200-mg tablets	400 mg TID (100-mg tablets can be dispersed in water; 200-mg tablet should be taken intact). Separate dosing from ddI or antacids by 1 hour, with or without food
Efavirenz (EFV; Sustiva, Bristol-Myers Squibb Oncology/Immunology; outside USA known as Stocrin)‡	50-, 100-, 200-mg capsules; 600-mg tablet	600 mg QD; best taken prior to bed to reduce incidence of CNS side effects

Table 3.2. Antiretroviral Agents Used for HIV Infection (cont'd)

Drug (abbreviation; trade name, manufacturer)	Formulations	Usual Adult Dosing[§]
NON-NUCLEOSIDE REVERSE TRANSCRIPTASE INHIBITORS (NNRTIs)* (cont'd)		
Etravirine (ETR; Intelence, Tibotec Therapeutics)	100-mg tablets	Two 100-mg tablets after a meal
Nevirapine (NVP; Viramune, Boehringer Ingelheim)[‡]	200-mg tablet; 50-mg/5 mL oral suspension (pediatric)	200 mg QD × 2 weeks, then 200 mg BID
COMBINATION NRTI/NNRTI		
Efavirenz/emtricitabine/ tenofovir (Atripla, Bristol-Myers Squibb & Gilead)	600/200/300-mg tablet	One 600/200/300-mg tablet daily
PROTEASE INHIBITORS (PIs)[†]		
Atazanavir sulfate (ATV; Reyataz, Bristol-Myers Squibb Virology)[‡]	100-, 150-, 200-, 300-mg capsules	400 mg QD, or 300 mg QD in combination with ritonavir 100 mg QD. For treatment-experienced patients, or when used with tenofovir or efavirenz or nevirapine use: 300 mg in combination with 100 mg of ritonavir. Take with food
Darunavir (DRV; Prezista, Tibotec Therapeutics)	400-, 600-mg tablets	600 mg BID with ritonavir 100 mg BID (treatment experienced); 800 mg QD with ritonavir 100 mg QD (treatment naïve)
Fosamprenavir (FPV; Lexiva, GlaxoSmithKline)[‡]	700-mg tablet	PI-naïve patients: 1400 mg BID, or 700 mg BID in combination with ritonavir 100 mg BID, or 1400 mg QD in combination with ritonavir 200 mg QD or 100 mg QD PI-experienced patients: 700 mg BID in combination with ritonavir 100 mg BID

Table 3.2. Antiretroviral Agents Used for HIV Infection (cont'd)

Drug (abbreviation; trade name, manufacturer)	Formulations	Usual Adult Dosing[§]
PROTEASE INHIBITORS (PIs)[†] (cont'd)		
Indinavir sulfate (IDV; Crixivan, Merck)[‡]	200-, 333-, 400-mg capsules	800 mg TID, or 800 mg BID in combination with ritonavir 100 mg or 200 mg BID <u>Administration</u>: *Unboosted*: Take 1 hour before or 2 hours after meals; may take with skim milk/low-fat meal *Boosted*: Take with or without food. Separate dosing from ddI by 1 hour
Lopinavir/ritonavir (LPV/r; Kaletra, Abbott)[‡]	200/50 mg tablet; 80/20-mg/mL oral solution	Two tablets (400/100 mg) BID; 5 mL oral solution BID. Four tablets (800/200 mg) QD an option for treatment-naïve patients <u>With EFV or NVP</u>: 3 tablets (600/150 mg) BID or 6.7 mL BID
Nelfinavir mesylate (NFV; Viracept, Agouron/Pfizer)	250-, 625-mg tablets; 50-mg/gm oral powder	750 mg TID or 1250 mg BID. Take with food
Ritonavir (RTV; Norvir, Abbott)[‡]	100-mg tablet or capsule; 600 mg/7.5 mL solution; 80 mg/mL oral solution	600 mg BID as sole PI; 100–400 mg daily in 1–2 divided doses as pharmacokinetic booster for other PIs <u>Administration</u>: Take with food or up to 2 hours after a meal to improve tolerability
Saquinavir (SQV; Invirase, Roche)[‡]	200-, 500-mg hard-gel capsules	1000 mg BID in combination with ritonavir 100 mg BID. Take with food
Tipranavir (TPV; Aptivus, Boehringer Ingelheim)[‡]	250-mg soft-gel capsule	500 mg BID in combination with ritonavir 200 mg BID. Take with food

Table 3.2. Antiretroviral Agents Used for HIV Infection (cont'd)

Drug (abbreviation; trade name, manufacturer)	Formulations	Usual Adult Dosing§
FUSION INHIBITOR		
Enfuvirtide (T-20; Fuzeon, Roche)‡	Injectable (lyophilized powder). Each single-use vial contains 108 mg of enfuvirtide to be reconstituted with 1.1 mL of sterile water for injection for delivery of approximately 90 mg/mL	90 mg BID IV. Administered subcutaneously into upper arm, anterior thigh, or abdomen
CCR5 ANTAGONIST		
Maraviroc (MVC; Selzentry, Pfizer)	150-, 300-mg tablets	150 mg, 300 mg or 600 BID depending on concomitant drugs (see p. 219 for details); may be taken with or without food
INTEGRASE INHIBITOR		
Raltegravir (RAL; Isentress, Merck)	400-mg tablet	One 400-mg tablet BID with or without food

* Nevirapine and efavirenz are cytochrome p450 CYP3A4 inducers; delavirdine is an inhibitor; etravirine has mixed effects. Consult package insert for full drug interaction profile.

† All protease inhibitors are hepatically metabolized by the cytochrome p450 system; they also are specific inhibitors of CYP3A4 and have induction effects on other enzymes. Consult package insert for full drug-drug interaction profile.

‡ Consult package insert for full drug interaction profile.

§ See Chapter 9 for dosing adjustments in renal or hepatic insufficiency. Unless otherwise stated, medication may be taken with or without food.

SELECTION OF AN OPTIMAL INITIAL ANTIRETROVIRAL REGIMEN (Tables 3.3–3.4)

Selection of the optimal initial antiretroviral regimen must take into consideration antiviral potency, tolerability, and safety. In the DHHS and IAS-USA Guidelines (Tables 3.4 and 3.5), all recommended regimens consist of three active agents: an NRTI pair (containing 3TC or FTC as one of the drugs) plus either an NNRTI or a ritonavir-boosted PI. As such, choosing a specific regimen therefore can be reduced to four major decisions (see Table 3.3).

Table 3.3. Major Decisions in Selecting the Initial Antiretroviral Regimen*

Decision	Comment
What is the optimal NRTI to pair with 3TC or FTC?	Because of the availability of once-daily, fixed-dose formulations and a low risk of lipoatrophy, many clinicians are currently choosing either TDF (co-formulated with FTC as Truvada) or ABC (co-formulated with 3TC as Epzicom). ABC therapy should be preceded by testing for HLA-B*5701 to reduce the risk of ABC hypersensitivity. Some studies have suggested that ABC treatment is associated with an increased risk of myocardial infarction (Lancet 2008 Apr 26;371[9622]: 1417–26; AIDS 2008 Sep 12;22[14]:F17–24). Furthermore, ABC/3TC had a higher rate of virologic failure compared with TDF/FTC in patients with a baseline HIV RNA greater than 100,000 copies per mL (N Engl J Med. 2009 Dec 3;361[23]:2230–40). Based on these data, the DHHS and IAS-USA guidelines list TDF/FTC as the preferred NRTI pair. Both guidelines still list ABC/3TC as an alternative option.
Should the third drug be an NNRTI or a PI or raltegravir?	NNRTI-based regimens—in particular those containing EFV—are in general simpler to take than PI-based treatments. EFV-based regimens have also demonstrated superior antiviral activity in prospective clinical trials (N Engl J Med 2008 May 15;358[20]:2095–106), although interestingly, immunologic response was better with the boosted PI. While PI-based regimens have a somewhat higher pill burden and more drug-drug interactions, they confer a lower risk of resistance in the case of virologic failure. The integrase strand transfer inhibitor (INSTI) raltegravir demonstrated comparable efficacy to EFV in a prospective clinical trial, with fewer drug-related adverse effects (Lancet 2009 Sep 5;37[9692]:796–806).
If an NNRTI-based regimen is chosen, which agent should be used?	In general, EFV is the preferred NNRTI due to comparable or superior antiviral activity to all comparators in prospective clinical trials. It is also available as a single-tablet triple regimen combined with TDF and FTC. However, EFV should be avoided in women of childbearing potential who may wish to become pregnant and may be difficult to tolerate for patients with psychiatric disease. In these contexts, NVP would be preferred, so long as the baseline CD4 cell count does not exceed 250/mm^3 in a woman or 400/mm^3 in a man.
If a PI-based regimen is chosen, which PI should be used?	There are more options for PI-based than for NRTI-or integrase inhibitor-based therapy. In general, RTV-boosted PIs provide the best combination of simplicity and antiviral potency. Comparative clinical trials have suggested more favorable tolerability and efficacy with ATV/r and DRV/r over LPV/r (Lancet 2008;372:646–55 and AIDS 2008;22:1389–97), and treatment guidelines hence list ATV/r and DRV/r as preferred.

* All recommended regimens consist of three active agents: an NRTI pair (containing 3TC or FTC as one of the drugs) plus either an NNRTI or a PI. Information on adverse drug reactions and drug-drug interactions highlight important differences between available agents. Combinations not listed as "Preferred" or "Alternative" regimens in Tables 3.4 and 3.5 should in general be avoided.

Table 3.4a. DHHS Guidelines: Antiretroviral Regimens Recommended for Treatment-Naïve Patients (Updated December 1, 2009)

Patients naïve to antiretroviral therapy should be started on one of the following three types of combination regimens:
- NNRTI + 2 NRTIs; or
- PI (preferably boosted with ritonavir) + 2 NRTIs; or
- INSTI + 2 NRTIs.

Selection of a regimen should be individualized based on virologic efficacy, toxicity, pill burden, dosing frequency, drug-drug interaction potential, resistance testing results, and comorbid conditions. The regimens in each category are listed in alphabetical order. Adapted from: Panel on Clinical Practices for Treatment of HIV Infection. Guidelines for the use of Antiretroviral Agents in HIV-Infected Adults and Adolescents. Department of Health and Human Services. December 1, 2009.

Preferred Regimens (Regimens with optimal and durable efficacy, favorable tolerability and toxicity profile, and ease of use) **The preferred regimens for non-pregnant patients are arranged by order of FDA approval of components other than nucleosides, thus, by duration of clinical experience.**

NNRTI-based Regimen • EFV/TDF/FTC[1] **PI-based Regimens** *(in alphabetical order)* • ATV/r + TDF/FTC[1] • DRV/r (once daily) + TDF/FTC[1] **INSTI-based Regimen** • RAL + TDF/FTC[1] **Preferred Regimen[2] for Pregnant Women** • LPV/r (twice daily) + ZDV/3TC[1]	**Comments** **EFV** should not be used during the first trimester of pregnancy or in women trying to conceive or not using effective and consistent contraception. **ATV/r** should not be used in patients who require >20mg omeprazole equivalent per day. Refer to <u>Table 14a</u> for dosing recommendations regarding interactions between ATV/r and acid-lowering agents.

Table 3.4a. DHHS Guidelines: Antiretroviral Regimens Recommended for Treatment-Naïve Patients (Updated December 1, 2009) (cont'd)

Alternative Regimens (Regimens that are effective and tolerable but have potential disadvantages compared with preferred regimens. An alternative regimen may be the preferred regimen for some patients.)

NNRTI-based Regimens *(in alphabetical order)*	**Comments**
• EFV + (ABC or ZDV)/3TC[1] **PI-based Regimens** *(in alphabetical order)* • ATV/r + (ABC or ZDV)/3TC[1] • FPV/r (once or twice daily) + either [(ABC or ZDV)/3TC[1]] or TDF/FTC[1] • LPV/r (once or twice daily) + either [(ABC or ZDV)/3TC[1]] or TDF/FTC[1] • SQV/r + TDF/FTC[1]	**NVP:** • Should not be used in patients with moderate to severe hepatic impairment (Child-Pugh B or C) • Should not be used in women with pre-ARV CD4 >250 cells/mm^3 or men with pre-ARV CD4 >400 cells/mm^3 **ABC:** • Should not be used in patients who test positive for HLA-B*5701 • Use with caution in patients with high risk of cardiovascular disease or with pre-treatment HIV-RNA >100,000 copies/mL (see text) **Once-daily LPV/r** is not recommended in pregnant women.

Acceptable Regimens (Regimens that may be selected for some patients but are less satisfactory than preferred or alternative regimens.)

NNRTI-based Regimen	**Comments**
• EFV + ddI + (3TC or FTC) **PI-based Regimen** • ATV + (ABC or ZDV)/3TC[1]	EFV + ddI + FTC or 3TC has only been studied in small clinical trials. ATV/r is generally preferred over ATV. Unboosted ATV may be used when ritonavir boosting is not possible.

[1]3TC may substitute for FTC or vice versa.
[2]For more detailed recommendations on antiretroviral use in an HIV-infected pregnant woman, refer to "*Recommendations for Use of Antiretroviral Drugs in Pregnant HIV-Infected Women for Maternal Health and Interventions to Reduce Perinatal HIV Transmission in the United States*," at http://aidsinfo.nih.gov/guidelines.

Abbreviations:
INSTI = integrase strand transfer inhibitor, NNRTI = non-nucleoside reverse transcriptase inhibitor, NRTI = nucleos(t)ide reverse transcriptase inhibitor, PI = protease inhibitor

ABC = abacavir, ATV = atazanavir, 3TC = lamivudine, ddI = didanosine, DRV = darunavir, EFV = efavirenz, FPV = fosamprenavir, FTC = emtricitabine, LPV = lopinavir, NVP = nevirapine, RAL = raltegravir, r = low dose ritonavir, SQV = saquinavir, TDF = tenofovir, ZDV = zidovudine

The following combinations in the recommended list above are available as fixed-dose combination formulations: ABC/3TC, EFV/TDF/FTC, LPV/r, TDF/FTC, and ZDV/3TC.

Table 3.4b. DHHS Guidelines: Antiretroviral Regimens that May be Acceptable and Regimens to be Used with Caution (Updated December 1, 2009)

Regimens that may be acceptable but more definitive data are needed	
CCR5-Antagonist-based Regimen • MVC + ZDV/3TC[1] **INSTI-based Regimen** • RAL + (ABC or ZDV)/3TC[1] **PI-based Regimen** • (DRV/r or SQV/r) + (ABC or ZDV)/3TC[1]	**Comment** With MVC, tropism testing required before treatment. Only patients found to have CCR-5 tropic-only virus (i.e., absence of CXCR4 tropic virus) are candidates for MVC.

Regimens to be Used with Caution (Regimens that have demonstrated virologic efficacy in some studies, but have safety, resistance, or efficacy concerns.)	
NNRTI-based Regimens • NVP + ABC/3TC[1]	**Comments** Use NVP and ABC together with caution because both can cause hypersensitivity reactions within first few weeks after initiation of therapy.
• NVP + TDF/FTC[1]	Early virologic failure with high rates of resistance has been reported in some patients receiving NVP + TDF + (3TC or FTC). Larger clinical trials are currently in progress.
PI-based Regimen • FPV + [(ABC or ZDV)/3TC[1] or TDF/FTC[1]]	FPV/r is generally preferred over unboosted FPV. Virologic failure with unboosted FPV-based regimen may select mutations that confer cross resistance to DRV.

[1]3TC maybe substituted with FTC or vice versa.

Abbreviations:
INSTI = integrase strand transfer inhibitor, NNRTI = non-nucleoside reverse transcriptase inhibitor, PI = protease inhibitor, ABC = abacavir, 3TC = lamivudine, DRV = darunavir, FPV = fosamprenavir, FTC = emtricitabine, MVC = maraviroc, NVP = nevirapine, RAL = raltegravir, r = low dose ritonavir, SQV = saquinavir, TDF = tenofovir, ZDV = zidovudine

Table 3.5a. IAS-USA Guidelines: Recommended Components of the Initial Antiretroviral Regimen[a]

Dual nRTI Component

Recommended

  Tenofovir/emtricitabine

    Available as fixed-dose combination alone and with efavirenz

    Once daily

    Low genetic barrier to resistance (emtricitabine)

    Renal dysfunction, decreased bone mineral density associated with tenofovir influence choice

Alternative

  Abacavir/lamivudine

    Available as fixed-dose combination

    Once daily

    Weaker antiviral efficacy in treatment-naive patients with baseline HIV-1 RNA >100,000 copies/mL than tenofovir/emtricitabine

    Low genetic barrier (lamivudine)

    Need to screen for HLA-B*5701[b] to reduce risk of abacavir hypersensitivity

    Abacavir may be associated with increased cardiovascular risk

Key Third Agent

Recommended

  Efavirenz[b]

    NNRTI class

    Available in fixed-dose combination with tenofovir/emtricitabine, which has become standard-of-care comparator regimen in most clinical trials

    Low genetic barrier

    Major psychiatric illness, first trimester of pregnancy, or intention to become pregnant influences choice

  Atazanavir/r[b]

    PI/r class

    Once daily

    Widely prescribed when PI/r is chosen for initial therapy

    Leaves options for future regimens

    Less lipidogenic potential than lopinavir/r

    Hyperbilirubinemia, need for acid-reducing agents, and risk of nephrolithiasis influence choice

  Darunavir/r[c]

    PI/r class

    Once daily in treatment-naive patients

    Limited experience in treatment-naive patients, presence of other options in most naive patients, and efficacy in patients with treatment experience, and multidrug-resistant virus influence choice

Table 3.5a. IAS-USA Guidelines: Recommended Components of the Initial Antiretroviral Regimen[a] (cont'd)

Key Third Agent (cont'd)

Raltegravir[c]

    INSTI class (only 1 FDA approved at present time)

    Twice daily

    Low drug interaction potential

    Rapid decline in HIV-1 RNA slope after initiation

    Low genetic barrier

    Limited experience in naive patients, presence of other options in most naive patients, and efficacy in treatment-experienced patients with multidrug-resistant virus influence choice

Alternatives

  Lopinavir/r

    PI/r class

    Extensive clinical experience

    Comparator PI/r in many trials

    Only PI coformulated with ritonavir (heat stable)

    Can be given once daily in naive patients

    Potential for hyperlipidemia and gastrointestinal adverse effects influences choice

  Fosamprenavir/r

    PI/r class

    Profile similar to lopinavir/r

    May be useful when other initial PI/r not tolerated

  Maraviroc

    CCR5 antagonist class

    Targets host protein (viral coreceptor)

    Need to perform viral tropism assay before use

    Limited clinical experience in treatment-naive patients

    Strategically, may be more useful in treatment-experienced patients or when primary (transmitted) drug resistance is present but viral population should be exclusively receptor 5

Abbreviations: CCR5, CC chemokine receptor 5; FDA, Food and Drug Administration; HIV, human immunodeficiency virus; INSTI, integrase strand transfer inhibitor; NNRTI, nonnucleoside reverse transcriptase inhibitor; nRTI, nucleoside or nucleotide analogue reverse transcriptase inhibitor; PI, protease inhibitor; /r, ritonavir boosted.

a Details, cautions, considerations, and supporting data[1,17,55–105] are described in the text.

b Based on extensive clinical experience.

c Based on antiviral efficacy and tolerability comparable to that of key third agents but more limited experience in treatment-naive patients.

Table 3.5b. IAS-USA Guidelines: Initial Antiretroviral Therapy (ART) and Considerations in Patients With Specific Conditions[a]

| Condition | Regimen Components | | Considerations |
	Possible Backbone Drugs	Third Agent	
High atherosclerotic cardiovascular risk	Emtricitabine, lamivudine, tenofovir	Efavirenz, nevirapine, atazanavir/r, raltegravir	Initiation of ART, regardless of CD4 cell count, is recommended. If possible avoid abacavir, fosamprenavir/r indinavir/r, lopinavir/r because of an associated increased risk of cardiovascular events.
Chronic kidney disease	Abacavir,[b] emtricitabine, lamivudine; avoid tenofovir (glomerular and tubular toxicity), atazanavir, and indinavir (nephrolithiasis).	Efavirenz, raltegravir, nevirapine, maraviroc, PI/r	Initiate ART regardless of CD4 cell count (BIIa). Avoid potentially nephrotoxic drugs (AIIa). When potentially nephrotoxic drugs must be used, monitor renal function closely. For patients with reduced estimated glomerular filtration rate, dose adjustment for drugs with renal metabolism (emtricitabine, lamivudine, tenofovir, maraviroc) should be considered.
Chronic HBV infection	Emtricitabine,lamivudine, tenofovir. Use 2 HBV-active drugs. Do not use abacavir or abacavir/lamivudine alone for treatment of HBV in coinfected patients.	Efavirenz, raltegravir, PI/r should be monitored for hepatotoxicity. Avoid nevirapine except for women with CD4 <250/μL and men with <400/μL. Maraviroc should be used with caution in patients with liver disease.	ART that includes tenofovir/emtricitabine should be used irrespective of CD4 cell count (BIIa). Monitor alanine aminotransferase after ART initiation and after withdrawal of suppressive therapy. In patients with moderate to severe liver impairment, dose adjustment for drugs metabolized by the liver should be considered. Alcohol should be avoided.
Chronic HCV infection requiring therapy	Emtricitabine, lamivudine, tenofovir	Efavirenz, raltegravir, PI/r should be monitored for hepatotoxicity.	ART should generally be initiated first in all patients with HCV coinfection regardless of CD4 cell count to slow liver disease progression (BIIa), except possibly in patients with HCV genotype 2 or 3 infection and a high CD4

Table 3.5b. IAS-USA Guidelines: Initial Antiretroviral Therapy (ART) and Considerations in Patients With Specific Conditions[a] (cont'd)

| Condition | Regimen Components | | Considerations |
	Possible Backbone Drugs	Third Agent	
		Avoid nevirapine except for women with CD4 <250/µL and men with <400/µL. Maraviroc should be used with caution in patients with liver disease.	cell count, for whom current HCV therapy has a higher probability of a sustained virologic response [26,28] (BIII). Avoid zidovudine, didanosine, zalcitabine, and stavudine, as well as abacavir. Alcohol should be avoided by all coinfected patients.
Pregnant women	Complete recommendations for the use of antiviral therapy in pregnant women are available at http://www.aidsinfo.nih.gov/ContentFiles/PerinatalGL.pdf, and http://www.europeanaidsclinicalsociety.org/guidelines.asp.		ART is recommended to prevent the transmission of the virus to the fetus or infant (AIa). Efavirenz should generally be avoided, especially in the first trimester of pregnancy (teratogenic effect).
Opportunistic infections, including tuberculosis	Any, according to the "What to Start" section	Choice of agent will be influenced by drug interactions, especially with rifampin and rifabutin.	ART should be initiated as soon as possible in patients with opportunistic infections, including tuberculosis, with attention to drug interactions and the potential for immune reconstitution inflammatory syndromes (AIa). Drug interactions likely to require dose adjustments; consult drug interaction dosing references (http://www.hiv-druginteractions.org, and http://hivinsite.ucsf.edu/insite?page=ar-00-02.

Abbreviations: ART, antiretroviral therapy; HBV, hepatitis B virus; HCV, hepatitis C virus; PI, protease inhibitor; /r, ritonavir boosted.

a   Details, cautions, considerations, and supporting data are described in the text. Levels of evidence are described in the eBox (available at http://www.jama.com).

b   In HLA B*5701–negative patients; has been associated with increased risk of myocardial infarction. Lower efficacy in patients with >100,000 copies/mL of HIV RNA at baseline (see text).

METABOLIC AND MORPHOLOGIC COMPLICATIONS OF THERAPY

The metabolic and morphologic changes that occur with HIV therapy are sometimes grouped under the term "lipodystrophy syndrome." Key features include *subcutaneous lipoatrophy*, which is most evident in the face, limbs, and buttocks; and *regional fat accumulation*, which may occur in the posterior or anterior portions of the neck, as well as in the midsection, as a manifestation of visceral adiposity. Patients may have predominantly lipoatrophy (the most common abnormality), fat accumulation, or both. These morphologic changes are often accompanied by metabolic derangements, including lipid dysregulation (increased triglycerides and total cholesterol; reduced HDL cholesterol) and insulin resistance. The etiology of the lipodystrophy syndrome is poorly understood, and there are clearly both host and treatment factors.

A. **Lipoatrophy**

1. **Overview.** Lipoatrophy is the most common morphologic abnormality in HIV disease. The most important host risk factor is the stage of HIV disease, as patients with more advanced HIV-related immunosuppression are at greatest risk. Among treatment-related factors, the leading hypothesis is that NRTI-induced mitochondrial toxicity induces fat cell apoptosis, and NRTIs with the highest *in vitro* inhibition of the mitochondrial enzyme polymerase gamma pose the greatest risk. Based on this hypothesis, a hierarchy of treatment-associated risk for lipoatrophy would be as follows: *highest risk* for dideoxynucleosides (stavudine, didanosine, and zalcitabine); *intermediate risk* for zidovudine; and *lowest risk* for tenofovir, abacavir, lamivudine, and emtricitabine. While one study showed a greater degree of mild lipoatrophy with efavirenz versus lopinavir/r treatment, (AIDS 2009;23:1109–18) in general the NNRTI class of medications has not been implicated in this process.

2. **Treatment.** Treatment strategies for lipoatrophy consist of drug substitutions, insulin-sensitizing agents, and plastic surgery. Substituting tenofovir or abacavir for stavudine or zidovudine leads to a gradual increase in limb fat that is often accompanied by a subjective improvement in facial appearance (AIDS 2006;20:2043–50). Such improvements occur slowly after antiretroviral switches and may not be evident to the patient for several months. The tenofovir substitution strategy may also improve lipid abnormalities. Substituting an NNRTI for the PI-component of the regimen has had no consistent effect on morphologic changes (AIDS 2005;19:917–25). Although there was initial optimism that insulin-sensitizing agents—in particular rosiglitazone—would help reverse lipoatrophy, the bulk of prospective data do not support a role for this approach, and it is not recommended in the absence of insulin resistance. Finally, plastic surgery for facial lipoatrophy can often dramatically improve appearance. The most common approach is injection of biologically inert substances such as polylactic acid (Sculptra). Patient satisfaction after polylactic acid injections is extremely high, and thus far the procedure appears safe. The major drawbacks to this treatment approach include the lack of long-term efficacy and safety data, relatively high cost, and lack of effect on lipoatrophy of the arms and legs. Patients should be informed that most insurance policies and state-funded programs will not cover the cost of polylactic acid injections.

B. Fat Accumulation

1. Overview. Fat accumulation occurs less commonly than fat atrophy, but can be highly disfiguring. The neck, upper body, and intra-abdominal (visceral) sites are most often involved. (Neck fat accumulation in the posterior compartment is often referred to as a buffalo hump.) Despite the similarity to Cushing's syndrome, serum cortisol levels are not elevated. While fat accumulation syndrome is anecdotally linked to PI-based therapy, cases have occurred in the absence of PIs as well; no definitive link between fat accumulation syndrome and PI's has been found.

2. Treatment. No treatment modification has consistently led to improvement. Exercise may reduce central fat accumulation, and weight loss may reduce neck fat, but improvements are generally modest. Recombinant growth hormone reduces central fat accumulation, but treatment is expensive and associated with a risk of other side effects, including glucose intolerance and carpal tunnel syndrome. The injectable growth hormone releasing factor tesamorelin appears safe and modestly effective for this indication (J Clin Endocrinol Metab. 2010 Jun 16); it is currently under FDA review for this indication. Liposuction of neck fat accumulation is the most rapidly effective technique, but recurrences are possible. Insurance coverage for neck liposuction can sometimes be deemed medically necessary if the fat accumulation leads to medical problems such as neck pain or sleep apnea.

C. Prevention of Lipodystrophy.

Since morphologic changes are only slowly reversible and may be permanent in some patients, the best strategy is to choose treatments that are least likely to induce these abnormalities. Of currently preferred NRTI combinations, tenofovir/emtricitabine and abacavir/lamivudine induce less fat atrophy than zidovudine/lamivudine (Table 3.6). In addition, providers should consider a proactive switching strategy for patients receiving long-term zidovudine/lamivudine. Regimens containing stavudine should be avoided unless there are no alternatives. The morphologic changes associated with didanosine + lamivudine are not well defined, but, as noted earlier, didanosine has a relatively high degree of mitochondrial toxicity *in vitro*, and this correlates with increased risk of fat atrophy.

Table 3.6. Treatment and Prevention of Body Habitus Changes Associated with Antiretroviral Therapy

Treatment	• Substitute tenofovir or abacavir for thymidine analogue • Polylactic acid injections for facial lipoatrophy • Weight loss and exercise for fat accumulation • Liposuction for dorsocervical fat accumulation
Prevention	• Start therapy before advanced HIV disease • Tesamorelin for central fat accumulation (investigational) • Select initial NRTI backbones less likely to induce lipoatrophy (i.e., emtricitabine/tenofovir or abacavir/lamivudine) • Consider proactive switch to tenofovir DF or abacavir for patients still on thymidine analogues (ZDV or d4T)

D. **Lipid Abnormalities.** Multiple abnormalities in lipid metabolism were reported in HIV-infected patients before the availability of PI-based antiretroviral therapy, including increased levels of very low-density lipoprotein (VLDL) cholesterol and triglycerides and decreased levels of high-density lipoprotein (HDL) cholesterol, low-density lipoprotein (LDL) cholesterol, and apolipoprotein B (JAMA 2003;289:2978–82). However, soon after the introduction of PIs, a dramatic increase in triglyceride levels and, to a lesser extent, total cholesterol levels were evident in PI-treated patients.

1. **Antiretroviral Therapy and Dyslipidemia.** The PIs are all associated to varying degrees with clinically significant dyslipidemia. Unboosted atazanavir is more lipid neutral; however, ritonavir boosting worsens lipid profile even of atazanavir, and ritonavir-boosted is generally recommended for optimal antiviral efficacy. Among recommended boosted PIs, atazanavir and darunavir appear to have the lowest risk of hyperlipidemia, possibly because they use only 100 mg/day of ritonavir. Other components of the antiretroviral regimen may also induce lipid disturbances: d4T, ZDV, and ABC are all more likely to raise lipids than tenofovir, and efavirenz increases lipids, especially triglycerides, more than nevirapine. Raltegravir and maraviroc both increase lipids less than efavirenz. Treatment of HIV may have the favorable effect of raising HDL cholesterol, particularly with nevirapine and efavirenz.

2. **Treatment of Dyslipidemia.** Various approaches can be taken to treat PI-associated dyslipidemia. As for HIV-negative patients, the first step consists of therapeutic lifestyle changes, including dietary counseling, reduction in alcohol intake, smoking cessation, and increased aerobic exercise. Unfortunately, lifestyle changes alone are often insufficient to reverse lipid abnormalities in patients with HIV. The two most widely used pharmacological strategies are substitution of the potentially offending antiretroviral agent with an alternative antiretroviral, or use of lipid-modifying drug therapy. In patients who are virologically suppressed and have no or little presumed antiretroviral resistance, the former strategy is generally safe but may not lower lipids into the desirable range (AIDS 2005;19:1051–8). When switching antiretroviral drugs it is important to weigh the risks of new treatment-related toxicities and virologic relapse against the risks of potential drug interactions and new treatment-related toxicities from lipid-lowering agents. Table 3.7 cites some potential switch strategies; if there is more than one possible offending agent, the changes should be made sequentially to ensure that the initial change is well tolerated. The use of lipid-lowering agents in HIV-infected patients is notable for a relative lack of efficacy and a high risk of drug interactions, particularly between the statins and PIs. Nonetheless, lipid abnormalities should be aggressively treated just as in HIV-negative patients, especially when other cardiac risk factors are present.

Elevations in LDL cholesterol will usually require statin therapy. Most of the statins, with the exception of pravastatin, fluvastatin, and rosuvastatin, are metabolized by the cytochrome P450 enzyme system via the 3A4 isoform (CYP3A4). Most PIs inhibit CYP3A4, potentially leading to elevated statin levels increasing the risk of statin-related toxicity, including rhabdomyolysis (Clin Infect Dis 2002;35:e111–2). Although pravastatin is recommended in some guidelines due to the relative absence of drug-drug interactions, it appears to reduce lipid levels less in HIV patients than other statins [Ann Intern Med 2009 Mar 3;150(5):301–13]. As a result, we generally prefer atorvastatin—a more potent agent—as an acceptable alternative, so long as the starting dose is 10 mg daily and the patient is closely monitored for hepatic/muscle toxicity. Fluvastatin and rosuvastatin, which are also not metabolized via CYP3A4, may be other acceptable options, although studies evaluating their use in HIV patients are more limited than with pravastatin or atorvastatin. Not all statin-ART drug-drug interactions are mediated through CYP3A4: rosuvastatin levels may increase significantly when given with lopinavir/r through unclear mechanisms, and darunavir appears to increase pravastatin levels. When hypertriglyceridemia is the predominant abnormality, a fibrate such as gemfibrozil or fenofibrate should be tried first. As for HIV-negative patients, refractory elevations in triglycerides may respond to fish oil preparations.

Table 3.7. Drug-Induced Dyslipidemia and Switch Therapy

Cause	Switch To	Comments
Protease inhibitors (PIs): ritonavir, indinavir, saquinavir, nelfinavir, lopinavir/r, tipranavir, fosamprenavir	Atazanavir or atazanavir/ ritonavir or darunavir/ ritonavir	Need to use boosted atazanavir if patient is also on tenofovir. Do not use unboosted atazanavir if there is any history of PI resistance or PI-related treatment failure. If patient is on a proton pump inhibitor, atazanavir should in general be avoided.
d4T or ZDV	Tenofovir	Use with caution in patients with impaired renal function; reduce dose per package insert guidelines
Efavirenz	Nevirapine	Avoid in women with CD4 > 250/mm³ or men with CD4 > 400/mm³ due to increased risk of hepatotoxicity

ANTIRETROVIRAL THERAPY ADVERSE EFFECTS

Although the tolerability and safety of antiretroviral therapy has improved substantially, adverse events have been reported with all the available agents. In addition, subjective side effects remain one of the most common causes of medication non-compliance and treatment failure. Certain drugs — such as d4T, ddI, and indinavir — are now rarely used in developed countries due to their relatively poor adverse event profile, but may still be used in resource-limited settings that do not have access to the newest agents. In addition, recently-approved compounds necessarily have less comprehensive data on side effects that are either particularly rare or might not occur except after prolonged exposure.

Clinicians should be particularly alert to potential side effects that may occur in patients who already have underlying disease processes, or who are taking concomitant medications with overlapping toxicities. For example, individuals co-infected with hepatitis B and C generally have higher rates of hepatotoxicity; those with psychiatric disease are more prone to the adverse CNS effects of efavirenz; and patients with pre-existing renal disease may be more likely to experience tenofovir nephrotoxicity. Table 3.8 was adapted from DHHS Guidelines for the Use of Antiretroviral Agents, last updated December, 2009.

Table 3.8. Antiretroviral Therapy-Associated Adverse Effects and Management Recommendations

Adverse Effects	Associated ARVs	Onset/Clinical Manifestation	Estimated Frequency	Risk Factors	Prevention/ Monitoring	Management
Bleeding events	TPV/r: reports of intracranial hemorrhage (ICH) PIs: ↑ bleeding in hemophiliac patients	Median time to ICH event: 525 days on TPV/r therapy Hemophiliac patients: ↑ spontaneous bleeding tendency–in joints, muscles, soft tissues, and hematuria	In 2006, 13 cases of ICH reported, w/ TPV/r use, including 8 fatalities (Dear Health Care Provider, Boehringer Ingelheim Pharmaceuticals, Inc. June 30, 2006) For hemophilia: frequency unknown	For ICH: • Patients with CNS lesions, head trauma, recent neurosurgery, coagulopathy, hypertension, alcohol abuse, or receiving anticoagulant or anti-platelet agents including vitamin E For hemophiliac patients: • PI use	Avoid Vitamin E supplements, particularly with the oral solution formulation of tipranavir For ICH: • Avoid use of TPV/r in patients at risk for ICH For hemophiliac patients: • Consider using NNRTI-based regimen • Monitor for spontaneous bleeding	For ICH: • Discontinue TPV/r; manage ICH with supportive care For hemophiliac patients: • May require increased use of Factor VIII products
Bone marrow suppression	ZDV	Onset: few weeks to months Laboratory abnormalities: • anemia (usually macrocytic) • neutropenia	Severe anemia (Hgb < 7 g/dL): 1.1%–4%	• Advanced HIV • High dose • Pre-existing anemia or neutropenia	• Avoid use in patients at risk • Avoid other bone marrow suppressants if possible	• Switch to another NRTI if there is an alternative option;

Symptoms: fatigue because of anemia; potential for increased bacterial infections because of neutropenia	Severe neutropenia (ANC < 500 cells/mm³): 1.8%–8%	Concomitant use of bone marrow suppressants (e.g., cotrimoxazole, ganciclovir, valganciclovir, etc.) or drugs that cause hemolytic anemia (e.g., ribavirin)	Monitor CBC with differential after the 1st few weeks, then at least every 3 months (more frequently in patients at risk)	Discontinue concomitant bone marrow suppressant if there is an alternative option; otherwise: For neutropenia: • Identify and treat other causes • Consider treatment with filgrastim For anemia: • Identify and treat other causes of anemia (if present) • Blood transfusion if indicated • Consider erythropoietin therapy

Table 3.8. Antiretroviral Therapy-Associated Adverse Effects and Management Recommendations (cont'd)

Adverse Effects	Associated ARVs	Onset/Clinical Manifestation	Estimated Frequency	Risk Factors	Prevention/ Monitoring	Management
Cardiovascular effects [including myocardial infarction (MI)] and cerebrovascular accidents (CVA)	MI & CVA: associated with PI use MI only: Observational cohort found possible association of recent ABC & ddI use, and MI in pts with high risk for cardiovascular events (D:A:D Study Group, Lancet, 2008. 371(9622): 1417-26)	<u>Onset:</u> months to years after beginning of therapy <u>Presentation:</u> premature coronary artery disease or CVA	3–6 per 1,000 patient-years CVA: ~ 1 per 1,000 patient-years	Other risk factors for cardiovascular disease, such as smoking, age, hyperlipidemia, hypertension, diabetes mellitus, family history of premature coronary artery disease, and personal history of coronary artery disease	• Assess cardiac disease risk factors • Monitor & identify patients with hyperlipidemia or hyperglycemia • Consider regimen with less adverse lipid effects • Life style modification: smoking cessation, diet, and exercise	• Early diagnosis, prevention, and pharmacologic management of other cardiovascular risk factors, such as hyperlipidemia, hypertension, and insulin resistance/ diabetes mellitus • Lifestyle modifications: diet, exercise, and/or smoking cessation • Switch to agents with less propensity for increasing cardiovascular risk factors

Central nervous system effects	EFV	<u>Onset:</u> begin with first few doses <u>Symptoms:</u> may include one or more of the following: drowsiness, somnolence, insomnia, abnormal dreams, dizziness, impaired concentration & attention span, depression, hallucination, exacerbation of psychiatric disorders, psychosis, suicidal ideation Most symptoms subside or diminish after 2–4 weeks	> 50% of patients may have some symptoms	• Pre-existing or unstable psychiatric illnesses • Use of concomitant drugs with CNS effects • Higher plasma EFV concentrations in people with G→T polymorphism at position 516 (516G→T) of CYP2B6 (Rodriguez-Novoa S, Barreiro P, Rendón A, et al. Clin Infect Dis. 2005. 40(9):1358-61)	• Take at bedtime or 2–3 hours before bedtime • Take on an empty stomach to reduce drug concentration & CNS effects • Warn patients regarding restriction of risky activities, such as operating heavy machinery during the 1st 2–4 weeks of therapy	• Symptoms usually diminish or disappear within 2–4 weeks • Consider switching to alternative agent if symptoms persist and cause significant impairment in daily function or exacerbation of psychiatric illness

Table 3.8. Antiretroviral Therapy-Associated Adverse Effects and Management Recommendations (cont'd)

Adverse Effects	Associated ARVs	Onset/Clinical Manifestation	Estimated Frequency	Risk Factors	Prevention/ Monitoring	Management
Gastrointestinal (GI) intolerance	All PIs, ZDV, ddI	Onset: within first doses Symptoms: • nausea, vomiting, abdominal pain with all listed agents • Diarrhea, most commonly seen with NFV	Varies with different agents	• All patients	• Taking with food may reduce symptoms (not recommended for ddI or unboosted IDV) • Some patients may require antiemetics or antidiarrheals pre-emptively to reduce symptoms	May spontaneously resolve or become tolerable with time; if not: For nausea & vomiting, consider: • Antiemetic prior to dosing • Switch to less emetogenic ARV For diarrhea, consider: • Bulk-forming agents, such as psyllium products • Antimotility agents, such as loperamide, diphenoxylate/ atropine • Calcium tablets • Pancreatic enzymes

		Onset/Symptoms	Frequency	Risk Factors	Prevention	Management
						• L-glutamate: may ↓ diarrhea, esp. when assoc. w/NFV or LPV/r _In case of severe GI loss:_ • Rehydration & electrolyte replacement as indicated
Hepatic failure	NVP	_Onset:_ Greatest risk within first 6 weeks of therapy; can occur through 18 weeks _Symptoms:_ Abrupt onset of flu-like symptoms (nausea, vomiting, myalgia, fatigue), abdominal pain, jaundice, or fever with or without skin rash; may	_Symptomatic hepatic events:_ • 4% overall (2.5%–11% from different trials) • In women: 11% in those w/pre-NVP CD4 > 250 cells/mm³ vs. 0.9% w/ CD4 < 250 cells/mm³	• Treatment-naive patients with higher CD4 count at initiation (> 250 cells/mm³ in women & > 400 cells/mm³ in men) • Females 3-fold higher risk than males	• Avoid initiation of NVP in women w/CD4 > 250 cells/mm³ or men w/CD4 > 400 cells/mm³ unless the benefit clearly outweighs the risk • Do not use NVP in HIV(-) individuals for post-exposure prophylaxis • Counsel patients re: signs &	• Discontinue ARVs, including NVP (caution should be taken in discontinuation of 3TC, FTC, or TDF in HBV-coinfected patients) • Discontinue all other hepatotoxic agents if possible • Rule out other causes of hepatitis

Table 3.8. Antiretroviral Therapy-Associated Adverse Effects and Management Recommendations (cont'd)

Adverse Effects	Associated ARVs	Onset/Clinical Manifestation	Estimated Frequency	Risk Factors	Prevention/Monitoring	Management
		progress to fulminant hepatic failure particularly in those with rash Approximately 1/2 of the cases have accompanying skin rash, some of which may present as part of DRESS syndrome (drug rash with eosinophilia and systemic symptoms)	• In men: 6.3% w/pre-NVP CD4 > 400 cells/mm³ vs. 2.3% w/ CD4 < 400 cells/mm³	• HIV (-) individuals when NVP is used for post-exposure prophylaxis • Possibly, high NVP concentrations	symptoms of hepatitis; stop NVP & seek medical attention if signs & symptoms of hepatitis, severe skin rash, or hypersensitivity reactions appear • Monitoring of ALT & AST (every 2 weeks x first month, then monthly x 3 months, then every 3 months) • Obtain AST & ALT in patients with rash • 2-week dose escalation may reduce incidence of hepatic events	• Aggressive supportive care as indicated **Note:** Hepatic injury may progress despite treatment discontinuation. Careful monitoring should continue until symptom resolution **Do not rechallenge patient with NVP** The safety of other NNRTIs (e.g., EFV, ETR, or DLV) in patients who experienced significant hepatic event from NVP is unknown; use with caution

| Hepatotoxicity (clinical hepatitis or asymptomatic serum transaminase elevation) | All NNRTIs; all PIs; most NRTIs; maraviroc | Varies with the different agents | Onset: NNRTIs: for NVP, 2/3 within 1st 12 weeks NRTIs: over months to years PIs: generally after weeks to months Symptoms/findings: NNRTIs: • Asymptomatic to non-specific symptoms, such as anorexia, weight loss, or fatigue. Approximately 1/2 of patients with NVP-associated symptomatic hepatic events present with skin rash NRTIs: • ZDV, ddI, d4T: may cause hepatotoxicity | • HBV or HCV coinfection • Alcoholism • Concomitant hepatotoxic drugs, particularly rifampin • Elevated ALT &/ or AST at baseline • For NVP-associated hepatic events: female w/ pre-NVP CD4 > 250 cells/mm³ or male w/pre-NVP CD4 > 400 cells/mm³ • Higher drug concentrations for PIs, particularly TPV | • NVP: monitor liver-associated enzymes at baseline, at 2 & 4 weeks, then monthly for 1st 3 months; then every 3 months • TPV/RTV: contraindicated in patients with moderate to severe hepatic insufficiency; for other patients follow frequently during treatment • Other agents: monitor liver-associated enzymes at least every 3–4 months or more frequently in patients at risk | • Rule out other causes of hepatotoxicity, such as alcoholism, viral hepatitis, chronic HBV w/3TC, FTC, or TDF withdrawal, HBV resistance, etc. For symptomatic patients: • Discontinue all ARVs and other potential hepatotoxic agents • After symptoms subside & serum transaminases return to normal, construct a new ARV regimen without the potential offending agent(s) |

Table 3.8. Antiretroviral Therapy-Associated Adverse Effects and Management Recommendations (cont'd)

Adverse Effects	Associated ARVs	Onset/Clinical Manifestation	Estimated Frequency	Risk Factors	Prevention/ Monitoring	Management
		associated with lactic acidosis with microvesicular or macrovesicular hepatic steatosis because of mitochondrial toxicity • 3TC, FTC, or TDF: HBV-coinfected patients may develop severe hepatic flare when these drugs are withdrawn or when resistance develops				For asymptomatic patients: • If ALT > 5–10x ULN, some may consider discontinuing ARVs, others may continue therapy with close monitoring unless direct bilirubin is also elevated • After serum transaminases return to normal, construct a new ARV regimen without the potential offending agent(s)

	PIs: • Clinical hepatitis & hepatic decompensation have been reported with TPV/r and also with other PIs to varying degrees. Underlying liver disease increases risk • Generally asymptomatic, some with anorexia, weight loss, jaundice, etc.				**Note:** Refer to information regarding NVP-associated symptomatic hepatic events & NRTI-associated lactic acidosis with hepatic steatosis in this table
Hyperlipidemia	All PIs (except unboosted ATV); EFV; NVP (to a less extent)	d4T	<u>Onset:</u> weeks to months after beginning of therapy <u>Presentation:</u> <u>All PIs (except unboosted ATV):</u> ↑ in LDL & total cholesterol	Varies with different agents <u>Swiss Cohort:</u> ↑ TC & TG: 1.7–2.3x higher in patients receiving (non-ATV) PI	• Underlying hyperlipidemia • Risk based on ARV therapy <u>PI:</u> All RTV-boosted PI may ↑ LDL & TG; ATV/r may
				• Assess cardiac disease risk factors • Use PIs and NNRTIs with less adverse effect on lipids and non–d4T-based regimen	• Lifestyle modification: diet, exercise, and/or smoking cessation • Switching to agents with less propensity for causing hyperlipidemia

Table 3.8. Antiretroviral Therapy-Associated Adverse Effects and Management Recommendations (cont'd)

Adverse Effects	Associated ARVs	Onset/Clinical Manifestation	Estimated Frequency	Risk Factors	Prevention/ Monitoring	Management
		(TC), & triglyceride (TG). Also: ↑ HDL seen w/ ATV, DRV, FPV, LPV, SQV when boosted w/RTV LPV/r (Molina J-M, Andrade-Villanueva J, Echevarria J, et al. Conference on Retroviruses and Opportunistic Infections; February 3-6, 2008; Boston, MA. Abstract 37) & FPV/r (Smith KY, Weinberg WG, Dejesus E, et al. AIDS Res Ther, 2008. 5(1):5) disproportionate ↑ in TG		produce less of an ↑ in LDL & TG. NNRTI: EFV > NVP (van Leth F, Phanuphak P, Ruxrungtham K, et al. Lancet, 2004. 363(9417):1253-1263) NRTI: d4T > ZDV > ABC > TDF (Pozniak AL, Gallant JE, DeJesus E, et al. J Acquir Immune Defic Syndr, 2006. 43(5):535-40) (Smith K, Fine D, Patel D, et al. Conference on Retroviruses and Opportunistic Infections; February 3-6,	• Fasting lipid profile at baseline, at 3–6 months after starting new regimen, then annually or more frequently if indicated (in high-risk patients or in patients with abnormal baseline levels)	Pharmacologic Management: • Per HIVMA/ ACTG guidelines (Dube MP, Stein JH, Aberg JA, et al. Clin Infect Dis, 2003. 37(5):613-27) & National Cholesterol Education Program ATP III guidelines (National Heart, Lung and Blood Institute, Third Report of the Expert Panel on Detection, Evaluation, and Treatment of High Blood Cholesterol in Adults)

					2008; Boston, MA. Abstract 774)	• HLA-B*5701 screening prior to initiation of ABC • Those patients tested (+) for HLA-B*5701 should be labelled as allergic to abacavir in medical records • Educate patients about potential signs and symptoms of HSR and need for reporting of symptoms promptly • Wallet card with warning	• Discontinue ABC and switch to another NRTI • Rule out other causes of symptoms (e.g., intercurrent illnesses such as viral syndromes, and other causes of skin rash) • Most signs and symptoms resolve 48 hours after discontinuation of ABC *More severe cases:* • Symptomatic support: antipyretic
Hypersensitivity reaction (HSR)	ABC	EFV & NVP (to a lesser extent): ↑ in LDL & TC, and slight ↑ TG; also ↑ HDL d4T & ZDV: ↑ in LDL, TC, & TG	Onset of 1st reaction: median onset, 9 days; approximately 90% within 1st 6 weeks Onset of rechallenge reactions: within hours of rechallenge dose Usually ≥ 2–3 acute symptoms seen with HSR (in descending frequency): high fever, diffuse skin rash, malaise,	Clinically suspected ≈ 8% in clinical trial (2%–9%); 5% in retrospective analysis; significantly reduced with pre-treatment HLA-B*5701 screening (Mallal S, Phillips E, Carosi G, et al. N Engl J Med, 2008. 358(6):568-79)		• HLA-B*5701, HLA-DR7, HLA-DQ3 • Higher incidence of grade 3 or 4 HSR with 600 mg once-daily dose than 300 mg twice-daily dose in one study (5% vs. 2%)	

Table 3.8. Antiretroviral Therapy-Associated Adverse Effects and Management Recommendations (cont'd)

Adverse Effects	Associated ARVs	Onset/Clinical Manifestation	Estimated Frequency	Risk Factors	Prevention/ Monitoring	Management
		nausea, headache, myalgia, chills, diarrhea, vomiting, abdominal pain, dyspnea, arthralgia, respiratory symptoms (pharyngitis, dyspnea/ tachypnea) With continuation of ABC, symptoms may worsen to include hypotension, respiratory distress, vascular collapse <u>Rechallenge reactions:</u> generally greater intensity than 1ˢᵗ reaction, can mimic anaphylaxis			information for patients • Note multiple names for products containing abacavir (ABC, ZIAGEN, EPZICOM or KIVEXA, TRIZIVIR)	fluid resuscitation, pressure support (if necessary) • **Do not rechallenge patients with ABC after suspected HSR, even in patients who are (-) for HLA-B*5701. There are cases of hypersensitivity in HLA-B*5701 (-) patients**

| Insulin resistance/ diabetes mellitus (DM) | Combination ART, thymidine analogs (ZDV, d4T), some PIs linked to insulin resistance and diabetes mellitus (but this may not be a class effect) | Onset: weeks to months after beginning of therapy

Presentation: Polyuria, polydipsia, polyphagia, fatigue, weakness; exacerbation of hyperglycemia in patients with underlying DM | Up to 3%–5% of patients developed diabetes in some series; D:A:D cohort incidence rate of 5.72 per 1,000 pt-yr f/up (95% CI: 5.31–6.13) (De Wit S, Sabin CA, Weber R, et al. Diabetes Care, 2008. 31(6):1224-9)

Incidence of DM in HIV (+) women in WHIS (2.5– 2.9 pt-yrs) not different from HIV(-) pts (Tien PC, Schneider MF, Cole SR, et al. AIDS, 2007. 21(13):1739-45) and associated with NRTIs | • Family history of DM | • Use non-thymidine analog containing regimens or NNRTIs
• Fasting blood glucose 1–3 months after starting new regimen, then at least every 3–6 months | • Diet and exercise
• Consider switching to non-thymidine analog-containing ART
• Consider switching PI to an alternative PI and/or NNRTI
• Pharmacotherapeutic management per American Diabetic Association and American Association of Clinical Endocrinologists guidelines (AACE Diabetes Mellitus Clinical Practice Guidelines |

Table 3.8. Antiretroviral Therapy-Associated Adverse Effects and Management Recommendations (cont'd)

Adverse Effects	Associated ARVs	Onset/Clinical Manifestation	Estimated Frequency	Risk Factors	Prevention/ Monitoring	Management
						Task Force. Endocr Pract, 2007. 13(Suppl 1):1-68) (American Diabetes Association. Clinical Practice Recommendations 2008)
Lactic acidosis/ hepatic steatosis +/- pancreatitis (severe mitochondrial toxicities)	NRTIs, esp. d4T, ddI, ZDV	Onset: months after initiation of NRTIs Symptoms: • Insidious onset with nonspecific GI prodrome (nausea, anorexia, abdominal pain, vomiting), weight loss, and fatigue; • Subsequent symptoms may be rapidly progressive,	Rare Depends on regimen and patient sex: U.S.: 0.85 cases per 1,000 pt-yrs (Falco V, Rodriguez D, Ribera E, et al. Clin Infect Dis, 2002. 34(6):838-46) South Africa: 16.1 per 1,000 pt-yrs in female & 1.2 cases per 1,000 pt-yrs in male patients	• d4T + ddI • d4T, ZDV, ddI use (d4T most frequently implicated) • Long duration of NRTI use • Female gender • Obesity • Pregnancy (esp. with d4T + ddI) • ddI + hydroxyurea or ribavirin	• Routine monitoring of lactic acid not recommended • Consider obtaining lactate levels in patients with low serum bicarbonate or high anion gap and with complaints consistent with lactic acidosis • Appropriate phlebotomy technique	• For mild cases, consider switching off offending drugs to safe alternatives • For severe lactic acidosis, discontinue all ARVs if this syndrome is highly suspected (diagnosis is established by clinical correlations, drug history,

and lactate level)
- Symptomatic support with fluid hydration
- Some patients may require IV bicarbonate infusion, hemodialysis or hemofiltration, parenteral nutrition, or mechanical ventilation
- IV thiamine and/or riboflavin, which resulted in rapid resolution of hyperlactatemia in some case reports

Note:
- Interpretation of high lactate level should be done in the context of clinical findings

for obtaining lactate level should be employed

with tachycardia, tachypnea, hyperventilation, jaundice, muscular weakness, mental status changes, or respiratory distress
- Some may present with multi-organ failure (e.g., hepatic failure, acute pancreatitis, encephalopathy, and respiratory failure)

<u>Laboratory findings:</u>
- Increased lactate (often > 5 mmol/L)
- Low arterial pH (some as low as < 7.0)
- Low serum bicarbonate

Table 3.8. Antiretroviral Therapy-Associated Adverse Effects and Management Recommendations (cont'd)

Adverse Effects	Associated ARVs	Onset/Clinical Manifestation	Estimated Frequency	Risk Factors	Prevention/ Monitoring	Management
		• Increased anion gap • Elevated serum transaminases, prothrombin time, bilirubin • Low serum albumin • Increased serum amylase & lipase in patients with pancreatitis • Histologic findings of the liver: microvesicular or macrovesicular steatosis Mortality up to 50% in some case series, esp in patients with serum lactate > 10 mmol/L				• The implication of asymptomatic hyperlactatemia is unknown at this point **ARV treatment options:** • Use NRTIs with less propensity for mitochondrial toxicity (e.g., ABC, TDF, 3TC, FTC) • Recommend close monitoring of serum lactate after restarting NRTIs • Consider NRTI-sparing regimens

Lipodystrophy	Lipoatrophy: NRTIs (d4T > ZDV > TDF, ABC, 3TC, FTC), especially when combined with EFV (Haubrich RH, Riddler S, DiRienzo G, et al. 14th Conference on Retroviruses and Opportunistic Infections; February 25-28, 2007; Los Angeles, CA. Abstract 38) Lipohypertrophy: Abdominal fat gain seen with	Onset: gradual: months after initiation of therapy Symptoms: • Lipoatrophy: peripheral fat loss manifested as facial thinning and as thinning of	High: exact frequency uncertain and dependent on regimen; increases with duration on offending agents	• Both lipoatrophy & Lipohypertrophy: low baseline body mass index	• Lipoatrophy: avoid thymidine analogs (esp. when combined with EFV), or switch from ZDV or d4T to ABC or TDF	Lipoatrophy: • Switch from thymidine analogs to TDF or ABC: may slow or halt progression; however, may not fully reverse effects

Table 3.8. Antiretroviral Therapy-Associated Adverse Effects and Management Recommendations (cont'd)

Adverse Effects	Associated ARVs	Onset/Clinical Manifestation	Estimated Frequency	Risk Factors	Prevention/ Monitoring	Management
	PI- or NNRTI-based regimens & with thymidine analogs (e.g., d4T, ZDV)	extremities and buttocks (d4T) • Lipo-hypertrophy: increase in abdominal girth, breast size, and dorsocervical fat pad (buffalo hump)			• _Lipohyper-trophy:_ pretreatment diet/exercise program may reduce incidence and extent	• Injectable poly-L-lactic acid or other injectable fillers for treatment of facial lipoatrophy _Lipohypertrophy:_ • Liposuction for dorsocervical fat pad enlargement (recurrence common) • Diet/exercise • Recombinant human growth hormone, under investigation
Nephrolithiasis/ urolithiasis/ crystalluria	IDV, ATV	_Onset:_ any time after beginning of therapy, especially at times of reduced fluid intake	IDV: 12.4% of nephrolithiasis reported in clinical trials (4.7%–34.4% in different trials) ATV: rare; case reports only	• History of nephrolithiasis • Patients unable to maintain adequate fluid intake • High peak IDV concentration	• Drink at least 1.5–2 liters of non-caffeinated fluid (preferably water) per day	• Increase hydration • Pain control • May consider switching to alternative agent or therapeutic drug

		Clinical manifestations		Risk factors	Prevention / Monitoring	Management
Nephrotoxicity	IDV, TDF	Laboratory abnormalities: pyuria, hematuria, crystalluria; rarely, rise in serum creatinine & acute renal failure Symptoms: flank pain and/or abdominal pain (can be severe), dysuria, frequency Onset: IDV: months after therapy; TDF: weeks to months after therapy Laboratory and other findings: IDV: ↑ serum creatinine, pyuria; hydronephrosis or renal atrophy	Severe toxicity is rare	(↑ ATV levels not found to correlate with risk) • ↑ duration of exposure • warmer climate IDV and TDF: • History of renal disease; elevated creatinine at baseline • Concomitant use of nephrotoxic drugs • TDF: advanced age, low body weight, low CD4 count	• Increase fluid intake at first sign of darkened urine • Monitor urinalysis and serum creatinine every 3–6 months • Avoid use of other nephrotoxic drugs • Adequate hydration if on IDV therapy • Monitor serum creatinine, urinalysis, serum potassium and phosphorus in patients at risk	monitoring (IDV) if treatment option is limited • Stent placement may be required • Stop offending agent, generally reversible • Supportive care • Electrolyte replacement as indicated

Table 3.8. Antiretroviral Therapy-Associated Adverse Effects and Management Recommendations (cont'd)

Adverse Effects	Associated ARVs	Onset/Clinical Manifestation	Estimated Frequency	Risk Factors	Prevention/ Monitoring	Management
		TDF: ↑ serum creatinine, proteinuria, hypophos- phatemia, glycosuria, hypokalemia, non-anion gap metabolic acidosis Symptoms: IDV: asymptomatic; rarely progresses to end-stage renal disease TDF: asymptomatic to signs of nephrogenic diabetes insipidus, Fanconi syndrome with weakness and myalgias				

| Neuromuscular weakness syndrome (ascending) | Most frequently implicated ARV: d4T | Rare | <u>Onset:</u> months after initiation of ARV; then dramatic motor weakness occurring within days to weeks

<u>Symptoms:</u> very rapidly progressive ascending demyelinating polyneuropathy, may mimic Guillain-Barré syndrome; some patients may develop respiratory paralysis requiring mechanical ventilation; has resulted in deaths in some patients

<u>Laboratory findings may include:</u>
• lactic acidosis reported in some cases | • Prolonged d4T use (found in 61 of 69 [88%] cases in one report) (HIV Neuromuscular Syndrome Study Group. AIDS, 2008. 18(10):1403-12) | • Early recognition and discontinuation of ARVs may avoid further progression | • Discontinuation of ARVs
• Supportive care, including mechanical ventilation if needed (as in cases of lactic acidosis listed previously)
• Other measures attempted with variable success: plasmapheresis, high-dose corticosteroid, intravenous immunoglobulin, carnitine, acetylcarnitine
• Recovery often takes months and ranges from complete recovery to substantial residual deficits
• Symptoms may be irreversible in some patients |

Table 3.8. Antiretroviral Therapy-Associated Adverse Effects and Management Recommendations (cont'd)

Adverse Effects	Associated ARVs	Onset/Clinical Manifestation	Estimated Frequency	Risk Factors	Prevention/ Monitoring	Management
						Do not rechallenge patient with offending agent
Osteonecrosis	Link to older PIs, but unclear whether it is caused by ARVs or by HIV	• Markedly increased creatine phosphokinase Clinical presentation (generally similar to non-HIV-infected population): • Insidious in onset, with subtle symptoms of mild to moderate periarticular pain • 85% of cases involving one or both femoral heads, but other bones may also be affected • Pain may be triggered by weight bearing or movement	Symptomatic osteonecrosis: 0.08%–1.33% Asymptomatic osteonecrosis: 4% from MRI reports	• Diabetes • Advanced HIV disease • Prior steroid use • Old age • Alcohol use • Hyperlipidemia • Role of ARVs and osteonecrosis is still controversial	• Risk reduction (e.g., limit steroid and alcohol use) • Asymptomatic cases w/< 15% bony head involvement: follow with MRI every 3–6 months x 1 yr, then every 6 months x 1 yr, then annually to assess for disease progression	Conservative management: • ↓ weight bearing on affected joint • Remove or reduce risk factors • Analgesics as needed Surgical Intervention: • Core decompression +/- bone grafting for early stages of disease • For more severe and debilitating disease. Total joint arthroplasty • Switch from potentially contributing ARVs (i.e., d4T or TDF) & stop other contributing drugs

| Osteopenia (defined as DEXA scan t-score of 1–2.5 SD from normal) or osteoporosis (t-score > 2.5 SD from normal) | Some evidence for early but not progressive bone loss after starting variety of ARVs; assoc/ with TDF or d4T; ↓ bone density and markers of bone turnover with TDF observed in randomized clinical trials | Onset: months to years after starting ART

Symptoms: generally asymptomatic, bone pain, increased risk of fractures | Wide range depending on methodology & patient population; rate appears much higher than seen in the general population: osteopenia: 20%–54%; osteoporosis: 2%–27% (Cazanave C, Dupon M, Lavignolle-Aurillac V, et al. AIDS,2008. 22(3):395-402) | General: low body weight, female, white, southeast Asian, older age, alcohol use, smoking, caffeine, hypogonadism, hyperthyroidism, corticosteroids, vitamin D deficiency, history of significant weight loss, TDF exposure

HIV: low CD4 T-cell count, duration of HIV, lipoatrophy, increased lactic acid levels | • Consider assessment of bone mineral density with DEXA scan (baseline and f/u if abnormal; proper interval in setting of HIV(+) not determined) (Qaseem A, Snow V, Shekelle P, et al. Ann Intern Med, 2008. 148(9):680-4)
• Weight-bearing exercise
• Calcium & vitamin D supplementation
• Hormone replacement | • Follow National Osteoporosis Foundation guidelines (National Osteoporosis Foundation. Clinician's Guide to Prevention and Treatment of Osteoporosis)
• Increase exercise, improve diet, decrease alcohol & tobacco use, increase calcium & vitamin D supplementation
• Bisphosphonate (e.g., once weekly alendronate)
• Judicious hormone replacement
• Intranasal calcitonin |

Table 3.8. Antiretroviral Therapy-Associated Adverse Effects and Management Recommendations (cont'd)

Adverse Effects	Associated ARVs	Onset/Clinical Manifestation	Estimated Frequency	Risk Factors	Prevention/ Monitoring	Management
Pancreatitis	ddI alone; ddI + d4T, hydroxyurea (HU), ribavirin (RBV), or TDF	<u>Onset</u>: usually weeks to months <u>Laboratory abnormalities</u>: increased serum amylase and lipase <u>Symptoms</u>: postprandial abdominal pain, nausea, vomiting	ddI alone: 1%–7% ddI with HU: ↑ by 4–5-fold ↑ frequency if ddI use w/d4T, TDF, or ribavirin	• High intracellular and/or serum ddI concentrations • History of pancreatitis • Alcoholism • Hypertriglyceridemia • Concomitant use of ddI with d4T, HU, or RBV • Use of ddI + TDF without ddI dose reduction	• ddI should not be used in patients with history of pancreatitis • Avoid concomitant use of ddI with d4T, TDF, HU, or RBV • Reduce ddI dose when used with TDF • Monitoring of amylase/lipase in asymptomatic patients is generally not recommended • Treat hypertriglyceridemia	• Discontinue offending agent(s) • Symptomatic management of pancreatitis: bowel rest, IV hydration, pain control, then gradual resumption of oral intake • Parenteral nutrition may be necessary in patients with recurrent symptoms upon resumption of oral intake
Peripheral neuropathy	ddI, d4T, ddC	<u>Onset</u>: weeks to months after initiation of therapy (may be sooner in patients with	ddI: 12%–34% in clinical trials d4T: 52% in monotherapy trial	• Pre-existing peripheral neuropathy; • Combined use of these NRTIs or	• Avoid using these agents in patients at risk, if possible	• Discontinue offending agent if alternative is available; may halt further progression, but

	pre-existing neuropathy) Symptoms: • Begins with numbness & paresthesia of toes and feet • May progress to painful neuropathy of feet and calf • Upper extremities less frequently involved • Can be debilitating for some patients • May be irreversible despite discontinuation of offending agent(s)	ddC: 22%–35% in clinical trials Incidence increases with prolonged exposure	concomitant use of other drugs that may cause neuropathy • Advanced HIV disease • High dose or concomitant use of drugs that may increase ddI intracellular activities (e.g., HU or RBV)	• Avoid combined use of these agents • Patient query at each encounter	symptoms may be irreversible • Substitute alternative ART without potential for neuropathy Pharmacologic management (with variable successes): • Gabapentin (most experience), tricyclic antidepressants, lamotrigine, oxycarbamazepine (potential for CYP interactions), topiramate, tramadol • Narcotic analgesics • Topical capsaicin • Topical lidocaine
Stevens-Johnson syndrome (SJS)/Toxic	NVP > EFV, DLV, ETR	Onset: first few days to weeks after initiation of	NVP: 0.3%–1%; DLV & EFV: 0.1%; ETR: < 0.1%	• NVP: Female, Black, Asian, Hispanic	• For NVP: 2-week lead-in period with 200 mg once	• Discontinue all ARVs and any other possible

Table 3.8. Antiretroviral Therapy-Associated Adverse Effects and Management Recommendations (cont'd)

Adverse Effects	Associated ARVs	Onset/Clinical Manifestation	Estimated Frequency	Risk Factors	Prevention/ Monitoring	Management
epidermal necrosis (TEN)	Also reported with APV, FPV, ABC, DRV, ZDV, ddI, IDV, LPV/r, ATV	therapy but can occur later Symptoms: • Skin eruption with mucosal ulcerations (may involve orogingival mucosa, conjunctiva, anogenital area) • Can rapidly evolve with blister or bullae formation • May eventually evolve to epidermal detachment and/or necrosis • For NVP, may occur with hepatic toxicity • Systemic symptoms (e.g., fever, tachycardia,	1–2 case reports for ABC, FPV, ddI, ZDV, IDV, LPV/r, ATV, DRV		daily, then escalate to 200 mg twice daily • Educate patients to report symptoms as soon as they appear • Avoid use of corticosteroid during NVP dose escalation: may increase incidence of rash	agent(s) (e.g., cotrimoxazole) <u>Aggressive symptomatic support may include:</u> • Intensive care support • Aggressive local wound care (e.g., in a burn unit) • Intravenous hydration • Parenteral nutrition, if needed • Pain management • Antipyretics • Empiric broad-spectrum antimicrobial therapy if superinfection is suspected

Controversial management strategies:
- Corticosteroid
- Intravenous immunoglobulin

Do not rechallenge patient with offending agent

- It is unknown whether patients who experienced SJS while on one NNRTI are more susceptible to SJS from another NNRTI. Most experts would suggest avoiding use of this class unless no other options are available

malaise, myalgia, arthralgia) may be present

Complications:
↓oral intake; fluid depletion; bacterial or fungal superinfection; multiorgan failure

REFERENCES AND SUGGESTED READINGS

AACE Diabetes Mellitus Clinical Practice Guidelines Task Force. American Association of Clinical Endocrinologists medical guidelines for clinical practice for the management of diabetes mellitus. *Endocr Pract*, 2007. 13 (Suppl 1):1–68.

American Diabetes Association. Clinical Practice Recommendations 2008. *Diabetes Care*, 2008. 31 (Suppl 1): S1–104.

Ann Intern Med, 2009. Mar 3;150(5):301–13.

Baylor MS, Johann-Liang R. Hepatotoxicity associated with nevirapine use. *J Acquir Immune Defic Syndr*, 2004. 35(5):538–9.

Bersoff-Matcha SJ, Miller WC, Aberg JA, et al. Sex differences in nevirapine rash. *Clin Infect Dis*, 2001. 32(1):124–9.

Bolhaar MG, Karstaedt AS. A high incidence of lactic acidosis and symptomatic hyperlactatemia in women receiving highly active antiretroviral therapy in Soweto, South Africa. *Clin Infect Dis*, 2007. 45(2):254–60.

Cazanave C, Dupon M, Lavignolle-Aurillac V, et al. Reduced bone mineral density in HIV-infected patients: prevalence and associated factors. *AIDS*, 2008. 22(3): 395–402.

D:A:D Study Group, Sabin CA, Worm SW, et al. Use of nucleoside reverse transcriptase inhibitors and risk of myocardial infarction in HIV-infected patients enrolled in the D:A:D study: a multi-cohort collaboration. *Lancet*, 2008. 371(9622):1417–26.

Dear Health Care Provider letter. Important safety information: intracranial hemorrhage in patients receiving Aptivus® (tipranavir) capsules. Boehringer Ingelheim Pharmaceuticals, Inc. June 30, 2006.

denBrinker M, Wit FW, Wertheim-van Dillen PM, et al. Hepatitis B and C virus co-infection and the risk for hepatotoxicity of highly active antiretroviral therapy in HIV-1 infection. *AIDS*, 2000. 14(18):2895–902.

De Wit S, Sabin CA, Weber R, et al. Incidence and risk factors for new-onset diabetes in HIV-infected patients: the Data Collection on Adverse Events of Anti-HIV Drugs (D:A:D) study. *Diabetes Care*, 2008. 31(6):1224–9.

Dieterich DT, Robinson PA, Love J, Stern JO. Drug-induced liver injury associated with the use of nonnucleoside reverse-transcriptase inhibitors. *Clin Infect Dis*, 2004. 38 (Suppl 2):S80–9.

Dube MP, Stein JH, Aberg JA, et al. Guidelines for the evaluation and management of dyslipidemia in human immunodeficiency virus (HIV)-infected adults receiving antiretroviral therapy: recommendations of the HIV Medical Association of the Infectious Disease Society of America and the Adult AIDS Clinical Trials Group. *Clin Infect Dis*, 2003. 37(5):613–27.

Fagot JP, Mockenhaupt M, Bouwes-Bavinck J-N, for the EuroSCAR study group. Nevirapine and the risk of Stevens-Johnson syndrome or toxic epidermal necrolysis. *AIDS*, 2001. 15(14):1843–8.

Falcó V, Rodríguez D, Ribera E, et al. Severe nucleoside-associated lactic acidosis in human immunodeficiency virus-infected patients: report of 12 cases and review of the literature. *Clin Infect Dis*, 2002. 34(6):838–46.

Fisac C, Fumero E, Crespo et al. Metabolic benefits 24 months after replacing a protease inhibitor with abacavir, efavirenz or nevirapine. *AIDS*, 2005. 19: 917–25.

Geddes R, Knight S, Moosa MY, et al. A high incidence of nucleoside reverse transcriptase inhibitor (NRTI)-induced lactic acidosis in HIV-infected patients in a South African context. *S Afr Med J*, 2006. 96(8):722–4.

Hare CB, Vu MP, Grunfeld C, Lampiris HW. Simvastatin-nelfinavir interaction implicated in rhabdomyolysis and death. *Clin Infect Dis*, 2002. 35:e111–2.

Hammer SM, et al. A controlled trial of two nucleoside analogues plus indinavir in persons with human immunodeficiency virus infection and CD4 cell counts of 200 per cubic milliliter or less. *N Engl J Med*, 1997 Sep 11. 337(11):725–33.

Haubrich RH, Riddler SA, DiRienzo AG, Komarow L, Powderly WG, et al. AIDS Clinical Trials Group (ACTG) A5142 Study Team. *AIDS*, 2009 Jun 1. 23(9):1109–18.

HIV Neuromuscular Syndrome Study Group. HIV-associated neuromuscular weakness syndrome. *AIDS*, 2004. 18(10):1403–12.

J Clin Endocrinol Metab, 2010 Jun 16.

Keiser O, Fellay J, Opravil M, et al. Adverse events to antiretrovirals in the Swiss HIV Cohort Study: effect on mortality and treatment modification. *Antivir Ther*, 2007. 12(8):1157–64.

Kitihata MM, et al. NA-ACCORD. *N Engl J Med*, 2009. 360:1815–26. *Lancet*, 2008. 372:646–55.

Lafeuillade A, Hittinger G, Chadapaud S. Increased mitochondrial toxicity with ribavirin in HIV/HCV coinfection. *Lancet*, 2001. 357(9252):280–1.

Mallal S, Phillips E, Carosi G, et al. HLA-B*5701 screening for hypersensitivity to abacavir. *N Engl J Med*, 2008. 358(6):568–79.

Molina J-M, Andrade-Villanueva J, Echevarria J, et al. Conference on Retroviruses and Opportunistic Infections; February 3–6, 2008. Boston, MA. Abstract 37.

Molina J-M, Andrade-Villanueva J, Echevarria J, et al. Efficacy and safety of once-daily atazanavir/ritonavir compared to twice-daily lopinavir/ritonavir, each in combination with tenofovir and emtricitabine in ARV-naïve HIV-1-infected subjects: The CASTLE Study, 48-week results. *Lancet*, 2008 Aug 23. 372(9639):604–6.

Moyle GJ, Sabin CA, Cartledge J, et al. A randomized comparative trial of tenofovir DF or abacavir as replacement for a thymidine analogue in persons with lipoatrophy. *AIDS*, 2006. 20:2043–50.

National Heart, Lung and Blood Institute. Third Report of the Expert Panel on Detection, Evaluation, and Treatment of High Blood Cholesterol in Adults (Adult Treatment Panel III). Available at http://www.nhlbi.nih.gov/guidelines/cholesterol/index.htm.

National Osteoporosis Foundation. Clinician's Guide to Prevention and Treatment of Osteoporosis. Available at http://www.nof.org/professionals/Clinicians_Guide.htm.

O'Brien ME, Clark RA, Besch CL, et al. Patterns and correlates of discontinuation of the initial HAART regimen in an urban outpatient cohort. *J Acquir Immune Defic Syndr*, 2003. 34(4):407–14.

Ortiz R, Dejesus E, Khanlou H, et al. Efficacy and safety of once-daily darunavir/ritonavir versus lopinavir/ritonavir in treatment-naive HIV-1-infected patients at week 48. *AIDS*, 2008. 22:1389–97.

Pozniak AL, Gallant JE, DeJesus E, et al. Tenofovir disoproxil fumarate, emtricitabine, and efavirenz versus fixed-dose zidovudine/lamivudine and efavirenz in antiretroviral-naïve patients: virologic, immunologic, and morphologic changes-a 96-week analysis. *J Acquir Immune Defic Syndr*, 2006. 43(5):535–40.

Qaseem A, Snow V, Shekelle P, et al. Screening for osteoporosis in men: a clinical practice guideline from the American College of Physicians. *Ann Intern Med*, 2008. 148(9):680–4.

Riddler SA, Smit E, Cole SR, et al. Impact of HIV infection and HAART on serum lipids in men. *JAMA*, 2003. 289:2978–82.

Rodriguez-Novoa S, Barreiro P, Rendón A, et al. Influence of 516G>T polymorphisms at the gene encoding the CYP450-2B6 isoenzyme on efavirenz plasma concentrations in HIV-infected subjects. *Clin Infect Dis*, 2005. 40(9):1358–61.

Saag M, Balu R, Phillips E, et al. High sensitivity of human leukocyte antigen-b*5701 as a marker for immunologically confirmed abacavir hypersensitivity in white and black patients. *Clin Infect Dis*, 2008. 46(7):1111–8.

Saves M, Raffi F, Clevenbergh P, et al. and the APROCO Study Group. Hepatitis B or hepatitis C virus infection is a risk factor for severe hepatic cytolysis after initiation of a protease inhibitor-containing antiretroviral regimen in human immunodeficiency virus-infected patients. *Antimicrob Agents Chemother*, 2000. 44(12):3451–5.

SMART Study Group; El-Sadr WM, Lundgren JD, Neaton JD, et al. CD4+ count-guided interruption of antiretroviral treatment. *N Engl J Med*, 2006. 355(22):2283–96.

Smith KY, Patel P, Fine D, Bellos N, Sloan L, Lackey P, Kumar PN, Sutherland-Phillips DH, Vavro C, Yau L, Wannamaker P, Shaefer MS; HEAT Study Team. *AIDS*, 2009 Jul 31. 23(12):1547–56.

Smith KY, Weinberg WG, Dejesus E, et al. Fosamprenavir or atazanavir once daily boosted with ritonavir 100 mg, plus tenofovir/emtricitabine, for the initial treatment of HIV infection: 48-week results of ALERT. *AIDS Res Ther*, 2008. 5(1):5.

Sulkowski MS, Thomas DL, Chaisson RE, Moore RD. Hepatotoxicity associated with antiretroviral therapy in adults infected with human immunodeficiency virus and the role of hepatitis C or B virus infection. *JAMA*, 2000. 283(1):74–80.

Thompson, MA, Aberg, JA, Cahn, P, et al. Antiretroviral treatment of adult HIV infection: 2010 recommendations of the International AIDS Society USA Panel. *JAMA*, 2010. 304(3):321–33.

Tien PC, Schneider MF, Cole SR, et al. Antiretroviral therapy exposure and incidence of diabetes mellitus in the Women's Interagency HIV Study. *AIDS*, 2007. 21(13):1739–45.

Van Leth F, Phanuphak P, Ruxrungtham K, et al. Comparison of first-line antiretroviral therapy with regimens including nevirapine, efavirenz, or both drugs, plus stavudine and lamivudine: a randomised open-label trial, the 2NN Study. *Lancet*, 2004. 363(9417):1253–63.

When to start consortium timing of initiation of antiretroviral therapy in AIDS-free HIV-1-infected patients: a collaborative analysis of 18 HIV cohort studies. *Lancet*, 2009. 373:1352–63.

Chapter 4

Treatment Failure and Resistance Testing

ANTIRETROVIRAL TREATMENT FAILURE (Table 4.1)

Antiretroviral treatment failure can be defined in various ways. These include **virologic failure** (inability to achieve virologic suppression, or occurrence of virologic rebound), **immunologic failure** (progressive CD4 decline), and **clinical failure** (HIV disease progression). Causes of treatment failure include inadequate adherence, preexisting drug resistance, regimen complexity, side effects, and suboptimal pharmacokinetics. All of these factors can lead to persistent viral replication and evolution of drug resistance.

Regimens for treatment-experienced patients need to be individualized, with the help of resistance testing. Such testing can identify drugs that are likely to be active in patients with prior treatment failures, although other factors, such as regimen tolerability, drug-drug interactions, and achievable plasma concentrations are also important. Choosing an individualized antiretroviral regimen, optimally containing at least two fully active agents, is critical in maximizing the chances for virologic suppression.

Poor medication adherence is the most common cause of treatment failure (J Infect Dis 2005;191:339–347). With poor adherence, subinhibitory drug levels occur, allowing ongoing viral replication and often the emergence of resistant virus. Such resistant variants are likely preexisting mutants that have escaped drug control or host immune failure. The level of adherence required to prevent treatment failure varies depending on the regimen used. In the early protease inhibitor (PI) era, there was a sharp increase in failure rates when adherence fell below 95% (Ann Intern Med 2000;133:21–30). More recent analyses suggest that lower levels of adherence are required when using NNRTI and boosted PI-based regimens, likely due to the longer plasma half-life of nevirapine and efavirenz compared with PIs (Clin Infect Dis 2006;43:939–41) and the higher barrier to resistance of boosted vs. non-boosted PIs (J Infect Dis 2005 Jun 15;191[12]:2046–52).

For patients with virologic failure due to noncompliance, the first step is to establish how much of the combination regimen is being taken. Pharmacy refill frequency has been shown to be a generally reliable proxy for adherence, often better than patient self-report [J Infect Dis 2006 Oct 15;194(8):1108–14]. Often a patient will have stopped an entire regimen simultaneously either due to poor tolerability or psychosocial issues. In this context, virologic failure usually occurs *without* the development of antiretroviral drug resistance, as viremia occurs in the absence of selective pressure of the antivirals. Starting a new regimen (one with the goal of fewer side effects) or restarting the same regimen with a renewed emphasis on the importance of adherence may result in treatment virologic suppression.

A. **Types of Treatment Failure**
   1. **Virologic Failure** is most strictly defined as the inability to achieve or maintain virologic suppression. In a treatment-naïve patient, the HIV RNA level should be < 400 copies/mL after 24 weeks or < 50 copies/mL by 48 weeks after starting therapy; most patients are < 50 copies/mL by 24 weeks except in those with very high baseline HIV RNA. Virologic rebound is seen when there is repeated detection of HIV RNA after virologic suppression in either treatment-naïve or treatment-experienced patients.

2. **Immunologic Failure** can occur in the presence or absence of virologic failure and is defined as a failure to increase the CD4 cell count by 25–50 cells/mm³ above baseline during the first year of therapy, or as a decrease in CD4 cell count to below baseline count while on therapy.

3. **Clinical Failure** is the occurrence or recurrence of HIV-related events after at least 3 months on potent antiretroviral therapy, excluding events related to an immune reconstitution syndrome.

4. **Usual Sequence of Treatment Failure.** Virologic failure usually occurs first, followed by immunologic failure, and finally by clinical progression (J Infect Dis 2000;181: 946–953). These events may be separated by months or years and may not occur in this order in all patients.

B. **Goals After Virologic Failure.** When patients have detectable HIV RNA on treatment, clinicians should attempt to identify the cause of their lack of response and set a treatment goal of achieving full virologic suppression (HIV RNA < 50 copies/mL). The availability of drugs from older classes with enhanced activity against resistant virus and newer agents from novel classes make this an attainable goal for virtually every treatment-experienced patient. In addition to improving clinical and immunologic outcomes, this strategy will also prevent the selection of additional resistance mutations (Ann Intern Med 2000;133:471–473; J Acquir Immune Defic Syndr 2005;40: 34–40). Provided that medication adherence issues and regimen tolerability have been addressed, the regimen should be changed sooner than later.

In rare cases, achieving an undetectable HIV RNA level in patients with an extensive prior treatment history may not be possible. The main goals in these patients should be partial suppression of HIV RNA below the pretreatment baseline level, which in turn leads to the preservation of immune function and the prevention of clinical progression. A likely explanation for this phenomenon is that continued antiretroviral therapy in the face of resistance selects for less fit virus, ultimately leading to less immediate immunologic damage (J Infect Dis 2000;181:946–953; AIDS 2004;18:1539–1548). It is well documented that such patients on treatment have a slower CD4 cell decline than those not on therapy who have wild-type virus (Lancet 2004;364:51–62). Consequently, even with extensive drug resistance and virologic rebound, antiviral therapy should be continued, since stopping therapy is associated with higher rates of disease progression (J Infect Dis 2002;186:189–197; N Engl J Med 2003;349:837–846).

C. **Antiretroviral Regimens After Virologic Failure**

1. **Timing of Switch.** The likelihood of achieving an undetectable HIV RNA level after virologic failure is greater when treatment is changed prior to the accumulation of multiple resistance mutations. Two additional important factors influencing the outcome of subsequent treatment are the level of virologic rebound and degree of CD4 decline (J Acquir Immune Defic Syndr 1999;22:132–138; HIV Clin Trials 2005;6:281–290). For example, in the TORO studies of enfuvirtide plus an optimized background regimen versus an optimized background regimen alone,

study participants with a CD4 cell count > 100/mm³ and/or an HIV RNA level < 100,000 copies/mL were significantly more likely to respond to therapy with or without enfuvirtide (HIV Clin Trials 2005;6:281–290). An additional predictor is having a greater number of active drugs in the optimized background regimen.

2. **Delayed Switch Strategy.** Patients with extensive triple-class drug resistance may be clinically stable, with relatively preserved CD4 cell counts. If 2 (or preferably 3) well-tolerated and active drugs are not available, deferring a switch to preserve active drug classes reduces the risk of selecting further resistance with sequential monotherapy. This delayed switch strategy is most defensible when the CD4 cell count is in a clinically safe range (> 200/mm³) and the patient is amenable and adherent to a strategy of regular clinical and laboratory monitoring. The risk of this approach is the selection of additional resistance mutations, which may compromise future options; a delayed switch was associated with worse clinical outcomes (AIDS 2008 Oct 18;22[16]:2097–106). Delayed switching of failing regimens should generally be avoided given the approval of several agents with activity against resistant viruses. If delayed switching is unavoidable, however, due to patient refusal to change therapy or other issues, providers should ensure that the regimen is less likely to select for additional resistance mutations (see "Holding" Regimens, below).

3. **"Holding" Regimens.** For patients who cannot switch therapy (adherence or financial barriers, no availability of at least 2 active agents), it is reasonable to continue a regimen chosen to maintain clinical stability—sometimes referred to as a "holding" regimen. In the face of incomplete viral suppression, holding regimens should have the following components: (1) at least 2 NRTIs, one of them 3TC or FTC; and (2) a boosted PI based on tolerability. The NRTIs seem particularly important in maintaining a low HIV RNA level in patients with incomplete viral suppression (J Infect Dis 2005;192: 1537–44). There is no evidence that NNRTIs continue to exert antiviral or other benefit after resistance develops, and continuing them may select for further NNRTI mutations, limiting subsequent response to new agents in this drug class, such as etravirine. The data on continued use of enfuvirtide after virologic rebound are conflicting in this regard; our practice is generally to discontinue enfuvirtide given the requirement for twice daily injections, the high cost of the medication, and the possibility of future fusion inhibitors with a similar mechanism of action and related resistance profiles.

4. **Blips.** It is important to emphasize that transient, low-level detectable HIV RNA levels—sometimes called "blips"—are often not indicative of virologic failure. In one study, 10 patients with virologic suppression (HIV RNA < 50 copies/mL) underwent intensive analysis with 36 visits over approximately 3 months (JAMA 2005;293:817–829). Of more than 700 viral load measurements, 26 samples showed transient low-level viremia. However, blips did not predict subsequent treatment failure or indicate underlying resistance. As a result, clinicians should not act based on single viral load measurements above the limit of detection but should confirm these results before changing treatment. In contrast, patients with persistent low-level viremia (> 400 and < 1000 HIV RNA copies/mL) have exhibited increases in immune activation and a higher risk of viral resistance evolution and subsequent virologic failure (AIDS

2004;18:981–989). Similarly, some sites have reported an increased frequency of detecting low-level HIV RNA since switching to from the Roche Amplicor to the newer real-time Taqman PCR [J Acquir Immune Defic Syndr 2009 Feb 25]. The clinical significance of this observation is unclear. For now our practice is not to switch treatments in patients who have newly detectable HIV RNA < 200 cop/mL on this newer assay especially if not confirmed with a second value.

D. Immunologic and Clinical Failure. Most cases of immunologic and clinical failure are seen after virologic rebound, in particular in patients who have completely stopped antiretroviral therapy. However, patients who have virologic suppression will rarely experience a limited CD4 response, or even a decline. Factors variably associated with poor immunologic response include older age, hepatitis C virus coinfection, cirrhosis, use of NNRTI- rather than PI-based therapy, use of zidovudine (which can reduce total white blood cell count), and the combination of tenofovir plus didanosine (J Infect Dis 2006;193:259–268; Clin Infect Dis 2005;41:901–905). These cases of poor CD4 response, even with virologic suppression, likely have a prominent host genetic component, and therefore are usually not related to any specific antiretroviral strategy (Ahuja et al, Nat Med 2008;14[4]:413–420). The management of patients with poor CD4 response despite virologic suppression is not well established, and no particular strategy has been proven to improve the CD4 cell count. Our practice is to modify the antiretroviral regimen only if there is a specific component known to reduce CD4 response (e.g., tenofovir + ddI, or ZDV-induced leukopenia). Importantly, the clinical prognosis for patients with virologic responses even without substantial CD4 increases is superior to those with comparable CD4 cell counts who do not have suppression of viremia (Ann Intern Med 2000;133:401–410). Actual clinical progression in the face of virologic suppression is rare, and often a manifestation of the immune reconstitution inflammatory syndrome (IRIS) rather than actual HIV disease progression. Such cases represent an enhanced immune response to a preexisting opportunistic process and not the acquisition of a new infection (Clin Infect Dis 2006;42:418–427). In cases of IRIS, usually the current antiretroviral therapy should be continued, with treatment of the underlying process and, if necessary, adjunctive anti-inflammatory therapy with corticosteroids.

Table 4.1. Management of Antiretroviral Treatment Failure

Type of Failure	Recommended Approach	Comments
Virologic failure *Limited or intermediate prior treatment*	Assess for adherence and regimen tolerability. Obtain genotype resistance test. Select new regimen based on resistance test results and tolerability	Usually associated with limited or no detectable resistance. If no resistance is found, consider re-testing for resistance 2–4 weeks after resuming antivirals. Stop NNRTIs if resistance is detected. Likelihood of virologic suppression is high if adherence is good

Table 4.1. Management of Antiretroviral Treatment Failure (cont'd)

Type of Failure	Recommended Approach	Comments
Extensive prior treatment	Assess for adherence and regimen tolerability. Obtain resistance test—consider phenotype, "virtual phenotype," or phenotype-genotype combination if level of resistance is likely to be high, especially to the protease inhibitor drug class. Obtain viral tropism assay to assess possible use of CCR5 antagonist. Select new regimen using at least 2 new active agents; if 2 new active agents not available, continue a "holding" regimen	In patients with resistance to NRTIs, NNRTIs, and PIs, the new regimen should generally contain: (1) at least one and if possible two drugs from a new drug class (integrase inhibitor, CCR5 antagonist, or fusion inhibitor); (2) a boosted PI with activity against resistant viruses (darunavir generally preferred over tipranavir); and (3) one or two NRTIs, one of them 3TC or FTC. For patients with documented PI resistance, the superiority of darunavir over other PIs has been demonstrated in several studies [Lancet 2007 Apr 7;369 (9568):1169–78; Lancet 2007 Jul 7;370 (9581):49–58]. The only exception would be those viruses with documented resistance to darunavir but preserved susceptibility to tipranavir. A holding regimen should always contain 3TC or FTC plus a boosted PI; NNRTIs should never be used.
Low-level HIV RNA (50–1000 copies)	Assess for adherence, drug-drug interactions, intercurrent illness, recent immunizations. Repeat test in 3–4 weeks	For low-level viremia followed by undetectable HIV RNA ("blip"), no treatment change is necessary. If HIV RNA is persistently detectable at > 500 copies/mL, obtain resistance test as described above, and treat accordingly. If HIV RNA is persistently detectable between 50–500 copies/mL, consider regimen "intensification" with use of an additional agent. Low-level detectable virus (48–500 cop/mL) using the newer Taqman RT-PCR assay is of unclear clinical significance.

Table 4.1. Management of Antiretroviral Treatment Failure (cont'd)

Type of Failure	Recommended Approach	Comments
Immunologic failure *Detectable HIV RNA*	Assess for adherence and tolerability. If non-adherent, resume treatment after barriers to adherence are addressed. If adherent, obtain resistance testing and alter therapy as described above.	If HIV RNA is back to pre-treatment baseline, non-adherence is the most likely explanation.
Suppressed HIV RNA	Investigate for modifiable conditions that may be associated with impaired CD4 response (chronic HCV, treatment with ZDV, TDF + ddl). If no modifiable conditions found, continue current regimen.	Prognosis for patients with suppressed HIV RNA and immunologic failure better than for those with comparable CD4 cell counts and detectable viremia.
Clinical failure *Detectable HIV RNA*	Treat OI with appropriate anti-infective therapy. Assess for antiretroviral adherence and tolerability. Send resistance test and choose new regimen based on results of test and other treatment options.	OIs (IRIS excluded) most commonly occur in those not on antiretroviral therapy due to poor compliance and/or regimen tolerability.
Suppressed HIV RNA	Continue current antiretrovirals. Treat OI with appropriate anti-infective therapy. If symptoms persist and IRIS is likely, use adjunctive corticosteroids.	IRIS most likely when baseline CD4 cell count is low (< 200/mm³); onset usually weeks-to-months after starting a potent regimen. IRIS been reported with virtually all OIs. True clinical progression with suppressed HIV RNA is unusual; IRIS should not be considered a sign of antiretroviral treatment failure.

IRIS = immune reconstitution inflammatory syndrome, OI = opportunistic infection

---

PRINCIPLES OF RESISTANCE TESTING

HIV drug resistance most commonly occurs as a result of non-suppressive antiretroviral regimens. Less commonly, resistance occurs as a result of transmission of a resistant strain. The prevalence of drug resistance among patients with sustained viral replication is high.

In a random sample of HIV-infected American adults, NRTI resistance was found in 71% of samples, PI resistance in 41%, NNRTI resistance in 25%, and triple-class resistance in 13% (AIDS 2004;18:1393–1401). Studies have demonstrated that the presence of resistance before starting a new antiretroviral regimen increases the likelihood that the regimen will fail, and that patients whose treatment is chosen with information from resistance testing have better short-term virologic outcomes than control subjects without use of resistance tests.

Resistance testing is a highly complex diagnostic strategy that for maximal effect requires both a thorough review of the patient treatment history and an understanding of the strengths and limitations of the resistance assays. Both genotypic and phenotypic criteria for resistance are under continuous evaluation and evolution. It is therefore important to consult with updated guidelines, such as those published by the International AIDS Society (Clin Infect Dis 2008;47:266–285).

In a patient's resistance testing history, the occurrence of a given mutation implies that this resistance will persist even when the selective pressure for this mutation is removed and the mutation is no longer detectable by conventional resistance testing. For example, the occurrence of the M184V mutation secondary to 3TC or FTC therapy may no longer appear on resistance tests after these drugs have been stopped. However, viruses that still harbor this mutation are "archived" and will re-emerge with resumption of these agents. Although there are literally hundreds of genotypic mutations described, certain mutations or patterns of mutations are more common or important than others. These are discussed below.

The correlation between the presence of resistance and response to a given combination of drugs is not always absolute. For example, even when viruses harbor several primary PI resistance mutations, ritonavir-boosted PIs may retain significant antiviral effect since achievable drug levels exceed levels required for inhibition of these strains; additionally, certain agents (notably darunavir, etravirine, and tipranavir) were specifically developed due to their retained activity against many viruses with resistance to other drugs within the same class. Among the NRTIs, it is well established that 3TC (and presumably FTC) continue to reduce HIV RNA even after development of substantial in vitro resistance to these drugs [Clin Infect Dis 2005 Jul 15;41(2):236–42]. As a result of these and other factors, continuing antiretroviral therapy even after widespread antiviral drug resistance leads to a better virologic, immunologic, and clinical outcome.

TYPES OF RESISTANCE TESTING

Two types of resistance testing can be ordered: genotypic and phenotypic. Genotype tests describe mutations known to be associated with resistance to specific drugs. Phenotype tests measure the ability of individual drugs to inhibit a recombinant virus that is derived from the patient's isolate. Advantages and disadvantages of the two types of resistance tests are described in Table 4.2.

Table 4.2. Genotype vs. Phenotype Resistance Testing

Method	Advantages	Disadvantages
Genotype testing	• Rapid turnaround (1–2 weeks) • Less expensive than phenotyping • Detection of mutations may precede phenotypic resistance • Widely available from multiple commercial and academic labs • More sensitive than phenotype for detecting mixtures of resistant and wild-type virus, especially for patients not on treatment • Two FDA-approved genotype assays (TRUGENE, ViroSeq)	• Indirect measure of resistance • Relevance of some mutations is unclear • Unable to detect minority variants (< 20–25% of viral sample) • Complex mutational patterns may be difficult to interpret • Interpretation of results variable depending on the laboratory
Phenotype testing	• Provides direct and quantitative measure of resistance • Methodology can be applied to any antiretroviral agent, including new drugs, for which genotypic correlates of resistance are unclear • Can assess interactions among mutations • Accurate with non-B HIV subtypes • May offer an estimate of the ability of resistant viruses to grow compared to wild-type strains ("replication capacity")	• Susceptibility cut-offs not standardized between assays • Clinical cut-offs not defined for some agents • Unable to detect minority variants (< 20–25% of viral sample) • Complex technology with longer turnaround (3–4 weeks) • More expensive than genotyping • Availability limited to two laboratories in USA (Monogram and Virco)

A. **Genotype Testing.** In most settings where resistance testing is indicated, genotype testing is preferred over phenotype testing, as a larger number of studies having validated the predictive value of genotype testing to help enhance treatment response. Genotype testing is also more easily standardized from lab-to-lab, less expensive, and has faster turnaround time.

B. **Phenotype Testing.** Phenotype testing, usually in conjunction with a genotype test, may be of particular value in the following clinical scenarios: (1) occurrence of certain viral strains that make sequencing difficult for the laboratory; (2) highly complex or contradictory genotype results, especially in multiple PI-resistant cases; and (3) when used in conjunction with therapeutic drug monitoring of protease inhibitors (rarely done in the United States currently). Phenotype testing is especially useful when deciding whether to use tipranavir or darunavir, as these are the most active agents against highly PI-resistant strains. In such a setting, predicting tipranavir or darunavir activity based on genotype testing is often difficult; in contrast, clinical cutoffs are provided by phenotype testing that detail whether these drugs are fully active, partially active, or inactive virologically.

C. **Other Options for Resistance Testing.** One of the companies that performs phenotype testing (Monogram) offers a combined phenotype/genotype test, called a "Phenosense GT." This test provides the most complete representation of resistance status, with a direct correlation between detected mutations and in vitro susceptibility. The combined test has the highest cost among commercially available assays. Another company (Virco) offers a test sometimes referred to as a "virtual" phenotype. Called "VircoType HIV," this test uses standard genotype results to predict drug susceptibility based on associations of detected mutations with existing phenotypes in a database. A benefit of this approach is that, similar to phenotyping, it indicates which drugs have partial activity. The cost is intermediate between genotype and phenotype testing.

D. **Co-Receptor Tropism Assay.** HIV enters the CD4 cell using both the CD4 receptor and either a CCR5 receptor (R5-tropic viruses) or a CXCR4 receptor (X4-tropic viruses). R5-tropic viruses are commonly transmitted and predominate in early infection. Over time, there is a shift in virus population to those that use both receptors (dual tropic) or to a mixture of R5 and X4 viruses. The CCR5 antagonist drug maraviroc is only active against R5-tropic viruses. As a result, when considering use of this agent, a co-receptor tropism assay should be ordered. It is reasonable to consider repeating this test for patients who experience virologic failure on maraviroc.

The best available tropism assay currently is a modification of the Monogram phenotype; results return in 3–4 weeks, and indicate whether the viral population is R5-tropic, of dual or mixed tropism (D/M), or X4-tropic. The report also provides a summary statement about whether CCR5 antagonist drugs will be active. In clinical studies of maraviroc in treatment-experienced patients, approximately 50% of patients screened had R5-tropic virus and hence were appropriate candidates for the drug. Notably, although the test is not 100% sensitive for X4-using viruses, a more sensitive assay was introduced in the summer of 2008, providing greater assurance about whether maraviroc would be active.

INDICATIONS FOR AND APPROACH TO RESISTANCE TESTING

Since the introduction of resistance testing in the late 1990s, indications for resistance testing have expanded significantly (Table 4.3). A suggested approach to HIV drug resistance testing is shown in Figure 4.1.

Table 4.3. Summary of Clinical Situations in Which Resistance Testing is Recommended

Clinical Setting	Comments
Before initiation of therapy Primary (acute and early) infection	Resistance testing is recommended. Initial therapy may be altered based on resistance test results
First evaluation of chronic HIV-1 infection	Resistance testing is recommended, including for patients for whom therapy is delayed, because plasma wild-type isolates may replace drug-resistant virus with time in the absence of treatment
Treatment initiation for chronic HIV-1 infection	Resistance testing is recommended because of a rising prevalence of baseline HIV-1 drug resistance in untreated patients with chronic infection, unless preexisting data or stored samples for testing are available
In antiretroviral-treated patients Treatment failure	Resistance testing is recommended. The decision to change therapy should integrate treatment history, new and prior resistance results (if available), and evaluation of adherence and possible drug interactions
In specific settings Pregnancy[a]	Resistance testing is recommended before initiation of therapy to effectively treat the mother and prevent mother-to-child transmission
Other considerations and general recommendations	Post-exposure prophylaxis should consider treatment history and resistance data from the source, when available. A sudden increase in HIV-1 plasma RNA may reflect superinfection, possibly with drug-resistant virus. Plasma samples to be tested for drug resistance should contain at least 500 HIV-1 RNA copies/mL to ensure successful PCR amplification required for all sequencing approaches. It is preferable that the blood sample for resistance testing be obtained while the patient is receiving the failing regimen, if possible Resistance testing should be performed by laboratories that have appropriate operator training, certification, and periodic proficiency assurance. Genotypic and phenotypic test results should be interpreted by individuals knowledgeable in antiretroviral therapy and drug resistance patterns. Inhibitory quotient testing is not recommended for clinical decision making.

Adapted from Clin Infect Dis 2008;47(2):266–285—Antiretroviral Drug Resistance Testing in Adult HIV-1 Infection: 2008 Recommendations of an International AIDS Society–USA Panel

a   If resistance test results are available from before the pregnancy, clinical judgment should guide whether retesting for resistance is necessary.

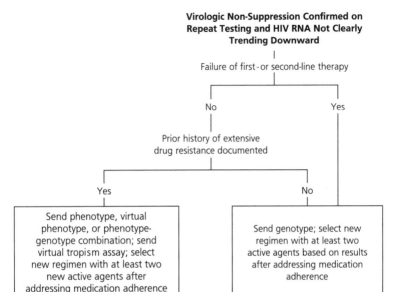

Figure 4.1. Approach to HIV Drug Resistance Testing

**IMPORTANT GENOTYPIC RESISTANCE PATTERNS
(SEE ALSO APPENDIX 1: DRUG RESISTANCE MUTATIONS IN HIV-1, P. 235)**

A. Nucleoside Reverse Transcriptase Inhibitors (NRTI's)

1. 3TC/FTC: M184V

- M184V emerges rapidly (days-weeks) in non-suppressive treatment regimens. This leads to a large reproducible increase in resistance of the virus to 3TC and FTC. On its own, M184V reduces the susceptibility of viruses to abacavir and ddI; however, these drugs do retain clinically significant antiviral activity even with M184V. One prospective study found that the incidence of M184V was lower in patients treated with tenofovir, FTC, and EFV than with ZDV/3TC and EFV (N Engl J Med 2006;43:535–540).

- Despite this resistance, significant antiviral activity of 3TC/FTC-containing regimens is often maintained for a prolonged period of time. Common explanations include: (1) M184V increases viral susceptibility to certain other NRTI's, notably ZDV, d4T, and tenofovir; (2) viruses with M184V have a lower replication capacity in vitro than wild-type viruses; and (3) 3TC/FTC exert an antiviral effect despite the presence of high-level phenotypic resistance.

- The combination of rapid development of resistance to 3TC/FTC, the potential benefits of the M184V mutation otherwise, and the excellent tolerability of these drugs leads to a clinical dilemma: should the drug be continued even in the face of resistance? Our practice is typically to continue the 3TC/FTC in patients who otherwise have extensive resistance and may benefit from the reduced viral fitness imparted by the M184V mutation. Supportive data for this approach is derived from studies in which patients receiving 3TC and having M184V experienced significant increases in HIV RNA after 3TC was discontinued (Clin Infect Dis 2005;41:236–42; AIDS 2006;20:795–803).

2. ZDV/d4T: Thymidine-Associated Mutations (TAMs)

- The thymidine-associated mutations are M41L, D67N, K70R, L210W, T215Y, and K219Q.

- TAMs emerge slowly and sequentially with ZDV and d4T-containing regimens. As ZDV and d4T are combined with 3TC or FTC for initial therapy, the M184V mutation generally evolves before the occurrence of TAMs.

- As with other non-suppressive regimens, in general the longer a patient is on an ZDV or d4T-containing regimen with a detectable HIV RNA, the greater the number of TAMs the patient will accumulate.

- The degree of resistance to ZDV and d4T as well as other NRTI's correlates with the total number of TAMs. Only 1 or 2 TAMs may reduce susceptibility to ZDV or d4T, whereas 3 or more TAMs are required to reduced susceptibility (and virologic response) to ABC, ddI, and TDF. (Note that M184V plus only 1 TAM will reduce viral susceptibility to ABC.)

- Often patients will evolve along one of two different TAM pathways: (1) M41L, L210W, T215Y: this occurs more commonly and is associated with broader resistance, including all other NRTI's as well as TDF; or (2) D67N, K70R, and K219Q: this induces a lower-level of resistance, and TDF treatment retains significant activity.

3. Tenofovir: K65R

- K65R reduces in vitro susceptibility to tenofovir, 3TC, ddI, and abacavir. In patients with prior ZDV or d4T treatment and associated TAMs, selection of K65R rarely occurs.

- As with the TAMs described above, in a typical combination regimen using TDF, 3TC or FTC, and EFV, the first mutations to appear are M184V (selected by 3TC and FTC) and NNRTI-associated mutations. In patients with continued non-suppressive therapy, K65R may also develop.

- The consequence of this pattern is broad NRTI resistance (analogous to multiple TAMs) and high-level NNRTI resistance (if NNRTI resistance mutations are present). Viruses harboring the K65R mutation remain susceptible to ZDV, and are sometimes "hypersusceptible," indicating that ZDV is more active vs. K65R mutants than against wild-type virus. Preliminary data suggest that patients with

K65R (plus M184V and NNRTI resistance) can usually be successfully treated with salvage regimens, generally in those containing boosted PI's.

- As with M184V, in vitro data suggest that K65R reduces replication capacity, and that both together reduce replication capacity more than either one alone.
- K65R also may develop in treatment-naïve patients placed on abacavir, ddI, or d4T-containing initial regimens. More commonly, however, d4T will select for TAMs, and ddI and abacavir for L74V.

4. **Abacavir, ddI: L74V**

- Virologic failure of initial therapy with abacavir or ddI (plus 3TC or FTC) most commonly selects initially for the M184V mutation, followed by L74V.
- L74V reduces susceptibility to ABC and ddI; ZDV remains fully active. The data on TDF activity are conflicting.

5. **Multinucleoside Resistance Patterns: Q151M and T69ins**

- Before the triple-therapy era, Q151M and T69 insertion mutation pattern (T69ins) developed in patients who were on prolonged ZDV/ddI or d4T/ddI-containing regimens with virologic failure.
- The occurrence of these mutational patterns is rare today.
- Q151M reduces susceptibility to all NRTI's except tenofovir.
- If the T69ins is accompanied by 1 or more TAMs, all NRTI's (including TDF) show reduced susceptibility.

B. **Non-Nucleoside Reverse Transcriptase Inhibitors (NNRTI's).** Unsuccessful treatment with NNRTI's leads rapidly to selection of NNRTI-associated resistance mutations. These mutations generally share two important properties: (1) a nearly complete loss of antiviral activity (contrast 3TC or FTC resistance); and (2) a high degree of cross-resistance between nevirapine, delavirdine, and efavirenz. As a result, sequencing of these older NNRTI's after resistance develops is not possible. The most common resistance mutation selected by efavirenz is K103N, and nevirapine often selects for Y181C, except when given with ZDV. Less common mutational patterns seen with NNRTI's are L100I, V106A/M, Y181C/I, Y188L, G190S/A, and M230L. As noted above, all may reduce susceptibility to all the drugs in the class. In vitro, efavirenz retains activity against viruses that have only the Y181C mutation selected by nevirapine. As a result, genotype reports may cite efavirenz viruses with Y181C as "possibly resistant" to efavirenz. However, clinical studies suggest that efavirenz efficacy will be reduced, possibly because of the presence of primary efavirenz resistance mutations that are below the level of detection of the genotype assay.

Etravirine is the first NNRTI with documented clinical activity against some NNRTI-resistant viruses. In the DUET studies, treatment-experienced patients with documented NNRTI resistance received either etravirine or placebo; they also received an optimized background regimen containing at least DRV/r, plus other agents selected by the investigators. At 24 weeks, viral load and CD4 cell count data significantly favored etravirine over placebo (Lancet 2007;370:39–48). In this study, response to etravirine was diminished only when patients had at least three of the following mutations (which are also included in the IAS–USA set): V90I, A98G, L100I, K101E/P, V106I, V179D/F,

Y181C/I/V, and G190A/S. Importantly, baseline presence of the K103N mutation—the most common mutation seen in patients with treatment failure on efavirenz—does not affect response to etravirine.

C. Protease Inhibitors (PI's)

1. Nelfinavir: D30N

- Virologic failure on a nelfinavir-containing regimen is most commonly associated with the D30N mutation, sometimes with N88D. While conferring high-level resistance to NFV, other PI's retain activity against these viruses.
- Clinical studies have confirmed that second PI's—especially when "boosted" with ritonavir—can be used to salvage virologic failures with D30N mutations. A potential disadvantage of this strategy is that 3TC and sometimes other NRTI-based mutations are often present as well.
- A minority of treatment failures with nelfinavir will select for the L90M mutation, which is associated with broader resistance to PI's than D30N. The L90M pathway is more common in non-subtype B viruses, which are considerably more prevalent outside of the United States and Western Europe.

2. Atazanavir: I50L

- In patients without prior PI treatment, unboosted atazanavir selects for the I50L mutation, usually after selection of 3TC or other NRTI resistance. As with D30N and nelfinavir, I50L reduces susceptibility to ATV but not to other PI's.
- On phenotype testing, viruses with I50L alone often demonstrate hypersusceptibility to other PI's—that is, non-ATV PI's appear to be more active against these viruses than against wild-type strains. The clinical significance of this phenomenon is unknown, as there are no controlled studies evaluating sequencing of PI's after ATV failure.
- PI-experienced patients treated with ATV rarely select for I50L, and more typical PI-mutations emerge.
- The resistance pattern selected by boosted ATV in treatment-naive patients is thus far unknown. One study showed no PI resistance mutations or virologic rebound on boosted ATV, analogous to other boosted PI's (presented at 13th CROY, Denver, CO, 2006 Abst. 107LB).

3. Fosamprenavir: I50V

- Use of unboosted FPV may select for the I50V mutation, generally occurring (as with NFV and ATV) along with some degree of NRTI resistance.
- I50V reduces susceptibility to lopinavir, ritonavir, and darunavir; other PI's retain activity, at least as measured by phenotype testing.
- Sequencing of PI's after development of I50V or other patterns of FPV failure has not been studied in controlled trials.

4. **General protease inhibitor resistance mutations: L10F/I/R/V, V32I, M46I/L, I54V/M/L, V82A/F/T/S, I84V/A/C, and L90M**

- The presence of an increasing number of mutations from the above list generally confers broad PI resistance to all FDA-approved PI's.
- With < 4 mutations from the above list, ritonavir-boosted atazanavir and lopinavir had similar virologic activity; with 4 or more such mutations, lopinavir was more active (AIDS 2006;20:847–53).
- When choosing a new regimen for patients with any PI resistance, phenotype testing is preferred. Tipranavir and darunavir are currently the PI's with the greatest activity against PI-resistant viruses and darunavir is generally preferred due to favourable tolerability and safety. To further increase the chances of achieving virologic suppression, all tipranavir- or darunavir-treated patients should also receive, at least one other fully active drug, along with the most active (often recycled) NRTI's. In most cases currently, this other active drug will be a drug from a newer drug class, such as an integrase inhibitor, CCR5 antagonist, or fusion inhibitor. See Figure 4.2 for the recommended approach.

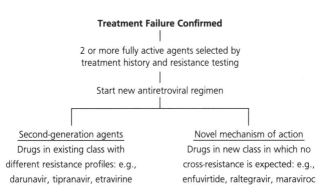

Treatment Failure Confirmed

2 or more fully active agents selected by
treatment history and resistance testing

Start new antiretroviral regimen

Second-generation agents	Novel mechanism of action
Drugs in existing class with different resistance profiles: e.g., darunavir, tipranavir, etravirine	Drugs in new class in which no cross-resistance is expected: e.g., enfuvirtide, raltegravir, maraviroc

Figure 4.2. Approach to Patients with Virologic Failure and Multiclass Resistance

From: Department of Health and Human Services Panel on Antiretroviral Guidelines for Adults and Adolescents. Aidsinfo.nih.gov

Chapter 5

Prophylaxis and Treatment of Opportunistic Infections

PROPHYLAXIS OF OPPORTUNISTIC INFECTIONS

Patients with HIV disease are at risk for infectious complications not otherwise seen in immunocompetent patients. Such opportunistic infections occur in proportion to the severity of immune system dysfunction (reflected by CD4 cell count depletion). While community acquired infections (e.g., pneumococcal pneumonia) can occur at any CD4 cell count, the "classic" HIV-related opportunistic infections (PCP, toxoplasmosis, cryptococcus, disseminated *M. avium* complex, CMV) do not occur until CD4 cell counts are dramatically reduced. Specifically, it is rare to encounter PCP in HIV patients with CD4 > 200/mm³, and CMV and disseminated MAC typically occur at median CD4 < 50/mm³. Indications for prophylaxis and specific prophylaxis regimens are summarized in Table 5.1 and detailed in Table 5.2. The US Public Health Service/Infectious Diseases Society of America guidelines for the prevention and treatment of opportunistic infections in persons infected with HIV can be found ataidsinfo. nih.gov, and were last updated in April 10, 2009 (see http://aidsinfo.nih.gov/Guidelines/ GuidelineDetail.aspx?MenuItem=Guidelines&Search=Off&GuidelineID=211&ClassID=4).

Table 5.1. Overview of Prophylaxis of Selected Opportunistic Infections (see Table 5.2 for details)

Infection	Indication for Prophylaxis	Intervention
PCP	CD4 < 200/mm³	TMP-SMX
TB *(M. tuberculosis)*	PPD > 5 mm (current or past) or contact with active case	INH
Toxoplasma	IgG Ab (+) and CD4 < 100/mm³	TMP-SMX
MAC	CD4 < 50/mm³	Azithromycin
S. pneumoniae	CD4 > 200/mm³	Pneumococcal vaccine
Hepatitis B	Susceptible patients	Hepatitis B vaccine
Hepatitis A	Susceptible patients	Hepatitis A vaccine
Influenza	All patients	Annual flu vaccine
VZV	CD4 > 200/mm³, VZV antibody negative	Varicella vaccine

Ab = antibody; HA = Hepatitis A; HCV = Hepatitis C virus; VZIG = varicella-zoster immune globulin; VZV = varicella-zoster virus; other abbreviations (p. ix)

Table 5.2 Prophylaxis to Prevent First Episode of Opportunistic Disease

Pathogen	Indication	First choice	Alternative
Pneumocystis pneumonia (PCP)	CD4+ count < 200 cells/µL or oropharyngeal candidiasis CD4+ < 14% or history of AIDS-defining illness CD4+ count > 200 but < 250 cells/µL if monitoring CD4+ count every 1–3 months is not possible	Trimethoprim-sulfamethoxazole (TMP-SMX), 1 DS PO daily; or 1 SS daily	TMP-SMX 1 DS PO tiw; **or** Dapsone 100 mg PO daily or 50 mg PO BID; **or** Dapsone 50 mg PO daily + pyrimethamine 50 mg PO weekly + leucovorin 25 mg PO weekly; **or** Aerosolized pentamidine 300 mg via Respigard II™ nebulizer every month; **or** Atovaquone 1,500 mg PO daily; **or** Atovaquone 1,500 mg + pyrimethamine 25 mg + leucovorin 10 mg PO daily
Toxoplasma gondii encephalitis	Toxoplasma IgG positive patients with CD4 + count < 100 cells/µL Seronegative patients receiving PCP prophylaxis not active against toxoplasmosis should have toxoplasma serology retested if CD4+ count decline to < 100 cells/µL Prophylaxis should be initiated if seroconversion occurred	TMP-SMX, 1 DS PO daily	TMP-SMX 1 DS PO tiw; **or** TMP-SMX 1 SS PO daily; Dapsone 50 mg PO daily + pyrimethamine 50 mg PO weekly + leucovorin 25 mg PO weekly; **or** (Dapsone 200 mg + pyrimethamine 75 mg + leucovorin 25 mg) PO weekly; (Atovaquone 1,500 mg +/- pyrimethamine 25 mg + leucovorin 10 mg) PO daily

Table 5.2 Prophylaxis to Prevent First Episode of Opportunistic Disease (cont'd)

Pathogen	Indication	First choice	Alternative
Mycobacterium tuberculosis infection (TB) (Treatment of latent TB infection or LTBI)	(+) diagnostic test for LTBI, no evidence of active TB, and no prior history of treatment for active or latent TB; (-) diagnostic test for LTBI, but close contact with a person with infectious pulmonary TB and no evidence of active TB; A history of untreated or inadequately treated healed TB (i.e., old fibrotic lesions) regardless of diagnostic tests for LTBI and no evidence of active TB	Isoniazid (INH) 300 mg PO daily or 900 mg PO biw for 9 months–both plus pyridoxine 50 mg PO daily; **or** For persons exposed to drug-resistant TB, selection of drugs after consultation with public health authorities	Rifampin (RIF) 600 mg PO daily x 4 months; **or** Rifabutin (RFB) (dose adjusted based on concomitant ART) x 4 months
Disseminated *Mycobacterium avium* complex (MAC) disease	CD4+ count < 50 cells/μL—after ruling out active MAC infection	Azithromycin 1,200 mg PO once weekly; **or** Clarithromycin 500 mg PO BID; or Azithromycin 600 mg PO twice weekly	RFB 300 mg PO daily (dosage adjustment based on drug-drug interactions with ART); rule out active TB before starting RFB
Streptococcus pneumoniae infection	CD4+ count > 200 cells/μL and no receipt of pneumococcal vaccine in the past 5 years CD4+ count < 200 cells/μL—vaccination can be offered In patients who received polysaccharide pneumococcal vaccination (PPV) when CD4+ count < 200 cells/μL, but has	23-valent PPV 0.5 mL IM x 1 Revaccination every 5 years may be considered	

Table 5.2 Prophylaxis to Prevent First Episode of Opportunistic Disease (cont'd)

Pathogen	Indication	First choice	Alternative
	increased to > 200 cells/μL in response to ARTs		
Influenza A and B virus infection	All HIV-infected patients	Inactivated influenza vaccine 0.5 mL IM annually	
Histoplasma capsulatum infection	CD4+ count ≤ 150 cells/μL and at high risk because of occupational exposure or live in a community with a hyperendemic rate of histoplasmosis (> 10 cases/100 patient-years)	Itraconazole 200 mg PO daily	
Coccidioidomycosis	Positive IgM or IgG serologic test in a patient from a disease-endemic area; and CD4+ count < 250 cells/μL	Fluconazole 400 mg PO daily Itraconazole 200 mg PO BID	
Varicella-zoster virus (VZV) infection	Pre-exposure prevention: Patients with CD4+ count ≥ 200 cells/μL who have not been vaccinated, have no history of varicella or herpes zoster, or who are seronegative for VZV Note: routine VZV serologic testing in HIV-infected adults is not recommended Post-exposure—close contact with a person who has active varicella or herpes zoster:	Pre-exposure prevention: Primary varicella vaccination (Varivax™), 2 doses (0.5 mL SQ) administered 3 months apart If vaccination results in disease because of vaccine virus, treatment with acyclovir is recommended Post-exposure therapy: Varicella-zoster immune globulin (VariZIG™) 125 IU per 10 kg (maximum of 625 IU) IM,	VZV-susceptible household contacts of susceptible HIV-infected persons should be vaccinated to prevent potential transmission of VZV to their HIV-infected contacts Alternative post-exposure therapy: Post-exposure varicella vaccine (Varivax) 0.5 mL SQ x 2 doses,

Table 5.2 Prophylaxis to Prevent First Episode of Opportunistic Disease (cont'd)

Pathogen	Indication	First choice	Alternative
	For susceptible patients (those who have no history of vaccination or of either condition, or are known to be VZV seronegative)	administered within 96 hours after exposure to a person with active varicella or herpes zoster Note: As of June 2007, VariZIG can be obtained only under a treatment IND (1-800-843-7477, FFF Enterprises)	3 months apart if CD4+ count > 200 cells/μL; **or** Pre-emptive acyclovir 800 mg PO 5x/day for 5 days These two alternatives have not been studied in the HIV population
Human Papillomavirus (HPV) infection	Women aged 15–26 yrs	HPV quadravalent vaccine 0.5 mL IM months 0, 2, and 6	
Hepatitis A virus (HAV) infection	HAV-susceptible patients with chronic liver disease, or who are injection-drug users, or men who have sex with men. Certain specialists might delay vaccination until CD4+ count > 200 cells/μL	Hepatitis A vaccine 1 mL IM x 2 doses-at 0 & 6–12 months IgG antibody response should be assessed 1 month after vaccination; non-responders should be revaccinated	
Hepatitis B virus (HBV) infection	All HIV patients without evidence of prior exposure to HBV should be vaccinated with HBV vaccine, including patients with CD4+ count < 200 cells/μL _Patients with isolated anti-HBc:_ (consider screening for HBV DNA before vaccination to rule out occult chronic HBV infection)	Hepatitis B vaccine IM (Engerix-B® 20 μg/mL or Recombivax HB® 10 μg/mL) at 0, 1, and 6 months Anti-HBs should be obtained one month after completion of the vaccine series	Some experts recommend vaccinating with 40 μg doses of either vaccine

Table 5.2 Prophylaxis to Prevent First Episode of Opportunistic Disease (cont'd)

Pathogen	Indication	First choice	Alternative
	Vaccine non-responders: Defined as anti-HBs < 10 IU/mL 1 month after a vaccination series For patients with low CD4+ count at the time of first vaccination series, certain specialists might delay revaccination until after a sustained increase in CD4+ count with ART.	Revaccinate with a second vaccine series	Some experts recommend revaccinating with 40 μg doses of either vaccine
Malaria	Travel to disease-endemic area	Recommendations are the same for HIV-infected and -uninfected patients. One of the following three drugs is usually recommended depending on location: atovaquone/proguanil, doxycycline, or mefloquine. Refer to the following website for the most recent recommendations based on region and drug susceptibility. http://www.cdc.gov/malaria/.	

Definitions of abbreviations: DS = double strength; PO = by mouth; SS = single strength; BID = twice daily; tiw = 3 times weekly; SQ = subcutaneous; IM = intramuscular

P. jiroveci (carinii) pneumonia (PCP)

Without prophylaxis, 80% of AIDS patients develop PCP, and 60–70% relapse within 1 year after the first episode. Prophylaxis with TMP-SMX also reduces the risk for toxoplasmosis and possibly bacterial infections. Among patients with prior non-life-threatening reactions to TMP-SMX, 55%

can be successfully rechallenged with 1 SS tablet daily, and 80% can be rechallenged with gradual dose escalation using TMP-SMX elixir (8 mg TMP + 40 mg SMX/mL) given as 1 mL × 3 days, then 2 mL × 3 days, then 5 mL × 3 days, then 1 SS tablet (PO) QD. Primary and secondary prophylaxis may be discontinued if CD4 cell counts increase to > 200/mm³ for 3 months or longer in response to antiretroviral therapy. Prophylaxis should be resumed if the CD4 cell count decreases to < 200/mm³.

Toxoplasmosis

Incidence of toxoplasmosis in seronegative patients is too low to warrant chemoprophylaxis. Primary prophylaxis can be discontinued if CD4 cell counts increase to > 200/mm³ for at least 3 months in response to antiretroviral therapy. Secondary prophylaxis (chronic maintenance therapy) may be discontinued in patients who responded to initial therapy, remain asymptomatic, and whose CD4 counts increase to > 200/mm³ for 6 months or longer in response to antiretroviral therapy. Prophylaxis should be restarted if the CD4 count decreases to < 200/mm³. Some experts would obtain an MRI of the brain as part of the evaluation prior to stopping secondary prophylaxis.

Tuberculosis *(M. tuberculosis)*

Consider prophylaxis for skin test-negative patients when the probability of prior TB exposure is > 10% (e.g., patients from developing countries, IV drug abusers in some cities, prisoners). However, a trial testing this strategy in the United States did not find a benefit for empiric prophylaxis. Rifamycins interact with PIs, NNRTIs, raltegravir, and maraviroc—use with caution.

M. avium complex (MAC)

Macrolide options (azithromycin, clarithromycin) preferable to rifabutin given greater efficacy, better tolerability, protection against other respiratory tract disease. Among macolide options, azithromycin is generally preferred over clarithromycin (fewer pills, fewer drug-drug interactions, better tolerated). Primary prophylaxis may be discontinued if CD4 cell counts increase to > 100/mm³ and HIV RNA suppresses for 3 months or longer in response to antiretroviral therapy. Resume MAC prophylaxis for CD4 < 100/mm³.

Pneumococcus *(S. pneumoniae)*

Incidence of invasive pneumococcal disease is > 100-fold higher in HIV patients. Efficacy of vaccine seen in multiple observational studies, though not all prospective randomized studies show protection. Vaccine may be offered to HIV pts with CD4 < 200/mm³; consider revaccination once CD4 has increased to > 200/mm³ due to antiviral therapy.

Influenza

Give annually (optimally between October and January). Intranasal live attenuated virus vaccine is contraindicated in immunosuppressed patients.

Hepatitis B

Check antibody response 1–3 months after completion of series. Response rate is lower than in HIV-negative controls. Repeat series if no response, especially if CD4 was low during initial series and has increased due to ART.

Vaccine non-responders: Defined as Anti-HBs < 10 IU/mL 1 month after a vaccination series. For patients with low CD4+ count at the time of first vaccination series, some experts might delay revaccination until after a sustained increase in CD4+ count with ART.

Management of patients with isolated antibody to hepatitis B core (i.e., "core alone") is not well defined—consider screen for HBV DNA to rule out occult chronic HBV prior to vaccination.

Hepatitis A
Response rate is lower than in HIV-negative controls; assess antibody response 1–3 months after vaccination. Some clinicians delay vaccination until CD4 is > 200 cells/mm³.

Measles, mumps, rubella
Single case of vaccine-strain measles pneumonia in severely immuno-compromised adult who received MMR; vaccine is therefore contraindicated in patients with severe immunodeficiency (CD4 < 200/mm³).

H. influenzae
Incidence of *H. influenzae* disease is increased in HIV patients, but 65% are caused by non-type B strains. Unclear whether vaccine offers protection; not generally recommended.

Travel vaccines*
All considered safe except oral polio, yellow fever, and live oral typhoid–each a live vaccine. Most could probably be given safely to patients with high CD4 cell counts (> 350/mm³), but data are limited.

Varicella zoster virus (VZV)
If vaccination results in disease due to vaccine virus, treatment with acyclovir is recommended

If exposure occurs and patient is non-immune, consider administration of varicella vaccine and pre-emptive acyclovir, 800 mg 5x/day for 5 days, or valacyclovir 1 gm TID × 5d or famciclovir 500 gm TID × 5d.

TREATMENT OF OPPORTUNISTIC INFECTIONS

Antiretroviral therapy (ART) and specific antimicrobial prophylaxis regimens have led to a dramatic decline in HIV-related opportunistic infections. Today, opportunistic infections occur predominantly in patients not receiving ART (due to undiagnosed HIV infection or nonacceptance of therapy), or in the period soon after starting ART (due to eliciting a previously absent inflammatory host response, called immune reconstitution inflammatory syndrome (IRIS)). Even when virologic failure occurs in clinical practice, the rate of opportunistic infections in patients compliant with ART remains low, presumably due to continued immunologic response despite virologic failure, a phenomenon that may be linked to impaired "fitness" (virulence) of resistant HIV strains. For patients on or off ART, the absolute CD4 cell count provides the best marker of risk for opportunistic infections. Guidelines for treatment of OIs in the post-potent antiretroviral therapy era were last updated April 10, 2009 (see aidsinfo.NIH.gov). Specific OI's are listed below in alphabetical order.

Aspergillosis, Invasive

Preferred Therapy, Duration of Therapy, Chronic Maintenance	Alternate Therapy	Other Options/Issues
Preferred therapy Voriconazole 6 mg/kg q12h × 1 day, then 4 mg/kg q12h IV, followed by voriconazole PO 200 mg q12h after clinical improvement Duration of therapy: until CD4+ count > 200 cells/μL and with evidence of clinical response	Alternative therapy Amphotericin B deoxycholate 1 mg/kg/day IV; **or** Lipid formulation of amphotericin B 5 mg/kg/day IV Caspofungin 70 mg IV × 1, then 50 mg IV daily Posaconazole 400 mg BID PO	Potential for significant pharmacokinetic interactions between PIs or NNRTIs with voriconazole; it should be used cautiously in these situations. Consider therapeutic drug monitoring and dosage adjustment if necessary.

Clinical Presentation: Pleuritic chest pain, hemoptysis, cough in a patient with advanced HIV disease. Additional risk factors include neutropenia and use of corticosteroids.

Diagnostic Considerations: Diagnosis by bronchoscopy with biopsy/culture. Open lung biopsy (usually video-assisted thorascopic surgery) is sometimes required. Radiographic appearance includes cavitation (sometimes with a characteristic "halo" around a nodule, called the air crescent sign), nodules, sometimes focal consolidation. Dissemination to CNS may occur and manifests as focal neurological deficits. As with HIV-negative patients, elevation in serum galactomannan generally occurs with invasive disease.

Pitfalls: Positive sputum culture for Aspergillus in advanced HIV disease should heighten awareness of possible infection. Watch for drug-drug interactions between voriconazole and antiretrovirals metabolized via the cytochrome p450 system (PIs, NNRTIs).

Therapeutic Considerations: Decrease/discontinue corticosteroids, if possible. If present, treat neutropenia with granulocyte-colony stimulating factor (G-CSF) to achieve absolute neutrophil count > 1000/mm³. There are insufficient data to recommend chronic suppressive or maintenance therapy.

Prognosis: Poor unless immune deficits can be corrected.

Bacterial Respiratory Diseases

Preferred Therapy, Duration of Therapy, Chronic Maintenance	Alternate Therapy	Other Options/Issues
Preferred empiric outpatient therapy (oral) A beta-lactam plus a macrolide (azithromycin or clarithromycin) *Preferred beta-lactams*: high-dose amoxicillin or amoxicillin/clavulanate *Alternative beta-lactams*: cefpodoxime or cefuroxime	Alternative empiric outpatient therapy (oral) A beta-lactam plus doxycycline *For penicillin-allergic patients or those with beta-lactam use in prior 3 months* A respiratory fluoroquinolone (levofloxacin 750 mg/day, gemifloxacin, or moxifloxacin)	Patients receiving macrolide for MAC prophylaxis should not receive macrolide monotherapy for empiric treatment of bacterial pneumonia Fluoroquinolones should be used with caution in patients where TB is suspected but is not being treated
Preferred empiric therapy for non-ICU inpatient A beta-lactam (IV) plus a macrolide *Preferred beta-lactams*: cefotaxime, ceftriaxone, or ampicillin-sulbactam	Alternative empiric therapy for non-ICU inpatient A beta-lactam (IV) plus doxycycline *For penicillin-allergic patients or those with beta-lactam use in prior 3 months* An IV respiratory fluoroquinolone (levofloxacin 750 mg or moxifloxacin)	Empiric therapy with a macrolide alone is not routinely recommended, because of increasing pneumococcal resistance Once the pathogen has been identified by a reliable microbiologic method, antibiotics should be directed at the pathogen
Preferred empiric ICU inpatient therapy A beta-lactam (IV) plus azithromycin IV or an IV respiratory fluoroquinolone (levofloxacin 750 mg or moxifloxacin) *Preferred beta-lactams*: cefotaxime, ceftriaxone, or ampicillin-sulbactam	Alternative empiric ICU therapy *For penicillin-allergic patients or those with beta-lactam use in prior 3 months* Aztreonam IV plus an IV respiratory fluoroquinolone	For patients begun on IV antibiotic therapy, switching to PO should be considered when patient is clinically improved and able to tolerate oral medications
Preferred empiric *Pseudomonas* therapy (if risks present) An antipneumococcal, antipseudomonal beta-lactam plus either ciprofloxacin or levofloxacin 750 mg/day	Alternative empiric Pseudomonas therapy An antipneumococcal, antipseudomonal beta-lactam plus an aminoglycoside plus azithromycin	Chemoprophylaxis may be considered for patients with frequent recurrences of serious bacterial respiratory infections

Bacterial Respiratory Diseases (cont'd)

Preferred Therapy, Duration of Therapy, Chronic Maintenance	Alternate Therapy	Other Options/Issues
Preferred beta-lactams: piperacillin-tazobactam, cefepime, imipenem, or meropenem	Above beta-lactam plus an aminoglycoside plus an antipneumococcal fluoroquinolone* *For penicillin-allergic patients or those with beta-lactam use in prior 3 months* Replace the beta-lactam with aztreonam	Clinicians should be cautious of using antibiotics to prevent recurrences, because of the potential for developing drug resistance and drug toxicities
<u>Preferred empiric methicillin-resistant *Staphylococcus aureus* (if risks present)</u> Add vancomycin (possibly plus clindamycin) or linezolid alone to above		

Clinical Presentation: HIV-infected patients with bacterial pneumonia present similar to those without HIV, with a relatively acute illness (over days) that is often associated with chills, rigors, pleuritic chest pain, and purulent sputum. Patients who have been ill over weeks to months are more likely have PCP, tuberculosis, or a fungal infection. Since bacterial pneumonia can occur at any CD4 cell count, this infection is frequently the presenting symptom of HIV disease, prompting initial HIV testing and diagnosis.

Diagnostic Considerations: The most common pathogens are *Streptococcus pneumoniae*, followed by *Haemophilus influenzae*, *Pseudomonas aeruginosa*, and *Staphylococcus aureus*. The pathogens of atypical pneumonia (*Legionella pneumophila*, *Mycoplasma pneumoniae*, and *Chlamydia pneumoniae*) are rarely encountered, even with extensive laboratory investigation; nonetheless, as with HIV-negative patients, these pathogens should be covered empirically unless a specific alternative diagnosis is made. A lobar infiltrate on chest radiography is a further predictor of bacterial pneumonia. Blood cultures should be obtained, as HIV patients have an increased rate of bacteremia compared to those without HIV.

Pitfalls: Sputum gram stain and culture are generally only helpful if collected prior to starting antibiotics, and only if a single organism predominates. HIV patients with bacterial pneumonia may rarely have a more subacute opportunistic infection concurrently, such as PCP or TB. Fluoroquinolones should be used with caution for treatment of suspected bacterial pneumonia if TB is a diagnostic consideration, as they may inadvertently select for quinolone-resistant TB.

Therapeutic Considerations: Once improvement has occurred, a switch to oral therapy is generally safe. Patients with advanced HIV disease are at greater risk of bacteremic pneumonia due to gram-negative bacilli, and should be covered empirically for this condition. Preventive therapy (for example daily trimethoprim-sulfa) may be considered for patients with frequent recurrent bacterial respiratory infections.

Prognosis: Response to therapy is generally prompt and overall prognosis is good.

Bartonella Infections

Preferred Therapy, Duration of Therapy, Chronic Maintenance	Alternate Therapy	Other Options/Issues
Preferred therapy for bacillary angiomatosis, peliosis hepatis, bacteremia, and osteomyelitis Erythromycin 500 mg PO or IV QID; **or** Doxycycline 100 mg PO or IV q12h Duration of therapy: at least 3 months CNS infections and severe infections Doxycycline 100 mg PO or IV q12h +/- rifampin 300 mg PO or IV q12h Duration of therapy: 4 months Long-term suppression With a macrolide or doxycycline for patients with relapse or reinfection as long as the CD4+ count remains < 200 cells/μL	Alternative therapy for bacillary angiomatosis infections, peliosis hepatis, bacteremia, and osteomyelitis Azithromycin 500 mg PO daily Clarithromycin 500 mg PO BID	Severe Jarisch-Herxheimer-like reaction can occur in the first 48 hours of treatment

Clinical Presentation: Skin lesions resemble Kaposi's sarcoma. CT of liver shows hepatomegaly and hypodense lesions. Bartonella can rarely present as a CNS mass lesion, similar to toxoplasmosis.

Diagnostic Considerations: Diagnosis by demonstrating organism by stain/culture of skin lesions or by blood culture after lysis-centrifugation.

Pitfalls: Requires lifelong suppressive therapy unless CD4 > 200 with ART. Does not grow in routine cultures.

Therapeutic Considerations: Fluoroquinolones have variable activity in case reports and in vitro; may be considered as alternative therapy. Azithromycin likely to be better tolerated than erythromycin with fewer drug-drug interactions. Long-term suppressive therapy should be given for patients with relapse or reinfection, especially if CD4 cell count remains < 200 cells/mm[3].

Prognosis: Related to extent of infection/degree of immunosuppression.

Campylobacteriosis

Preferred Therapy, Duration of Therapy, Chronic Maintenance	Alternate Therapy	Other Options/Issues
<u>For mild disease</u> Might withhold therapy unless symptoms persist for several days <u>For mild-to-moderate disease</u> Ciprofloxacin 500 mg PO BID; **or** Azithromycin 500 mg PO daily Consider addition of an aminoglycoside in bacteremic patients Duration of therapy: Mild-to-moderate disease: 7 days Bacteremia: at least 2 weeks		There is an increasing rate of fluoroquinolone resistance Antimicrobial therapy should be modified based on susceptibility reports

Clinical Presentation: Acute onset of diarrhea, sometimes bloody; constitutional symptoms may be prominent.

Diagnostic Considerations: Diagnosis by stool culture; bacteremia may rarely occur, so blood cultures also indicated. Suspect campylobacter in AIDS patient with diarrhea and curved gram-negative rods in blood culture. Non-jejuni species may be more strongly correlated with bacteremia.

Therapeutic Considerations: Optimal therapy not well defined. Treat with quinolone or azithromycin; modify therapy based on susceptibility testing. Quinolone resistance can occur and correlates with treatment failure. Imipenem is sometimes used for bacteremia.

Prognosis: Depends on underlying immune status; prognosis is generally good.

Candidiasis (Mucosal)

Preferred Therapy, Duration of Therapy, Chronic Maintenance	Alternate Therapy	Other Options/Issues
<u>Preferred therapy oropharyngeal candidiasis: initial episodes (7–14 day treatment)</u> Fluconazole 100 mg PO daily; **or** Clotrimazole troches 10 mg PO 5 times daily; **or** Nystatin suspension 4–6 mL QID or 1–2 flavored pastilles 4–5 times daily	<u>Alternative therapy oropharyngeal candidiasis: initial episodes (7–14 day treatment)</u> Itraconazole oral solution 200 mg PO daily; **or** Posaconazole oral solution 400 mg PO BID × 1, then 400 mg daily	Chronic or prolonged use of azoles might promote development of resistance Higher relapse rate of esophageal candidiasis with echinocandins than with fluconazole has been reported

Candidiasis (Mucosal) (cont'd)

Preferred Therapy, Duration of Therapy, Chronic Maintenance	Alternate Therapy	Other Options/Issues
Miconazole mucoadhesive tablet PO daily		Patients with fluconazole refractory oropharyngeal or esophageal candidiasis who responded to echinocandin should be started on voriconazole or posaconazole for secondary prophylaxis until ART produces immune reconstitution.
<u>Preferred therapy esophageal candidiasis (14–21 days)</u> Fluconazole 100 mg (up to 400 mg) PO or IV daily Itraconazole oral solution 200 mg PO daily	<u>Alternative therapy esophageal candidiasis (14–21 days)</u> Voriconazole 200 mg PO or IV BID Posaconazole 400 mg PO BID Caspofungin 50 mg IV daily Micafungin 150 mg IV daily Anidulafungin 100 mg IV × 1, then 50 mg IV daily Amphotericin B deoxycholate 0.6 mg/kg IV daily	Suppressive therapy is usually not recommended unless patients have frequent or severe recurrences. If decision is to use suppressive therapy:
<u>Preferred therapy uncomplicated vulvovaginal candidiasis</u> Oral fluconazole 150 mg for 1 dose Topical azoles (clotrimazole, butoconazole, miconazole, tioconazole, or terconazole) for 3–7 days	<u>Alternative therapy uncomplicated vulvovaginal candidiasis</u> Itraconazole oral solution 200 mg PO daily for 3–7 days <u>Alternative therapy fluconazole-refractory oropharyngeal candidiasis or esophageal candidiasis</u> Amphotericin B deoxycholate 0.3 mg/kg IV daily	<u>Oropharyngeal candidiasis</u> Fluconazole 100 mg PO tiw Itraconazole oral solution 200 mg PO daily Fluconazole 100–200 mg PO daily Posaconazole 400 mg PO BID
<u>Preferred therapy fluconazole-refractory oropharyngeal candidiasis or esophageal candidiasis</u> Itraconazole oral solution ≥ 200 mg PO daily Posaconazole oral solution 400 mg PO BID	Lipid formulation of amphotericin B 3–5 mg/kg IV daily Anidulafungin 100 mg IV × 1, then 50 mg IV daily Caspofungin 50 mg IV daily Micafungin 150 mg IV daily Voriconazole 200 mg PO or IV BID *Fluconazole-refractory oropharyngeal candidiasis (not esophageal)*	<u>Vulvovaginal candidiasis</u> Fluconazole 150 mg PO once weekly Daily topical azole

Candidiasis (Mucosal) (cont'd)

Preferred Therapy, Duration of Therapy, Chronic Maintenance	Alternate Therapy	Other Options/Issues
	Amphotericin B oral suspension 100 mg/mL (not available in U.S.) 1 mL PO QID	
Preferred therapy complicated (severe or recurrent) vulvovaginal candidiasis Fluconazole 150 mg q72h × 2–3 doses Topical antifungal ≥ 7 days		

Oral Thrush *(Candida)*
Clinical Presentation: Dysphagia/odynophagia. More common/severe in advanced HIV disease.
Diagnostic Considerations: Pseudomembranous (most common), erythematous, and hyperplastic (leukoplakia) forms. Pseudomembranes (white plaques on inflamed base) on buccal muscosa/tongue/gingiva/palate scrape off easily, hyperplastic lesions do not. Diagnosis of oral thrush most commonly by clinical appearance. KOH/gram stain of scraping showing yeast/pseudomycelia. Other oral lesions in AIDS patients include herpes simplex, aphthous ulcers, Kaposi's sarcoma, oral hairy leukoplakia.
Pitfalls: Patients may be asymptomatic.
Therapeutic Considerations: Fluconazole is superior to topical therapy in preventing relapses of thrush and treating *Candida* esophagitis. Continuous treatment with fluconazole may lead to fluconazole-resistance, which is best treated initially with itraconazole suspension and, if no response, with IV caspofungin (or other echinocandin) or amphotericin. Chronic suppressive therapy is usually only considered for severely immunosuppressed patients.
Prognosis: Improvement in symptoms are often seen within 24–48 hours.

Candida Esophagitis
Clinical Presentation: Dysphagia/odynophagia, almost always in the setting of oropharyngeal thrush. Fever is uncommon.
Diagnostic Considerations: Most common cause of esophagitis in HIV disease. For persistent symptoms despite therapy, endoscopy with biopsy/culture is recommended to confirm diagnosis and assess azole-resistance.
Pitfalls: May extend into stomach. Other common causes of esophagitis include CMV, herpes simplex, and aphthous ulcers. Rarely, Kaposi's sarcoma, non-Hodgkin's lymphoma, zidovudine, dideoxycytidine, and other infections may cause esophageal symptoms.
Therapeutic Considerations: Systemic therapy is preferred over topical therapy. Failure to improve on empiric therapy mandates endoscopy to look for other causes, especially herpes viruses/aphthous ulcers. Consider maintenance therapy with fluconazole for frequent relapses, although the risk of fluconazole resistance is increased. Fluconazole resistance is best treated initially with itraconazole suspension and, if no response, with IV echinocandin (caspofungin, micafungin, anidulafungin) or amphotericin. Patients with fluconazole refractory oropharyngeal or esophageal candidiasis who responded to echinocandin should be started on voriconazole or posaconazole for secondary prophylaxis until ART produces immune reconstitution.
Prognosis: Relapse rate is related to degree of immunosuppression.

Chagas Disease (American Trypanosomiasis)

Preferred Therapy, Duration of Therapy, Chronic Maintenance	Alternate Therapy	Other Options/Issues
Preferred therapy for acute, early chronic, and reactivated disease Benznidazole 5–8 mg/kg/day PO in 2 divided doses for 30–60 days (not commercially available in the US, contact the CDC Drug Service at 404–639–3670 or drugservice@ cdc.gov)	Alternative therapy Nifurtimox 8–10 mg/kg/day PO for 90–120 days (Contact the CDC Drug Service at 404–639–3670 or drugservice@cdc.gov)	Duration of therapy has not been studied in HIV-infected patients Initiation or optimization of ART in patients undergoing treatment for Chagas disease, once the patient is clinically stable

Clostridium difficile Diarrhea/Colitis

Preferred Therapy	Alternate Therapy	Other Options/Issues
Preferred therapy for mild disease Metronidazole 500 mg (PO) q8h*—10–14 days. Avoid use of other antibacterials if possible Preferred therapy for moderate-severe disease (fever, WBC, colitis) Vancomycin 125 mg (PO) q6h*—10–14 days. Avoid use of other antibacterials if possible	Nitazoxanide 500 mg BID × 7–10 days	Severe disease with illeus/ toxic mega-colon IV metronidazole Vancomycin per rectum Surgical consultation for possible colectomy

Clinical Presentation: Diarrhea and abdominal pain following antibiotic therapy. Diarrhea may be watery or bloody. Proton pump inhibitors increase the risk. Among antibiotics, clindamycin, quinolones, and beta-lactams are most frequent. Rarely occurs after aminoglycosides, linezolid, doxycycline, TMP-SMX, daptomycin, vancomycin.

Diagnostic Considerations: Most common cause of bacterial diarrhea in United States among HIV patients (Clin Infect Dis 2005;41:1620–7). Diagnosed with positive *C. difficile* toxin in stool specimen. *C. difficile* stool toxin test is sufficiently sensitive/specific; cultures not useful. After therapy completed, no indication for retesting if the patient is doing well clinically. *C. difficile* virulent epidemic strain is type B1 (toxinotype III), which produces 20-times the amount of toxin A/B compared to less virulent strains.

Pitfalls: *C. difficile* toxin may remain positive in stools for weeks following treatment; do not treat positive stool toxin unless patient has symptoms.

Therapeutic Considerations: Initiate therapy for mild disease with metronidazole; symptoms usually begin to improve within 2–3 days. For moderate or severe disease, or with evidence of colitis clinically (leukocytosis, fever, colonic thickening on CT scan), vancomycin has become the preferred agent due to concern for the more virulent strain, and based on the results of some studies suggesting vancomycin is more effective. In severe disease, surgical consultation should be obtained; if ileus and/or systemic toxicity occur, then colectomy may be indicated. The duration of therapy should be extended beyond 14 days if other systemic antibiotics must be continued. Relapse occurs in 10–25% of patients, and rates may be higher in patients with HIV due to the frequent need for other antimicrobial therapy. First relapses can be treated with a repeat of the initial regimen of metronidazole or vancomycin. For multiple relapses, a long-term taper of vancomycin is appropriate: week 1, give 125 mg 4x/day; week 2, give 125 mg 2x/day; week 3 , give 125 mg once daily; week 4, give 125 mg every other day; weeks 5 and 6, give 125 mg every 3 days. Every effort should be made to resume a normal diet and to avoid other antibacterial therapies. Probiotic treatments (such as lactobacillus or *Saccharomyces boulardii*) have not yet been shown to reduce the risk of relapse in controlled clinical trials.

Prognosis: Prognosis with *C. difficile* colitis is related to severity of the colitis.

Coccidioidomycosis

Preferred Therapy, Duration of Therapy, Chronic Maintenance	Alternate Therapy	Other Options/Issues
Preferred therapy for mild infections (focal pneumonia or positive coccidiodal serologic test alone) Fluconazole 400 mg PO daily; **or** Itraconazole 200 mg PO TID × 3 days, then 200 mg BID		Certain patients with meningitis may develop hydrocephalus and require CSF shunting
Preferred therapy for severe, nonmeningeal infection (diffuse pulmonary or severely ill patients with extrathoracic disseminated disease): acute phase Amphotericin B deoxycholate 0.7–1.0 mg/kg IV daily Lipid formulation amphotericin B 4–6 mg/kg IV daily Duration of therapy: until clinical improvement, then switch to azole	Alternative therapy for severe nonmeningeal infection (diffuse pulmonary or disseminated disease): acute phase Certain specialists add triazole to amphotericin B therapy and continue triazole once amphotericin B is stopped	Therapy should be continued indefinitely for patients with diffuse pulmonary or disseminated diseases as relapse can occur in 25%–33% in HIV-negative patients Therapy should be lifelong in patients with meningeal infections as relapse occurred in 80% of HIV-infected patients after discontinuation of triazole therapy
Preferred therapy for meningeal infections Fluconazole 400–800 mg PO or IV daily	Alternative therapy for meningeal infections Itraconazole 200 mg PO TID × 3 days, then 200 mg PO BID	

Coccidioidomycosis (cont'd)

Preferred Therapy, Duration of Therapy, Chronic Maintenance	Alternate Therapy	Other Options/Issues
Maintenance therapy (for all cases) Fluconazole 400 mg PO daily; **or** Itraconazole 200 mg PO BID	Intrathecal amphotericin B when triazole antifungals are not effective	Case reports of successful therapy with voriconazole and posaconazole are available

Clinical Presentation: Typically a complication of advanced HIV infection (CD4 cell count < 200/mm^3). Most patients present with disseminated disease, which can manifest as fever, diffuse pulmonary infiltrates, adenopathy, skin lesions (multiple forms—verrucous, cold abscesses, ulcers, nodules), and/or bone lesions. Approximately 10% will have spread to the CNS in the form of meningitis (fever, headache, altered mental status).

Diagnostic Considerations: Consider the diagnosis in any patient with advanced HIV-related immunosuppression who has been in a *C. immitis* endemic area (Southwestern United States, Northern Mexico) and presents with a systemic febrile syndrome. Diagnosis can be made by culture of the organism, visualization of characteristic spherules on histopathology, or a positive complement-fixation antibody (≥ 1:16). In meningeal cases, CSF profile shows low glucose, high protein, and lymphocytic pleocytosis.

Pitfalls: Antibody titers are often negative on presentation. CSF profile of meningitis can be similar to TB. CSF fungal cultures may be negative.

Prognosis: Related to extent of infection and degree of immunosuppression. Clinical response tends to be slow, especially with a high disease burden and advanced HIV disease. Meningeal disease is treated with lifelong fluconazole regardless of CD4 recovery.

Cryptococcal Meningitis

Preferred Therapy, Duration of Therapy, Chronic Maintenance	Alternate Therapy	Other Options/Issues
Preferred induction therapy Amphotericin B deoxycholate 0.7 mg/kg IV daily plus flucytosine 100 mg/kg PO daily in 4 divided doses for at least 2 weeks; **or** Lipid formulation amphotericin B 4–6 mg/kg IV daily (consider for persons who have renal dysfunction on therapy or have high likelihood of renal failure) plus flucytosine 100 mg/kg PO daily in 4 divided doses for at least 2 weeks	Alternative induction therapy Amphotericin B (deoxycholate or lipid formulation, dose as preferred therapy) plus fluconazole 400 mg PO or IV daily Amphotericin B (deoxycholate or lipid formulation, dose as preferred therapy) alone	Addition of flucytosine to amphotericin B has been associated with more rapid sterilization of CSF and decreased risk for subsequent relapse

Cryptococcal Meningitis (cont'd)

Preferred Therapy, Duration of Therapy, Chronic Maintenance	Alternate Therapy	Other Options/Issues
	Fluconazole 400–800 mg/day (PO or IV) plus flucytosine 100 mg/kg PO daily in 4 divided doses for 4–6 weeks; for persons unable to tolerate or unresponsive to amphotericin B	Patients receiving flucytosine should have blood levels monitored; peak level 2 hours after dose should not exceed 75 µg/mL. Dosage should be adjusted in patients with renal insufficiency
Preferred consolidation therapy (after at least 2 weeks of successful induction—defined as significant clinical improvement & negative CSF culture) Fluconazole 400 mg PO daily for 8 weeks	Alternative consolidation therapy Itraconazole 200 mg PO BID for 8 weeks, or until CD4+ count > 200 cells/µL for > 6 months as a result of ART	Opening pressure should always be measured when a lumbar puncture (LP) is performed. Repeated LPs or CSF shunting are essential to effectively manage increased intracranial pressure
Preferred maintenance therapy Fluconazole 200 mg PO daily lifelong or until CD4+ count ≥ 200 cells/µL for > 6 months as a result of ART	Alternative maintenance therapy Itraconazole 200 mg PO daily lifelong unless immune reconstitution as a result of potent ART; for patients intolerant of or who failed fluconazole	

Clinical Presentation: Often indolent onset of fever, headache, subtle cognitive deficits. Occasional meningeal signs and focal neurologic findings, though non-specific presentation is most common.

Diagnostic Considerations: Diagnosis usually by cryptococcal antigen of serum and/or CSF; India ink stain of CSF is less sensitive. Diagnosis is essentially excluded with a negative serum cryptococcal antigen (sensitivity of test in AIDS patients approaches 100%). If serum cryptococcal antigen is positive, CSF antigen may be negative in disseminated disease without spread to CNS/meninges. Brain imaging is often normal, but CSF analysis is usually abnormal with elevated opening pressure.

Pitfalls: Be sure to obtain a CSF opening pressure, since reduction of increased intracranial pressure is critical for successful treatment. Remove sufficient CSF during the initial lumbar puncture (LP) to reduce closing pressure to < 200 mm H_2O or 50% of opening pressure. Increased intracranial pressure requires repeat daily lumbar punctures until CSF pressure stabilizes; persistently elevated pressure should prompt placement of a lumbar drain or ventriculo-peritoneal shunting. Adjunctive corticosteroids and acetazolamide are not recommended.

Therapeutic Considerations: Optimal total dose/duration of amphotericin B prior to fluconazole switch depends on clinical response and rapidity of CSF sterilization (2–3 weeks is reasonable if patient is doing well). Addition of flucytosine to amphotericin B associated with more rapid sterilization of CSF and decreased risk for subsequent relapse. If available, flucytosine levels should be monitored– peak level 2 hours after dose should not exceed 75 mcg/mL. Flucytosine dose must be reduced in renal insufficiency. Fluconazole is preferred over itraconazole for lifelong maintenance therapy. Consider discontinuation of chronic maintenance therapy in patients who remain asymptomatic with CD4 > 100–200/mm³ for > 6 months due to ART.

Prognosis: Variable. Mortality up to 40%. Adverse prognostic factors include increased intracranial pressure, abnormal mental status.

Cryptosporidiosis

Preferred Therapy, Duration of Therapy, Chronic Maintenance	Alternate Therapy	Other Options/Issues
Preferred therapy Initiate or optimize ART for immune restoration Symptomatic treatment of diarrhea Aggressive oral or IV rehydration & replacement of electrolyte loss	Alternative therapy for cryptosporidiosis A trial of nitazoxanide 500–1,000 mg PO BID with food for 14 days + optimized ART, symptomatic treatment and rehydration & electrolyte replacement	Use of antimotility agents such as loperamide or tincture of opium might palliate symptoms

Clinical Presentation: High-volume watery diarrhea with weight loss and electrolyte disturbances, especially in advanced HIV disease.

Diagnostic Considerations: Spore-forming protozoa. Diagnosis by AFB smear of stool demonstrating characteristic oocyte. Malabsorption may occur.

Pitfalls: No fecal leukocytes; organisms are not visualized on standard ova and parasite exams (need to request special stains).

Therapeutic Considerations: Anecdotal reports of antimicrobial success. Nitazoxanide may be effective in some settings, but no increase in cure rate for nitazoxanide if CD4 < 50/mm³. Immune reconstitution in response to antiretroviral therapy is the most effective therapy, and may induce prolonged remissions and cure. Anti-diarrheal agents (Lomotil, Pepto-Bismol) are useful to control symptoms. Hyperalimentation may be required for severe cases.

Prognosis: Related to degree of immunosuppression/response to antiretroviral therapy.

Cytomegalovirus (CMV) Disease

Preferred Therapy, Duration of Therapy, Chronic Maintenance	Alternate Therapy	Other Options/Issues
Preferred therapy for CMV retinitis *For immediate sight-threatening lesions* Ganciclovir intraocular implant + valganciclovir 900 mg PO (BID for 14–21 days, then once daily) One dose of intravitreal ganciclovir may be administered immediately after diagnosis until ganciclovir implant can be placed *For small peripheral lesions* Valganciclovir 900 mg PO BID for 14–21 days, then 900 mg PO daily	Alternative therapy for CMV retinitis Ganciclovir 5 mg/kg IV q12h for 14–21 days, then 5 mg/kg IV daily; **or** Ganciclovir 5 mg/kg IV q12h for 14–21 days, then valganciclovir 900 mg PO daily; **or** Foscarnet 60 mg/kg IV q8h or 90 mg/kg IV q12h for 14–21 days, then 90–120 mg/kg IV q24h; **or** Cidofovir 5 mg/kg/week IV for 2 weeks, then 5 mg/kg every other week with saline hydration before and after therapy and probenecid 2 g PO 3 hours before the dose followed by 1 g PO 2 shours after the dose, and 1 g PO 8 hours after the dose (total of 4 g) **Note:** This regimen should be avoided in patients with sulfa allergy because of cross hypersensitivity with probenecid	The choice of initial therapy for CMV retinitis should be individualized, based on location and severity of the lesion(s), level of immunosuppression, and other factors such as concomitant medications and ability to adhere to treatment Initial therapy in patients with CMV retinitis, esophagitis, colitis, and pneumonitis should include initiation or optimization of ART In patients with CMV neurological disease, localized morbidity might occur because of IRIS, a brief delay in initiation of ART until clinical improvement might be prudent Maintenance therapy for CMV retinitis can be safely discontinued in patients with inactive disease and sustained CD4+ count (> 100 cells/mm^3 for ≥ 3–6 months); consultation with ophthalmologist is advised
Preferred chronic maintenance therapy (secondary prophylaxis) for CMV retinitis Valganciclovir 900 mg PO daily; **or** Ganciclovir implant (may be replaced every 6–8 months if	Alternative chronic maintenance (secondary prophylaxis) for CMV retinitis Ganciclovir 5 mg/kg IV 5–7 times weekly; **or**	

Cytomegalovirus (CMV) Disease (cont'd)

Preferred Therapy, Duration of Therapy, Chronic Maintenance	Alternate Therapy	Other Options/Issues
CD4+ count remains < 100 cells/µL + valganciclovir 900 mg PO daily until immune recovery	Foscarnet 90–120 mg/kg body weight IV once daily; **or** Cidofovir 5 mg/kg body weight IV every other week with saline hydration and probenecid as above	Patients with CMV retinitis who discontinued maintenance therapy should undergo regular eye examination, optimally every 3 months, for early detection of relapse or immune recovery uveitis (IRU)
Preferred therapy for CMV esophagitis or colitis Ganciclovir IV or foscarnet IV for 21–28 days or until resolution of signs and symptoms Oral valganciclovir may be used if symptoms are not severe enough to interfere with oral absorption Maintenance therapy is usually not necessary, but should be considered after relapses		IRU might develop in the setting of immune reconstitution. Treatment of IRU: periocular corticosteroid or short courses of systemic steroid
Preferred therapy CMV pneumonitis Treatment should be considered in patients with histologic evidence of CMV pneumonitis and who do not respond to treatment of other pathogens The role of maintenance therapy has not been established		
Preferred therapy CMV neurological disease *Treatment should be initiated promptly* Combination of ganciclovir IV + foscarnet IV to stabilize disease and maximize response, continue until symptomatic improvement Maintenance therapy (with valganciclovir PO + IV foscarnet) should be continued for life unless evidence of immune recovery is evident		

CMV Retinitis

Clinical Presentation: Blurred vision, scotomata, field cuts common. Often bilateral, even when initial symptoms are unilateral.

Diagnostic Considerations: Diagnosis by characteristic hemorrhagic ("tomato soup and milk") retinitis on funduscopic exam. Consult ophthalmology in suspected cases.

Pitfalls: May develop immune reconstitution vitreitis after starting antiretroviral therapy.

Therapeutic Considerations: Oral valganciclovir is the preferred option for initial and maintenance therapy. Lifelong maintenance therapy for CMV retinitis is required for CD4 counts $< 100/mm^3$, but may be discontinued if CD4 counts increase to $> 100–150/mm^3$ for 6 or more months in response to antiretroviral therapy (in consultation with ophthalmologist). Patients with CMV retinitis who discontinue therapy should undergo regular eye exams to monitor for relapse. Ganciclovir intraocular implants might need to be replaced every 6–8 months for patients who remain immunosuppressed with CD4 $< 100–150/mm^3$. Immune recovery uveitis (IRU) may develop in the setting of immune reconstitution due to ART and be treated by ophthalmologist with periocular corticosteroid, sometimes systemic corticosteroid.

Prognosis: Good initial response to therapy. High relapse rate unless CD4 improves with antiretroviral therapy.

CMV Encephalitis/Polyradiculitis

Clinical Presentation: Encephalitis presents as fever, mental status changes, and headache evolving over 1–2 weeks. True meningismus is rare. CMV encephalitis occurs in advanced HIV disease (CD4 $< 50/mm^3$), often in patients with prior CMV retinitis. Polyradiculitis presents as rapidly evolving weakness/sensory disturbances in the lower extremities, often with bladder/bowel incontinence. Anesthesia in "saddle distribution" with $\downarrow$ sphincter tone possible.

Diagnostic Considerations: CSF may show lymphocytic or neutrophilic pleocytosis; glucose is often decreased. For CMV encephalitis, characteristic findings on brain MRI include confluent periventricular abnormalities with variable degrees of enhancement. Diagnosis is confirmed by CSF CMV PCR (preferred), CMV culture, or brain biopsy.

Pitfalls: For CMV encephalitis, a wide spectrum of radiographic findings are possible, including mass lesions (rare). Obtain ophthalmologic evaluation to exclude active retinitis. For polyradiculitis, obtain sagittal MRI of the spinal cord to exclude mass lesions, and CSF cytology to exclude lymphomatous involvement (can cause similar symptoms).

Therapeutic Considerations: For any established CMV disease, optimization of antiretroviral therapy is important along with initiating anti-CMV therapy. Ganciclovir plus foscarnet may be beneficial as initial therapy for severe cases. Consider discontinuation of valganciclovir maintenance therapy if CD4 increases to $> 100–150/mm^3 \times 6$ months or longer in response to antiretroviral therapy.

Prognosis: Unless CD4 cell count increases in response to antiretroviral therapy, response to anti-CMV treatment is usually transient, followed by progression of symptoms.

CMV Esophagitis/Colitis

Clinical Presentation: Localizing symptoms, including odynophagia, abdominal pain, diarrhea, sometimes bloody stools.

Diagnostic Considerations: Diagnosis by finding CMV inclusions on biopsy. CMV can affect the entire GI tract, resulting in oral/esophageal ulcers, gastritis, and colitis (most common). CMV colitis varies greatly in severity, but typically causes fever, abdominal cramping, and sometimes bloody stools.

Pitfalls: CMV colitis may cause colonic perforation and should be considered in any AIDS patient presenting with an acute abdomen, especially if radiography demonstrates free intraperitoneal air.

Therapeutic Considerations: Initial therapy for any CMV disease should include optimization of antiretroviral therapy. Duration of therapy is dependent on clinical response, typically 3–4 weeks. Consider chronic suppressive therapy for recurrent disease. Screen for CMV retinitis.

Prognosis: Relapse rate is greatly reduced with immune reconstitution due to antiretroviral therapy.

Hepatitis B Virus (HBV)

Preferred Therapy, Duration of Therapy, Chronic Maintenance	Alternate Therapy	Other Options/Issues
Therapy for patients who require ART Patients should be treated with agents active against both HIV and HBV or with agents with independent activity against each virus Consider tenofovir + emtricitabine as part of HIV and HBV regimen *Lamivudine or emtricitabine-naïve patients* [Lamivudine 150 mg PO BID (or 300 mg PO daily) or emtricitabine 200 mg PO daily] + tenofovir (TDF) 300 mg PO daily (+ additional agent[s] active against HIV) *Lamivudine or emtricitabine-experienced patients with detectable HBV DNA (assume lamivudine-resistance)* *If not on TDF*: Add TDF 300 mg PO daily as part of an ART regimen + lamivudine or emtricitabine; **or** Adefovir 10 mg PO daily + lamivudine or emtricitabine + other combination ART; **or** Entecavir 1 mg PO daily can be considered in patients with complete HIV suppression (while on ART) who do not demonstrate YMDD (M204V/I) motif mutations in HBV DNA	Treatment for patients who do not require ART Use agents with sole activity against HBV and with the least potential of selecting HIV resistance mutations Consider early initiation of ART, especially for patients with high HBV DNA *For patients with CD4+ count > 350 cells/µL, HBeAg (-), HBV DNA > 2,000 IU/mL (> 20,000 copies/mL)* Adefovir 10 mg PO daily *For patients with CD4+ count > 350 cells/µL, HBeAg (+), HBV DNA > 20,000 IU/mL (> 200,000 copies/mL), and elevated ALT* Peginterferon alfa-2a 180 µg SQ weekly × 48 weeks—with careful follow-up of HBeAg conversion	Emtricitabine, entecavir, lamivudine, or tenofovir should not be used for the treatment of HBV infection in patients who are not receiving combination ART Among patients coinfected with HIV, HBV, and HCV, consideration of starting ART should be the first priority. If ART is not required, an interferon-based regimen, which suppresses both HCV & HBV, should be considered If IFN-based treatment for HCV has failed, treatment of chronic HBV with nucleoside or nucleotide analogs is recommended Cross-resistance to emtricitabine or telbivudine should be assumed in patients with suspected or proven 3TC resistance When changing ART regimens, continue agents with anti-HBV activity because of the risk of IRIS If anti-HBV therapy is discontinued and a flare occurs, therapy should be reinstituted, as it can be potentially life saving

Hepatitis B Virus (HBV) (cont'd)

Preferred Therapy, Duration of Therapy, Chronic Maintenance	Alternate Therapy	Other Options/Issues
Duration of therapy: Because of the high rates of relapse, certain specialists recommend continuing therapy indefinitely		

Epidemiology: Hepatitis B virus (HBV) infection is relatively common in patients with HIV, with approximately 60% showing some evidence of prior exposure. Chronic hepatitis B infection interacts with HIV infection in several important ways:

- HBV increases the risk of liver-related death and hepatotoxicity from antiretroviral therapy (Lancet 2002;360:1921–6; Hepatology 2002;35:182–9).
- 3TC, FTC, and tenofovir each have anti-HBV activity. Thus selection of antiretroviral therapy for patients with HBV can have clinical and resistance implications for HBV as well as HIV. This is most notable with 3TC and FTC, as a high proportion of coinfected patients will develop HBV-associated resistance to these drugs after several years of therapy. This resistance reduces response to subsequent non-3TC or FTC anti-HBV therapy.
- Cessation of anti-HBV therapy may lead to exacerbations of underlying liver disease; in some cases, these flares have been fatal (Clin Infect Dis 1999;28:1032–5; Scand J Infectious Diseases 2004;36:533–5).
- Immune reconstitution may lead to worsening of liver status, presumably because HBV disease is immune mediated. This is sometimes associated with loss of HBEAg.
- Entecavir can no longer be recommended for HIV/HBV coinfected patients, as it has anti-HIV activity and may select for HIV resistance mutation M184V (N Engl J Med 2007;356: 2614–21). If needed, it should be used only with a fully suppressive HIV regimen.

Diagnostic Consideration: Obtain HBSAb, HBSAg, and HBCAb at baseline in all patients. If negative, hepatitis B vaccination is indicated. If chronic HBV infection (positive HBSAg) is identified, obtain HBEAg, HBEAb, and HBV DNA levels. As with HCV infection, vaccination with hepatitis A vaccine and counseling to avoid alcohol are important components of preventive care. Isolated Hepatitis B Core Antibody: Many patients with HIV have antibody to hepatitis B core (anti-HBc) but are negative for both HBSAg and HBSAb. This phenomenon appears to be more common in those with HCV coinfection (Clin Infec Dis 2003 36:1602–6). In this scenario, diagnostic considerations include: (1) recently acquired HBV, before development of HBSAb; (2) chronic HBV, with HBSAg below the levels of detection; (3) immunity to HBV, with HBSAb below the levels of detection; (4) false-positive anti-HBV core. As the incidence of HBV is relatively low in most populations and anti-HBc alone is usually a stable phenomenon over years, recent acquisition of HBV is rarely the explanation. We recommend checking HBV DNA in this situation: If positive, this indicates chronic HBV; if negative, then low-level immunity or false-positive anti-HBV core remain as possible explanations; since distinguishing between these possibilities cannot be done, we recommend immunization with the hepatitis B vaccine series. It is useful to measure HBV serologic markers periodically in this population, as improvement in immune status due to ART may lead to increasing titers of HBSAb and subsequently confirm immunity (Clin Infect Dis 2007;45:1221–9).

Therapeutic Considerations: The optimal treatment for HBV infection is in evolution. Current guidelines suggest treatment of HBV in all patients with active HBV replication, defined as a detectable HBEAg or HBV DNA. Pending long-term studies defining optimal management, the recommendations set forth in the grid above are reasonable. Patients being treated with regimens for HBV should be monitored for ALT every 3–4 months. HBV DNA levels provide a good marker for efficacy of therapy and should be added to regular laboratory monitoring. The goal of therapy is to reduce HBV DNA to as low a level as possible, preferably below the limits of detection. The duration of HBV therapy is not well established; with development of HBEAb, while some individuals without HIV can stop therapy after reversion of HBEAg to negative, there are no clear stopping rules for HIV-coinfected patients.

Hepatitis C virus (HCV)

Preferred Therapy, Duration of Therapy, Chronic Maintenance	Alternate Therapy	Other Options/Issues
Genotype 1, 4, 5, or 6 Peginterferon alfa-2a 180 μg SQ weekly, **or** Peginterferon alfa-2b 1.5 mg/kg SQ weekly + Ribavirin PO (wt-based dosing) < 75 kg: 600 mg qAM and 400 mg qPM; ≥ 75 kg: 600 mg qAM and 600 mg qPM	In patients for whom ribavirin is contraindicated (e.g. unstable cardiopulmonary disease, pre-existing anemia unresponsive to erythropoietin, renal failure, or hemoglobinopathy) Peginterferon alfa-2a 180 μg SQ weekly, **or** Peginterferon alfa-2b 1.5 μg/kg SQ weekly	For patients with CD4+ count < 200 cells/μL, initiation of ART may be considered before HCV treatment Didanosine + ribavirin may lead to increased mitochondrial toxicities; concomitant use is contraindicated
Genotype 2 or 3 Peginterferon alfa-2a 180 μg SQ weekly, **or** Peginterferon alfa-2b 1.5 mg/kg SQ weekly + Ribavirin (fixed dose) PO 400 mg qAM and 400 mg qPM Duration of therapy: 48 weeks–genotypes 1 or 4, 5 or 6 and genotypes 2 and 3 At least 24 weeks–treatment of acute HCV infection (< 6 months from HCV exposure)	In patients with decompensated liver disease Liver transplantation if feasible	HCV therapy is not recommended in patients with hepatic decompensation. Liver transplantation, if feasible, should be the primary treatment option Interferon is abortifacient in high doses and ribavirin is teratogenic. HCV treatment is not recommended in pregnant women or women who are not willing to use birth control

Epidemiology: Hepatitis C virus (HCV) infection is transmitted primarily through blood exposure; sexual and perinatal transmission are also possible but less efficient. A notable exception is sexually transmitted HCV among gay men. Since modes of transmission of HIV and HCV are similar, there are high rates of HCV coinfection in HIV—an estimated 16% of HIV patients overall, including 80% or more of IDUs and 5–10% of gay men (Clin Infect Dis 2002;34:831–7). Genotype 1 accounts for 75% of HCV in the United States. HIV accelerates the progression of chronic HCV infection to cirrhosis, liver failure, and hepatocellular carcinoma (J Infect Dis 2001;183:1112–5; Clin Infect Dis 2001;33:562–569). Data are conflicting regarding the independent effect of HCV on HIV disease progression, but several studies have shown a markedly higher rate of antiretroviral therapy-induced hepatotoxicity in those with chronic HCV. In some series, liver failure from HCV is one of the leading causes of death in HIV/HCV coinfected individuals (Clin Infect Dis 2001;32:492–7).

Clinical Presentation: Persistently elevated liver transaminases; usually asymptomatic.

Diagnostic Considerations: All HIV-positive patients should be tested for HCV antibody. If the antibody test is negative but the likelihood of HCV infection is high (IDU, unexplained increase in LFTs), obtain an HCV RNA since false-negative antibody tests may occur, especially in advanced HIV disease (J Clin Microbiol 2000;38:575–7). Since LFT elevation does not correlate well with underlying HCV activity, a liver biopsy is the best way to assess the degree of fibrosis and inflammation.

Therapeutic Considerations:

Once Diagnosis is Established. Advise patients to abstain from alcohol and administer vaccinations for hepatitis A and B (if non-immune). Also obtain HCV RNA levels with genotype assessment. HCV RNA levels do not have prognostic significance for underlying degree of liver disease, but higher levels make treatment for cure less likely. Genotype results also correlate with cure rates (reported cure rates: 60–75% for genotypes 2 and 3; 15–25% for genotype 1). Some clinicians elect to treat HCV without a liver biopsy due to: the risks, costs, and discomfort of the test; the potential to underestimate the degree of HCV activity due to sampling error; and the high rate of treatment success for genotypes 2 and 3.

Optimal Patient Characteristics for HCV Treatment in HIV include no active psychiatric disease or substance abuse; stable HIV disease with undetectable HIV RNA and higher CD4 cell count; receiving an antiretroviral regimen that does not contain ddI (in particular), d4T, or ZDV; and adherent to medications, follow-up visits, and blood test monitoring. Only a small proportion of patients will meet all these criteria; therefore, to maximize treatment effect, it is important to optimize clinical status prior to starting HCV therapy. Patients should be fully educated regarding the goals and risks of treatment, with provision of written information about side effects, local support groups, and whom to contact with questions. It is useful to administer the first dose of treatment in the office in order to provide instructions on injection techniques.

Choice of Drug Therapy. The treatment of choice for HCV infection is pegylated interferon plus ribavirin. All patients should also receive hepatitis A vaccine and counseling to avoid alcohol use.

- _Pegylated Interferon_. Two different formulations of pegylated interferon are available for treatment of HCV infection: (1) peginterferon alfa-2a (Pegasys), supplied as a pre-mixed solution and administered subcutaneously as a fixed dose of 180 mcg once a week; and (2) peginterferon alfa-2b (Peg-Intron), supplied as a powder that is reconstituted in saline and administered subcutaneously as a weight-based dose once a week. Efficacy and toxicity of these two peginterferon preparations appear to be similar. Three clinical trials have shown that pegylated interferon plus ribavirin is more effective than standard interferon plus ribavirin (N Engl J Med 2004;351:451–9; N Engl J Med 2004;351:438–50; JAMA 2004;292:2839–48). Interferon has numerous side effects, the most important of which are listed in Table 5.3.

- <u>Ribavirin</u>. Ribavirin is available in 200-mg capsules. Although the dose used in clinical trials was 800 mg daily (400 mg BID), it appears that a higher initial dose is associated with greater efficacy. Standard dose is now 400 mg qAM and 600 mg qPM for weight < 75 kg, and 600 mg qAM and 600 mg qPM for weight > 75 kg. Ribavirin causes hemolytic anemia that predictably leads to a measurable decline in hemoglobin; this stabilizes by week 4–8 of treatment. Hemolytic anemia may be exacerbated in patients receiving ZDV; if possible an alternative NRTI should be chosen, with preference for tenofovir or abacavir. For symptomatic anemia or patients with coexisting conditions exacerbated by anemia, erythropoietin is used to maintain hemoglobin levels > 10 gm/dL or higher as needed. The typical starting dose of erythropoietin is 40,000 units SQ once a week. ddI is contraindicated during ribavirin administration due to an increased risk of mitochondrial toxicity and hepatic decompensation (Clin Infect Dis 2004;38:e79–e80). d4T should also be avoided because of its potential for inducing mitochondrial toxicity itself. Finally, some data suggest that ABC may interact with ribavirin, reducing efficacy of HCV therapy. Another common side effect of ribavirin is GI distress, which can overlap with a similar effect of interferon. Ribavirin is pregnancy category × (potent teratogen), and can only be used in sexually active women of childbearing potential if they are using 2 forms of birth control. Pregnancy should be avoided until at least 6 months after stopping ribavirin.

Monitoring. The monitoring plan for HIV/HCV coinfected patients consists of both safety and efficacy evaluations (Table 5.4). Results of HCV RNA testing are used to decide between completing 48 weeks of HCV therapy vs. discontinuing treatment at 12 or 24 weeks due to low probability of cure (Figure 5.1).

Table 5.3. Adverse Effects Associated with Interferon

Side Effect	Comments
Fatigue and flu-like symptoms (fever, chills, muscle aches, headache)	Dose at night so that some initial symptoms can be slept through. Symptoms may not peak until 48–78 hours after weekly dose and can be managed with acetaminophen (maximum 1300 mg/day) or ibuprofen plus good hydration. Fatigue is sometimes a manifestation of thyroid dysregulation or anemia; monitor thyroid function tests and CBC
Depression	Interferon can aggravate life-threatening psychiatric conditions. Low threshold for initiating anti-depressant therapy. Patients with a preexisting history of depression or other psychiatric disease should be followed closely by mental health professionals during HCV treatment
Leukopenia, thrombocytopenia, anemia	Cytopenias are more common in HIV/HCV co-infection. Can treat with G-CSF 300 mcg 3x/week if absolute neutrophil count is < 500/mm³. If neutropenia persists, decrease dose of interferon. If platelet count falls to < 80,000/mm³, also consider decreasing interferon dose (some clinicians tolerate counts down to 50,000/mm³). Low threshold for use of erythropoietin (EPO) 40,000 U/week for anemia (see section on ribavirin)

Table 5.3. Adverse Effects Associated with Interferon (cont'd)

Side Effect	Comments
Mouth ulcers	Topical viscous lidocaine or sucralfate is helpful in some
Gastrointestinal symptoms	Nausea and anorexia are the most common, often leading to weight loss. Advise patients to eat several small meals daily rather than a few large meals
Hair loss	Reversible after completion of therapy

Table 5.4. Monitoring Plan During Treatment for HCV Infection

	Weeks of Treatment								
	Baseline	2	4	8	12	16	20	24	24–48
CBC	X	X	X	X	X	X	X	X	q4 weeks
LFTs + metabolic panel	X		X	X	X	X	X	X	q4 weeks
HCV RNA	X		X¶		X*			X**	q12 weeks
HIV RNA + CD4 profile	X				X†			X	q12 weeks
TSH	X				X			X	q12 weeks
Depression	X	X	X	X	X	X	X	X	ongoing
Ophthalmologic exam	X‡				X			X	q12 weeks
PT	X					X			q12 weeks
Pregnancy test	Perform at regular intervals if appropriate								

*   Patients who have not dropped ≥ 2 logs from baseline HCV RNA at 12 weeks (early virologic response) have < 3% chance of obtaining a sustained viral response (undetectable HCV RNA 6 months post-treatment). Optimally, the HCV RNA will be undetectable by week 12 ("complete" early virologic response). One proposed strategy for patients with low-level detectable HCV RNA at week 12 ("partial" early virologic response) is to lengthen the course of therapy to 72 weeks or longer to reduce the risk of relapse; this is currently under investigation.

** If undetectable HCV RNA at 24 weeks, continue therapy for an additional 24 weeks (if known genotype 2 or 3 discuss option to stop, but some experts agree co-infected patients should continue treatment for 48 weeks to decrease risk of relapse). If HCV RNA is positive at 24 weeks, consider discontinuing HCV therapy. Even in patients without viral response, treatment may improve liver histology. Also see Figure 5.1.

†   *Anticipate decrease in absolute cell count but stable CD4%.*

‡   Necessary for patients with a history of retinopathy; IFN package insert recommends screening for all patients prior to treatment. Many clinicians choose to defer the initial exam and monitor for disturbances in vision and loss of color perception.

¶   Check HCV RNA at week 4; if no decline in HIV RNA is seen, response is extremely unlikely. In contrast, ≥ 1 log decline can be very motivating and treatment should be continued. Best chance at cure is with an undetectable HIV RNA at 4 weeks, sometimes called a "rapid virologic response."

Adapted from: Brown, et al. Clinician's Guide to HIV/HCV Coinfection, June, 2004.

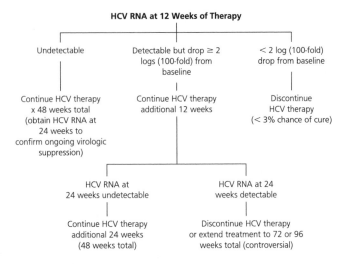

HCV RNA at 12 Weeks of Therapy

Undetectable	Detectable but drop ≥ 2 logs (100-fold) from baseline	< 2 log (100-fold) drop from baseline
Continue HCV therapy x 48 weeks total (obtain HCV RNA at 24 weeks to confirm ongoing virologic suppression)	Continue HCV therapy additional 12 weeks	Discontinue HCV therapy (< 3% chance of cure)

HCV RNA at 24 weeks undetectable	HCV RNA at 24 weeks detectable
Continue HCV therapy additional 24 weeks (48 weeks total)	Discontinue HCV therapy or extend treatment to 72 or 96 weeks total (controversial)

Figure 5.1. Management of HCV Infection Based on HCV RNA Testing

HCV RNA should be assessed at week 12. If the HCV viral load has not dropped by more than 2 logs (100-fold), then the likelihood of achieving a cure is extremely low. Many patients and providers will elect to discontinue therapy at this point. HCV RNA should be measured at weeks 24 and 48. If undetectable at week 48, additional measurements should be obtained at weeks 4, 12, and 24 after stopping treatment. An undetectable HCV RNA at week 24 post-treatment is the current standard for assessing a "sustained virologic response" (SVR), which can be equated with cure. Importantly, patients cured of HCV are susceptible to reacquisition and should be cautioned about resuming high-risk behavior.

Internet Resources:

- AIDSinfo: aidsinfo.nih.gov
- Chronic Hepatitis C: Current Disease Management: http://digestive.niddk.nih.gov/ddiseases/pubs/chronichepc/
- Hep C Connection: www.hepc-connection.org
- HIV and Hepatitis.com: www.hivandhepatitis.com
- Johns Hopkins Hepatitis C and HIV Coinfection Information: www.hopkins-hivguide.org/diagnosis/opportunistic_infections/viral/full_hepatitis_c.html
- National HIV/AIDS Clinicians' Consultation Center: www.nccc.ucsf.edu/
- The National AIDS Treatment Advocacy Project: www.natap.org
- Projects in Knowledge: www.projectsinknowledge.com

Herpes Simplex Virus (HSV) Disease

Preferred Therapy, Duration of Therapy, Chronic Maintenance	Alternate Therapy	Other Options/Issues
<u>Preferred therapy for orolabial lesions and initial or recurrent genital HSV</u> Valacyclovir 1 g PO BID, famciclovir 500 mg PO BID, or acyclovir 400 mg PO TID Duration of therapy: Orolabial HSV: 5–10 days Genital HSV: 5–14 days <u>Preferred therapy for severe mucocutaneous HSV infections</u> Initial therapy acyclovir 5 mg/kg IV q8h After lesions began to regress, change to PO therapy as above. Continue therapy until lesions have completely healed <u>Preferred therapy for acyclovir-resistant mucocutaneous HSV infections</u> Foscarnet 80–120 mg/kg/day IV in 2–3 divided doses until clinical response		
	<u>Alternative therapy for acyclovir-resistant mucocutaneous HSV infections</u> Topical trifluridine Topical cidofovir Topical imiquimod Duration of therapy: 21–28 days or longer	Topical formulations of neither trifluridine nor cidofovir are commercially available in the US Extemporaneous compounding of topical products can be prepared using trifluridine ophthalmic solution and the intravenous formulation of cidofovir
<u>Preferred therapy for HSV encephalitis</u> Acyclovir 10 mg/kg IV q8h for 21 days <u>Suppressive therapy (For patients with frequent or severe recurrences of genital herpes)</u> Valacyclovir 500 mg PO BID Famciclovir 500 mg PO BID Acyclovir 400 mg PO BID		

Herpes Simplex (genital/oral)

Clinical Presentation: Painful, grouped vesicles on an erythematous base that rupture, crust, and heal within 2 weeks. Lesions may be chronic, severe, ulcerative with advanced immunosuppression.

Diagnostic Considerations: Diagnosis by viral culture of swab from lesion base/roof of blister; alternative diagnostic techniques include Tzanck prep or immunofluorescence staining.

Pitfalls: Acyclovir prophylaxis is not required in patients receiving ganciclovir or foscarnet.

Therapeutic Considerations: In refractory cases, consider acyclovir resistance and treat with foscarnet. Topical trifluridine ophthalmic solution (Viroptic 1%) may be considered for direct application to small, localized areas of refractory disease; clean with hydrogen peroxide, then debride lightly with gauze, apply trifluridine, and cover with bacitracin/polymyxin ointment and nonadsorbent gauze; topical cidofovir (requires compounding) also may be tried. Chronic suppressive therapy with oral acyclovir, famciclovir, or valacyclovir may be indicated for patients with frequent recurrences, dosing similar to HIV-negative patients.

Prognosis: Responds well to treatment except in severely immunocompromised patients, in whom acyclovir resistance may develop.

Herpes Encephalitis (HSV-1)

Clinical Presentation: Acute onset of fever and change in mental status.

Diagnostic Considerations: EEG is abnormal early (< 72 hours), showing unilateral temporal lobe abnormalities. Brain MRI is abnormal before CT scan, which may require several days before a temporal lobe focus is seen. Definitive diagnosis is by CSF PCR for HSV-1 DNA. Profound decrease in sensorium is characteristic of HSV meningoencephalitis. CSF may have PMN predominance and low glucose levels, unlike other viral causes of meningitis. A different clinical entity is HSV meningitis, which is usually associated with HSV-2 and can recur with lymphocytic meningitis. HSV encephalitis is surprisingly rare in HIV patients, but when it occurs, residual neurologic deficits are common; by contrast, HSV meningitis (usually in association with genital HSV outbreaks) has an excellent prognosis.

Pitfalls: Rule out non-infectious causes of encephalopathy. Surprisingly, HSV encephalitis is a relatively rare cause of encephalitis in patients with HIV.

Therapeutic Considerations: Treat as soon as possible since neurological deficits may be mild and reversible early on, but severe and irreversible later.

Prognosis: Related to extent of brain injury and early antiviral therapy.

HHV-6 Infection

Preferred Therapy, Duration of Therapy, Chronic Maintenance	Alternate Therapy	Other Options/Issues
If HHV-6 has been identified as cause of disease in HIV-infected patients, use same drugs and doses as treatment for CMV disease Ganciclovir (or valganciclovir) Foscarnet		

HHV-8 Infection*

Preferred Therapy, Duration of Therapy, Chronic Maintenance	Alternate Therapy	Other Options/Issues
Initiation or optimization of ART should be done for all patients with KS, PEL, or MCD Preferred therapy for visceral KS, disseminated cutaneous KS, and PEL Chemotherapy + ART Oral valganciclovir or IV ganciclovir might be useful as adjunctive therapy in PEL Preferred therapy for MCD Valganciclovir 900 mg PO BID; **or** Ganciclovir 5 mg/kg IV q12h	Alternative therapy for MCD Rituximab, 375 mg/m^2 given weekly × 4–8 weeks, may be an alternative to antiviral therapy	

* (Kaposi's Sarcoma [KS], primary effusion lymphoma [PEL], multicentric Castleman's disease [MCD])

Histoplasma capsulatum

Preferred Therapy, Duration of Therapy, Chronic Maintenance	Alternate Therapy	Other Options/Issues
Preferred therapy for moderately severe to severe disseminated disease *Induction therapy* (for 2 weeks or until clinically improved) Liposomal amphotericin B at 3 mg/kg IV daily Maintenance therapy Itraconazole 200 mg PO TID for 3 days, then BID Preferred therapy for less severe disseminated disease *Induction and maintenance therapy* Itraconazole 200 mg PO TID for 3 days, then 200 mg PO BID	Alternative therapy moderately severe to severe disseminated disease *Induction therapy* (for 2 weeks or until clinically improved) Amphotericin B deoxycholate 0.7 mg/kg IV daily Amphotericin B lipid complex 5 mg/kg IV daily *Maintenance therapy* same as "Preferred therapy"	Itraconazole levels should be obtained in all patients to ensure adequate absorption. Serum concentrations of itraconazole + hydroxyitraconazole should be > 1 μg/mL Itraconazole oral solution is preferred over capsule by certain specialists because of improved absorption

Histoplasma capsulatum (cont'd)

Preferred Therapy, Duration of Therapy, Chronic Maintenance	Alternate Therapy	Other Options/Issues
Duration of therapy: at least 12 months Preferred therapy for meningitis *Induction therapy (4–6 weeks)* Liposomal amphotericin B 5 mg/kg/day *Maintenance therapy* Itraconazole 200 mg PO BID-TID for ≥ 1 year and until resolution of abnormal CSF findings Preferred therapy for long-term suppression therapy In patients with severe disseminated or CNS infection and in patients who relapse despite appropriate therapy Itraconazole 200 mg PO daily		Acute pulmonary histoplasmosis in HIV-infected patients with CD4+ count > 300 cells/μL should be managed as non-immunocompromised host

Clinical Presentation: Two general forms: Mild disease with fever/lymph node enlargement (e.g., cervical adenitis), or severe disease with fever, wasting—also may have diarrhea/meningitis/GI ulcerations.

Diagnostic Considerations: Diagnosis by urine/serum histoplasmosis antigen, sometimes by culture of bone marrow/liver or isolator blood cultures. May occur in patients months to years after having lived/moved from an endemic area.

Pitfalls: Relapse is common after discontinuation of therapy. Cultures may take 7–21 days to turn positive. Itraconazole has many drug-drug interactions with antiretrovirals, especially PIs.

Therapeutic Considerations: Initial therapy depends on severity of illness on presentation. Extremely sick patients should be started on amphotericin B deoxycholate, with duration of IV therapy dependent on response to treatment. Mildly ill patients can be started on itraconazole. Regardless of disease severity, itraconazole levels should be obtained to ensure adequate absorption. Serum concentrations of itraconazole + hydroxyitraconazole should be > 1 μg/mL. All patients require chronic suppressive therapy, with possible discontinuation for immune reconstitution with CD4 counts > 100/mm³ for at least 6 months. HIV patients with CD4 > 500/mm³ and acute pulmonary histoplasmosis might not require therapy, but a short course of itraconazole (4–8 weeks) is reasonable to prevent systemic spread.

Prognosis: Usually responds to treatment, except in fulminant cases.

Human Papillomavirus (HPV) Disease

Preferred Therapy, Duration of Therapy, Chronic Maintenance	Alternate Therapy	Other Options/Issues
Treatment of condyloma acuminata (genital warts)		
Patient-applied therapy Podofilox 0.5% solution or 0.5% gel—apply to all lesions BID × 3 consecutive days, followed by 4 days of no therapy, repeat weekly for up to 4 cycles; **or** Imiquimod 5% cream—apply to lesion at bedtime and remove in the morning on 3 nonconsecutive nights weekly for up to 16 weeks. Each treatment should be washed with soap and water 6–10 hours after application	Provider-applied therapy Cryotherapy (liquid nitrogen or cryoprobe)—apply until each lesion is thoroughly frozen; repeat every 1–2 weeks. Some providers allow the lesion to thaw, then freeze a 2nd time in each session. Trichloroacetic acid or bicloroacetic acid cauterization—80%–90% aqueous solution, apply to each lesion, repeat weekly for 3–6 weeks Surgical excision or laser surgery Podophyllin resin 10%–25% suspension in tincture of benzoin—apply to all lesions, then wash off a few hours later, repeat weekly for 3–6 weeks	Intralesional interferon-alpha is usually not recommended because of high cost, difficult administration, and potential for systemic side effects The rate of recurrence of genital warts is high, despite treatment

Genital/Perianal Warts (Condyloma Acuminata)

Clinical Presentation: Single/multiple verrucous genital lesions ± pigmentation usually without inguinal adenopathy.

Diagnostic Considerations: Diagnosis by clinical appearance. Genital warts are usually caused by HPV types 11, 16. Anogenital warts caused by HPV types 16, 18, 31, 33, 35 are associated with cervical neoplasia.

Pitfalls: Most HPV infections are asymptomatic.

Therapeutic Considerations: First-line therapy is ablative (cryotherapy or cauterization); if no response to standard treatment, attempt to treat with surgery or cidofovir. Intralesional interferon-alfa generally is not recommended.

Prognosis: The rate of recurrence of anogenital warts is high despite treatment.

Isospora belli Infection

Preferred Therapy, Duration of Therapy, Chronic Maintenance	Alternate Therapy	Other Options/Issues
Preferred therapy for acute infection: TMP-SMX (160 mg/800 mg) PO (or IV) QID for 10 days; **or** TMP-SMX (160 mg/800 mg) PO (or IV) BID for 7–10 days May increase daily dose and/ or duration (up to 3–4 weeks) if symptoms worsen or persist	Alternative therapy for acute infection Pyrimethamine 50–75 mg PO daily plus leucovorin 10–25 mg PO daily; **or** Ciprofloxacin 500 mg PO BID × 7 days–as a second line alternative	Fluid and electrolyte management in patients with dehydration Nutritional supplementation for malnourished patients Immune reconstitution with ART may result in fewer relapses
Preferred chronic maintenance therapy (secondary prophylaxis) In patients with CD4+ count < 200/μL, TMP-SMX (160 mg/800 mg) PO tiw	Alternative chronic maintenance therapy (secondary prophylaxis) TMP-SMX (160 mg/800 mg) PO daily or (320 mg/ 1600 mg) tiw Pyrimethamine 25 mg PO daily + leucovorin 5–10 mg PO daily Ciprofloxacin 500 mg tiw–as a second line alternative	

Clinical Presentation: Severe chronic diarrhea without fever/fecal leukocytes.

Diagnostic Considerations: Spore-forming protozoa *(Isospora belli)*. Oocyst on AFB smear of stool larger that cryptosporidium (20–30 microns vs. 4–6 microns). More common in HIV patients from tropical areas. Less common than cryptosporidium or microsporidia**.** Malabsorption may occur with severe cases. Can be associated with eosinophilia.

Pitfalls: Multiple relapses are possible.

Therapeutic Considerations: Chronic suppressive therapy may be required if CD4 cell count does not increase.

Prognosis: Related to degree of immunosuppression/response to antiretroviral therapy.

Comments: Immune reconstitution with ART results in fewer relapses.

Leishmaniasis, Cutaneous

Preferred Therapy, Duration of Therapy, Chronic Maintenance	Alternate Therapy	Other Options/Issues
Preferred therapy for acute infection Liposomal amphotericin B 2–4 mg/kg IV daily for 10 days or interrupted schedule (e.g., 4 mg/kg on days 1–5, 10, 17, 24, 31, 38) to achieve total dose of 20–60 mg/kg; **or** Sodium stibogluconate 20 mg/kg IV or IM daily for 3–4 weeks	Alternative therapy for acute infection Choice dependent on species of _Leishmania_ Other options include oral miltefosine, topical paromomycin, intralesional pentavalent antimony, and local heat therapy	

Leishmaniasis, Visceral

Preferred Therapy, Duration of Therapy, Chronic Maintenance	Alternate Therapy	Other Options/Issues
Preferred therapy for initial infection Liposomal amphotericin B or amphotericin B lipid complex 2–4 mg/kg IV daily × 10 days; or interrupted schedule (e.g., 4 mg/kg on days 1–5, 10, 17, 24, 31, 38) to achieve total dose of 20–60 mg/kg	Alternative therapy for initial infection Amphotericin B deoxycholate 0.5–1.0 mg/kg IV daily for total dose of 1.5–2.0 grams; **or** Sodium stibogluconate (pentavalent antimony) 20 mg/kg body weight IV or IM daily for 3–4 weeks. (Contact the CDC Drug Service at 404-639-3670 or drugservice@cdc.gov)	ART should be initiated or optimized Parenteral paromomycin has been proven effective in HIV-negative patients in India-may be available as an alternative in India in the future
Preferred chronic maintenance therapy (secondary prophylaxis)—especially in patients with CD4+ count < 200 cells/µL Liposomal amphotericin B 4 mg/kg every 2–4 weeks	Alternative chronic maintenance therapy (secondary prophylaxis) Amphotericin B lipid complex 3–4 mg/kg evesry 2–4 weeks Sodium stibogluconate 20 mg/kg IV or IM every 4 weeks	Alternative regimens for treatment failure Miltefosine 100 mg PO daily for 4 weeks (available in Europe via compassionate use)

Malaria*

Preferred Therapy, Duration of Therapy, Chronic Maintenance	Alternate Therapy	Other Options/Issues
All regions use the following regimens (except for Papua New Guinea and Indonesia, in which case treat as for chloroquine-resistant *P. falciparum* malaria as below) Chloroquine phosphate 1000 mg PO × 1, then 500 mg PO at 6, 24, and 48 hours, total dose = 2,500 mg; then Anti-relapse therapy (after checking G6PD status): primaquine 30 mg base PO daily × 14 days		G6PD status should be checked before initiation of primaquine

* from: *P. vivax, P. ovale, P. malariae*

Malaria, severe, from all regions

Preferred Therapy, Duration of Therapy, Chronic Maintenance	Alternate Therapy	Other Options/Issues
Preferred therapy Quinidine gluconate 10 mg/kg IV over 1–2 hours, then 0.02 mg/kg/min infusion (quinidine 6.25 mg base/kg IV over 1–2 hours, then 0.0125 mg/kg/min) for ≥ 24 hours with cardiac monitoring + Doxycycline 100 mg PO or IV q12h × 7 days; **or** Clindamycin 20 mg base/kg/day (in 3 divided doses) PO or 10 mg base/kg loading dose IV followed by 5 mg base/kg IV q8h; switch to PO clindamycin (dose as above) as soon as patient can take PO medication for a total course of 7 days	Alternative therapy Artesunate 2.4 mg/kg IV bolus at 0, 12, and 24 hours, then daily Duration of therapy: 7 days for Southeast Asia and Oceania and 3 days for other areas When able to take PO, switch to: Atovaquone-proquanil, mefloquine, or doxycycline (doses as listed above)	Intravenous artesunate is available from CDC quarantine stations (CDC Malaria Hotline 770-488-7788)

Malaria, uncomplicated, from *Plasmodium falciparum* or unknown malaria species

Preferred Therapy, Duration of Therapy, Chronic Maintenance	Alternate Therapy	Other Options/Issues
Preferred therapy for chloroquine-sensitive infection (north of the Panama Canal) Chloroquine phosphate 1,000 mg PO (=600 mg chloroquine base) once, then 500 mg PO (=300 mg chloroquine base) at 6, 24, and 48 hours Total dose = chloroquine phosphate 2,500 mg Preferred therapy for chloroquine-resistant infections (all other malaria areas or unknown region) Atovaquone-proguanil (250 mg/100 mg)—4 tablet PO daily × 3 days	Alternative therapy for chloroquine-sensitive infection (north of the Panama Canal) No alternative listed Alternative therapy for chloroquine-resistant infections (all other malaria areas or unknown region) Mefloquine 750 mg PO × 1, then 500 mg administered 12 hrs later, total dose = 1,250 mg Quinine sulfate 650 mg PO q8h × 3 days (infections acquired outside of southeast Asia) to 7 days (infections acquired in southeast Asia) + (doxycycline 100 mg PO q12h × 7 days or clindamycin 20 mg base/kg/day [in 3 divided doses] PO × 7 days)	Treatment recommendations for HIV-infected patients are the same as HIV non-infected patients For most updated treatment recommendations for specific region, clinicians should refer to the following web link: http://www.cdc.gov/malaria/ or call the CDC Malaria Hotline: 770-488-7788: M-F 8 AM-4:30 PM ET 770-488-7100: after hours

Microsporidiosis

Preferred Therapy, Duration of Therapy, Chronic Maintenance	Alternate Therapy	Other Options/Issues
Initiate or optimize ART; immune restoration to CD4+ count > 100 cells/μL is associated with resolution of symptoms of enteric microsporidiosis		Severe dehydration, malnutrition, and wasting should be managed by fluid support and nutritional supplement

Microsporidiosis (cont'd)

Preferred Therapy, Duration of Therapy, Chronic Maintenance	Alternate Therapy,	Other Options/Issues
Preferred therapy for gastrointestinal infections caused by *Enterocytozoon bienuesi* Fumagillin 20 mg PO TID (not available in US) TNP-470 (a synthetic analog of fumagillin) might also be effective (not available in US)	Alternative therapy for gastrointestinal infections caused by *E. bienuesi* Nitazoxanide 1,000 mg BID with food for 60 days—effects might be minimal for patients with low CD4+ count	Antimotility agents can be used for diarrhea control if required
Preferred therapy for disseminated (not ocular) and intestinal infection attributed to microsporidia other than *E. bienuesi* and *Vittaforma corneae* Albendazole 400 mg PO BID, continue until CD4+ count > 200 cells/μL for > 6 months after initiation of ART	Alternative therapy for disseminated disease Itraconazole 400 mg PO daily plus albendazole 400 mg PO BID for disseminated disease attributed to *Trachipleistophora* or *Anncaliia*	
For ocular infection Topical fumagillin bicylohexylammonium (Fumidil B) 3 mg/mL in saline (fumagillin 70 μg/mL) eye drops—2 drops every 2 hours for 4 days, then 2 drops QID (investigational use only in US) plus albendazole 400 mg PO BID for management of systemic infection Treatment should be continued indefinitely to prevent recurrence or relapse		

Clinical Presentation: Most commonly, intermittent chronic diarrhea without fever/fecal leukocytes; also can disseminate and cause disease in other organs (eyes, lungs).

Diagnostic Considerations: Spore-forming protozoa *(S. intestinalis, E. bienuesi)*. Diagnosis by modified trichrome or fluorescent antibody stain of stool. Microsporidia can rarely disseminate to sinuses/cornea. Severe malabsorption may occur.

Pitfalls: Microsporidia cannot be detected by routine microscopic examination of stool due to small size.

Therapeutic Considerations: Key to successful resolution is optimizing ART to improve immune function. Albendazole is less effective for *E. bieneusi* than *S. intestinalis*, but speciation is usually not possible. Consider treatment discontinuation for CD4 > 200/mm³ if patient remains asymptomatic (no signs or symptoms of microsporidiosis). If ocular infection is present, continue treatment indefinitely.

Prognosis: Related to degree of immunosuppression/response to antiretroviral therapy.

Mycobacterium avium Complex (MAC) Disease

Preferred Therapy, Duration of Therapy, Chronic Maintenance	Alternate Therapy	Other Options/Issues
<u>Preferred therapy for disseminated MAC</u> At least 2 drugs as initial therapy with Clarithromycin 500 mg PO BID + ethambutol 15 mg/kg PO daily Addition of rifabutin may also be considered: Rifabutin 300 mg PO daily (dosage adjusted may be necessary based on drug-drug interactions) <u>Chronic maintenance therapy (secondary prophylaxis)</u> Same as treatment drugs and regimens Duration: Lifelong therapy, unless in patients with sustained immune recovery on ART	<u>Alternative therapy for disseminated MAC (e.g., when drug interactions or intolerance precludes the use of clarithromycin)</u> Azithromycin 500–600 mg + ethambutol 15 mg/kg PO daily Addition of a third or fourth drug should be considered for patients with advanced immunosuppression (CD4+ count < 50 cells/μL), high mycobacterial loads (> 2 log CFU/mL of blood), or in the absence of effective ART Amikacin 10–15 mg/kg IV daily; **or** Streptomycin 1 gm IV or IM daily; **or** Ciprofloxacin 500–750 mg PO BID; **or** Levofloxacin 500 mg PO daily; **or** Moxifloxacin 400 mg PO daily	Testing of susceptibility to clarithromycin and azithromycin is recommended In ART-naïve patients, may consider withholding initiation of ART until after 2 weeks of MAC treatment to lessen drug interactions, reduce pill burden, and potentially lower occurrence of IRIS NSAIDs may be used for patients who experience moderate to severe symptoms attributed to ART-associated IRIS If immune reconstitution inflammatory syndrome (IRIS) symptoms persist, short term (4–8 weeks) of systemic corticosteroid (equivalent to 20–40 mg of prednisone) can be used

Clinical Presentation: Typically presents as a febrile wasting illness in advanced HIV disease (CD4 < 50/mm^3). Focal invasive disease is possible, especially in patients with advanced immunosuppression after starting antiretroviral therapy. Focal disease likely reflects restoration of pathogen-specific immune response to subclinical infection ("immune reconstitution inflammatory syndrome" [IRIS]), and typically manifests as lymphadenitis (mesenteric, cervical, thoracic) or rarely disease in the spine mimicking Pott's disease. Immune reconstitution syndrome usually occurs within weeks to months after starting antiretroviral therapy for the first time, but may occur a year or more later.

Diagnostic Considerations: Diagnosis by isolation of organism from a normally sterile body site (blood, lymph node, bone marrow, liver biopsy). Lysis centrifugation (DuPont isolator) is the preferred blood culture method. Anemia/↑ alkaline phosphatase are occasionally seen.

Pitfalls: Isolator blood cultures may be negative, especially in immune reconstitution inflammatory syndrome initially.

Therapeutic Considerations: Some studies suggest benefit for addition of rifabutin 300 mg (PO) QD, others do not. Rifabutin may require dosage adjustment with NNRTIs and PIs (see p. 135). Monitor carefully for rifabutin drug toxicity (arthralgias, uveitis, leukopenia). Treat IRIS initially with NSAIDs; if symptoms persist, systemic corticosteroids (prednisone 20–40 mg daily) for 4–8 weeks can be used. Some patients will require a more prolonged course of corticosteroids with a slow taper over months. Azithromycin is often better tolerated than clarithromycin and has fewer drug-drug interactions. Optimal long-term management is unknown, though most studies suggest that treatment can be discontinued in asymptomatic patients with > 12 months of therapy and CD4 > 100/mm^3 for > 6 months.

Prognosis: Depends on immune reconstitution in response to antiretroviral therapy. Adverse prognostic factors include high-grade bacteremia or severe wasting.

Mycobacterium tuberculosis

Preferred Therapy, Duration of Therapy, Chronic Maintenance	Alternate Therapy	Other Options/Issues
Empiric treatment should be initiated and continued in HIV-infected persons in whom TB is suspected until all diagnostic work-up is complete		Directly observed therapy (DOT) is recommended for all HIV patients undergoing treatment for active TB
Treatment of drug-susceptible active TB disease Initial phase (2 months) Isoniazid (INH)† + [rifampin (RIF) or rifabutin (RFB)] + pyrazinamide (PZA) + ethambutol (EMB); if drug susceptibility report shows sensitivity to INH & RIF and PZA, then EMB may be discontinued before 2 months of treatment is completed	**Treatment for drug-resistant active TB** Resistant to INH Discontinue INH (and streptomycin, if used) (RIF or RFB) + EMB + PZA for 6 months; **or** (RIF or RFB) + EMB for 12 months (preferably with	Initial phase of TB treatment may also be administered 5 days weekly (40 doses), or tiw (24 doses) by DOT For CNS disease, corticosteroid should be initiated as early as possible and continued for 6–8 weeks

Mycobacterium tuberculosis (cont'd)

Preferred Therapy, Duration of Therapy, Chronic Maintenance	Alternate Therapy	Other Options/Issues
Continuation phase INH + (RIF or RFB) daily or tiw or biw (if CD4+ count > 100/μL) Duration of therapy: *Pulmonary TB—6 months* *Pulmonary TB w/ cavitary lung lesions & (+) culture after 2 months of TB treatment—9 months* *Extrapulmonary TB w/ CNS, bone, or joint infections—9 to 12 months;* *Extrapulmonary TB in other sites—6 to 9 months*	PZA during at least the first 2 months) A fluoroquinolone may strengthen the regimen for patients with extensive disease <u>Resistant to rifamycins</u> INH + PZA + EMB + a fluoroquinolone for 2 months, followed by 10–16 additional months with INH + EMB + fluoroquinolone Amikacin or capreomycin may be included in the first 2–3 months for patients with rifamycin resistance & severe disease <u>Multidrug resistant (MDR, i.e., INH & RIF resistant) or extensively drug resistant (XDR, i.e., resistance to INH & RIF, fluoroquinolone & at least 1 injectable agent) TB</u> Therapy should be individualized based on resistance pattern and with close consultation with experienced specialist	RIF is not recommended for patients receiving HIV protease inhibitors (PI) because of its induction of PI metabolism RFB is a less potent CYP 3A4 inducer than RIF and is preferred in patients receiving PIs Rifapentine administered once weekly can result in development of resistance in HIV-infected patients and is not recommended Therapeutic drug monitoring should be considered in patients receiving rifamycin and interacting ART Paradoxical reaction that is not severe may be treated with nonsteroidal anti-inflammatory drugs (NSAIDs) without a change in anti-TB or anti-HIV therapy For severe paradoxical reaction, may consider prednisone or methylprednisolone 1 mg/kg of body weight, gradually reduced after 1–2 weeks

† All patients receiving INH should receive pyridoxine 25–50 mg PO daily

Clinical Presentation: May present atypically. HIV patients with high (> 500/mm³) CD4 cell counts are more likely to have a typical pulmonary presentation, but patients with advanced HIV disease may have a diffuse interstitial pattern, hilar adenopathy, or a normal chest x-ray. Tuberculin skin testing (TST) is helpful if positive, but unreliable if negative due to anergy.

Diagnostic Considerations: In many urban areas, TB is one of the most common HIV-related respiratory illnesses. In other areas, HIV-related TB occurs infrequently except in immigrants or patients arriving from highly TB endemic areas. Maintain a high Index of suspicion for TB in HIV patients with unexplained fevers/pulmonary infiltrates.

Pitfalls: Extrapulmonary and pulmonary TB often coexist, especially in advanced HIV disease.

Therapeutic Considerations: Treatment by directly observed therapy (DOT) is strongly recommended for all HIV patients. If patients have cavitary disease or either positive sputum cultures or lack of clinical response at 2 months, total duration of therapy should be increased up to 9 months or longer depending on clinical response. For CNS disease (meningitis or mass lesions), corticosteroid should be initiated as early as possible (along with TB treatment) and continued for 6–8 weeks. If hepatic transaminases are elevated (AST ≥ 3 times normal) before treatment initiation, treatment options include: (1) standard therapy with frequent monitoring; (2) rifamycin (rifampin or rifabutin) + EMB + PZA for 6 months; or (3) INH + rifamycin + EMB for 2 months, then INH + rifamycin for 7 months. Once-weekly rifapentine is not recommended for HIV patients. Non-severe immune reconstitution inflammatory syndrome (IRIS) may be treated with nonsteroidal anti-inflammatory drugs (NSAIDs); severe cases should be treated with corticosteroids. In all cases of IRIS, antiretroviral therapy should be continued if possible. Monitor carefully for signs of rifabutin drug toxicity (arthralgias, uveitis, leukopenia).

Prognosis: Usually responds to treatment. Relapse rates are related to the degree of immunosuppression and local risk of re-exposure to TB.

Penicilliosis

Preferred Therapy, Duration of Therapy, Chronic Maintenance	Alternate Therapy	Other Options/Issues
Acute infection in severely ill patients Amphotericin B deoxycholate 0.6 mg/kg/day IV for 2 weeks; followed by itraconazole 400 mg PO daily for 10 weeks Mild disease Itraconazole 400 mg PO daily for 8 weeks Chronic maintenance therapy (secondary prophylaxis) Itraconazole 200 mg PO daily		ART should be administered according to standard of care in the community; consideration should be given to simultaneously initiating ART and treatment for penicilliosis

Penicilliosis (*Penicillium marneffei*)

Clinical Presentation: Papules, pustules, nodules, ulcers, or abscesses. Mostly seen in advanced HIV/AIDS in residents/visitors of Southeast Asia or Southern China.

Diagnostic Considerations: Diagnosis by demonstrating organism by stain/culture in tissue. specimen. An early presumptive diagnosis can be made several days before the results of fungal cultures are available by microscopic examination of the Wright-stained samples of skin scrapings, bone marrow aspirate, or lymph-node biopsy specimens. Many intracellular and extracellular basophilic, spherical, oval, and elliptical yeast-like organisms can be seen, some with clear central septation, which is a characteristic feature of *P. marneffei*.

Pitfalls: Lesions commonly become umbilicated and resemble molluscum contagiosum.

Therapeutic Considerations: ART should be administered according to standard of care in the community. Requires lifelong suppressive therapy with itraconazole unless CD4 increases to > 100 for ≥ 6 months in response to ART.

Prognosis: Dependent on degree of immune recovery secondary to ART. Without HIV treatment, prognosis is poor, as most affected patients have advanced immunosuppression.

Pneumocystis Pneumonia (PCP)

Preferred Therapy, Duration of Therapy, Chronic Maintenance	Alternate Therapy	Other Options/Issues
Preferred treatment for moderate to severe PCP Trimethoprim-sulfamethoxazole (TMP-SMX): [15–20 mg TMP and 75–100 mg SMX]/kg/day IV administered q6h or q8h, may switch to PO after clinical improvement Duration of therapy: 21 days	Alternative therapy for moderate to severe PCP Pentamidine 4 mg/kg IV daily infused over ≥ 60 minutes, certain specialists reduce dose to 3 mg/kg IV daily because of toxicities; **or** Primaquine 15–30 mg (base) PO daily plus clindamycin 600–900 mg IV q6h to q8h or clindamycin 300–450 mg PO q6h to q8h	Indications for corticosteroids PaO_2 < 70 mmHg at room air or alveolar-arterial O_2 gradient > 35 mmHg Prednisone dosses (beginning as early as possible and within 72 hours of PCP therapy): Days 1–5 40mg PO BID Days 6–10 40mg PO daily Days 11–21 20 mg PO daily
Preferred treatment for mild to moderate PCP Same daily dose of TMP-SMX as above, administered PO in 3 divided doses; **or** TMP-SMX (160 mg/800 mg or DS) 2 tablets TID Duration of therapy: 21 days	Alternative therapy for mild-to-moderate PCP Dapsone 100 mg PO daily and TMP 15 mg/kg/day PO (3 divided doses); **or** Primaquine 15–30 mg (base) PO daily plus clindamycin 300–450 mg PO q6h to q8h; **or** Atovaquone 750 mg PO BID with food	IV methylprednisolone can be administered as 75% of prednisone dose

Pneumocystis Pneumonia (PCP) (cont'd)

Preferred Therapy, Duration of Therapy, Chronic Maintenance	Alternate Therapy	Other Options/Issues
Preferred secondary prophylaxis TMP-SMX (160 mg/800 mg or DS) tablet PO daily; **or** TMP-SMX (80 mg/400 mg or SS) tablet PO daily	Alternative secondary prophylaxis TMP-SMX (160 mg/800 mg or DS) PO tiw Dapsone 50 mg PO BID or 100 mg PO daily; **or** Dapsone 50 mg PO daily plus pyrimethamine 50 mg PO weekly plus leucovorin 25 mg PO weekly; **or** Dapsone 200 mg PO plus pyrimethamine 75 mg PO plus leucovorin 25 mg PO weekly; **or** Aerosolized pentamidine 300 mg every month via Respirgard II™ nebulizer; **or** Atovaquone 1,500 mg PO daily; **or** Atovaquone 1,500 mg + pyrimethamine 25 mg + leucovorin 10 mg PO daily	Benefits of corticosteroid if started after 72 hours of treatment is unknown, but a majority of clinicians will use it in patients with moderate to severe PCP Whenever possible, patients should be tested for G6PD deficiency before use of primaquine

Clinical Presentation: Fever, cough, dyspnea; often indolent presentation. Physical exam is usually normal. Chest x-ray is variable, but commonly shows a diffuse interstitial pattern. Elevated LDH and exercise desaturation are highly suggestive of PCP.

Diagnostic Considerations: Diagnosis by immunofluorescent stain of induced sputum or bronchoscopy specimen. Check ABG if O_2 saturation is abnormal or respiratory rate is increased. Serum 1, 3 beta-glucan is usually elevated and may provide additional supportive evidence for the diagnosis of PCP, even if the induced sputum is negative (Clin Infect Dis 2008 Jun 15;46[12]:1928–30).

Pitfalls: Slight worsening of symptoms is common after starting therapy, especially if not treated with steroids. Benefits of corticosteroid if started after 72 hours of treatment is unknown, but majority of clinicians will still use it if clinically warranted even after 72 hours. Do not overlook superimposed bacterial pneumonia or other secondary infections, especially while on pentamidine. Patients receiving second-line agents for PCP prophylaxis—in particular aerosolized pentamidine—may present with atypical radiographic findings, including apical infiltrates, multiple small-walled cysts, pleural effusions, pneumothorax, or single/multiple nodules.

Therapeutic Considerations: Outpatient therapy is possible for mild-moderate disease, but only when close follow-up is assured. Adverse reactions to TMP-SMX (rash, fever, GI symptoms, hepatitis, hyperkalemia, leukopenia, hemolytic anemia) occur in 25–50% of patients, many of whom will need a second-line regimen to complete therapy (e.g., trimethoprim-dapsone or atovaquone). Unless an adverse reaction to TMP-SMX is particularly severe (e.g., Stevens-Johnson syndrome or other life-threatening problem), TMP-SMX may later be considered for PCP prophylaxis, since prophylaxis requires a much lower dose (only 10–15% of treatment dose). Patients being treated for severe PCP with TMP-SMX who do not improve after one week may be switched to pentamidine or clindamycin plus primaquine, although there are no prospective data to confirm this approach. In general, patients receiving antiretroviral therapy when PCP develops should have their treatment continued, since intermittent antiretroviral therapy can lead to drug resistance. For newly diagnosed or antiretroviral-naïve HIV patients, antiretroviral therapy should be started as soon as feasible, preferably within 2 weeks. Steroids should be tapered, not discontinued abruptly. Adjunctive steroids increase the risk of thrush/herpes simplex infection, but probably not CMV, TB, or disseminated fungal infection. Patients should be tested for G6PD deficiency prior to use of primaquine and dapsone.

Prognosis: Usually responds to treatment. Adverse prognostic factors include ↑ A-a gradient, hypoxemia, ↑ LDH.

Progressive Multifocal Leukoencephalopathy (PML)

Preferred Therapy, Duration of Therapy, Chronic Maintenance	Alternate Therapy	Other Options/Issues
Initiate antiretroviral therapy in ART-naïve patients Optimize ART in patients who develop PML in phase of HIV viremia on antiretroviral therapy		Some patients might experience a remission after initiation of ART. Although their neurological deficits frequently persist, disease progression remits. Corticosteroids may be used in patients with progressive clinical deficits and neuroimaging features suggesting inflammatory disease (e.g., edema, swelling, and contrast enhancement) as a result of initiating ART.

Clinical Presentation: Hemiparesis, ataxia, aphasia, other focal neurologic defects, which may progress over weeks to months. Usually alert without headache or seizures on presentation.

Diagnostic Considerations: Demyelinating disease caused by reactivation of the latent papovavirus JC virus. Diagnosis by clinical presentation and MRI showing patchy demyelination of white matter, usually without enhancement. Any region of the CNS may be involved, most commonly the occipital lobes (with hemianopia), frontal and parietal lobes (hemiparesis and hemisensory deficits), and cerebellar peduncles and deep white matter (dysmetria and ataxia). JC virus PCR of CSF is useful for non-invasive diagnosis. In confusing or atypical presentation, biopsy may be needed to distinguish PML from other opportunistic infections, CNS lymphoma, or HIV encephalitis/encephalopathy.

Pitfalls: Primary HIV-related encephalopathy may have a similar appearance on MRI.

Therapeutic Considerations: Most effective therapy is antiretroviral therapy with immune reconstitution. Treatment should be started immediately if the patient is not on therapy. Some patients experience worsening neurologic symptoms once ART is initiated due to immune reconstitution induced inflammation. ART should be continued, with consideration of adjunctive steroids especially if neuroimaging shows evidence of inflammation (enhancement or edema). Randomized controlled trials have evaluated cidofovir and vidarabine—neither is effective nor recommended.

Prognosis: Rapid progression of neurologic deficits over weeks to months is common. Best chance for survival is immune reconstitution in response to antiretroviral therapy, although some patients will have progressive disease despite immune recovery. (J Infect Dis 2009;199:77)

Salmonellosis

Preferred Therapy, Duration of Therapy, Chronic Maintenance	Alternate Therapy	Other Options/Issues
Most specialists recommend treatment for all HIV-infected patients with salmonellosis due to the high risk of bacteremia in these patients		The role of long-term secondary prophylaxis for patients with recurrent bacteremia is not well established. Must weigh the benefit against the risks of long-term antibiotic exposure
Preferred therapy for _Salmonella gastroenteritis with or without symptomatic bacteremia_ Ciprofloxacin 500–750 mg PO BID (or 400 mg IV BID)	Alternative therapy for _Salmonella_ gastroenteritis with or without symptomatic bacteremia Levofloxacin 750 mg or moxifloxacin TMP-SMX PO or IV—if susceptible Third generation cephalosporin such as ceftriaxone (IV) or cefotaxime (IV)—if susceptible	
Duration for mild gastroenteritis with or without bacteremia If CD4+ count ≥ 200/μL: 7–14 days If CD4+ count < 200/μL: 2–6 weeks If recurrent symptomatic septicemia– may need 6 months or more		

Clinical Presentation: Patients with HIV are at markedly increased risk of developing salmonellosis. Three different presentations may be seen: (1) self-limited gastroenteritis, as typically seen in immunocompetent hosts; (2) a more severe and prolonged diarrheal disease, associated with fever, bloody diarrhea, and weight loss; or (3) *Salmonella* septicemia, which may present with or without gastrointestinal symptoms.

Diagnostic Considerations: The diagnosis is established through cultures of stool and blood. Given the high rate of bacteremia associated with *Salmonella* gastroenteritis—especially in advanced HIV disease—blood cultures should be obtained in any HIV patient presenting with diarrhea and fever.

Pitfalls: A distinctive feature of *Salmonella* bacteremia in patients with AIDS is its propensity for relapse (rate > 20%).

Therapeutic Considerations: The mainstay of treatment is a fluoroquinolone; greatest experience is with ciprofloxacin, but newer quinolones (moxifloxacin, levofloxacin) may also be effective. For uncomplicated salmonellosis in an HIV patient with CD4 > 200/mm^3, 1–2 weeks of treatment is reasonable to reduce the risk of extraintestinal spread. For patients with advanced HIV disease (CD4 < 200/mm^3) or who have *Salmonella* bacteremia, at least 2–6 weeks of treatment is required. Chronic suppressive therapy, given for several months or until antiretroviral therapy-induced immune reconstitution ensues, is indicated for patients who relapse after cessation of therapy. Consider using ZDV as part of the antiretroviral regimen (ZDV is active against salmonella).

Prognosis: Usually responds well to treatment. Relapse rate in AIDS patients with bacteremia is > 20%.

Shigellosis

Preferred Therapy, Duration of Therapy, Chronic Maintenance	Alternate Therapy	Other Options/Issues
Preferred therapy for Shigella infection Fluoroquinolone IV or PO Duration of therapy: *for gastroenteritis:* 3–7 days *for bacteremia:* 14 days	Alternative therapy depending on antibiotic susceptibility *For gastroenteritis* TMP-SMX DS 1 tab PO BID for 3–7 days; **or** Azithromycin 500 mg PO on day 1, then 250 mg PO daily for 4 days	Therapy is indicated both to shorten the duration of illness and to prevent spread of infection Shigella infections acquired outside of United States have high rates of TMP-SMX resistance

Clinical Presentation: Acute onset of bloody diarrhea/mucus.

Diagnostic Considerations: Diagnosis by demonstrating organism in stool specimens. Shigella ulcers in colon are linear, serpiginous, and rarely lead to perforation. More common in gay men.

Therapeutic Considerations: Shigella dysentery is more acute/fulminating than amebic dysentery. Shigella has no carrier state, unlike entamoeba. Shigella infections acquired outside of United States have high rates of TMP-SMX resistance. Therapy is indicated to shorten the duration of illness and to prevent spread of infection.

Prognosis: Good if treated early. Severity of illness related to shigella species: *S. dysenteriae* (most severe) > *S. flexneri* > *S. boydii/S. sonnei* (mildest).

Toxoplasma gondii Encephalitis

Preferred Therapy, Duration of Therapy, Chronic Maintenance	Alternate Therapy	Other Options/Issues
<u>Preferred therapy</u> Pyrimethamine 200 mg PO × 1, then 50 mg (< 60 kg) to 75 mg (≥ 60 kg) PO daily plus sulfadiazine 1,000 mg (< 60 kg) to 1,500 mg (≥ 60 kg) PO q6h plus leucovorin 10–25 mg PO daily (can increase 50 mg) <u>Duration for acute therapy</u> At least 6 weeks; longer duration if clinical or radiologic disease is extensive or response is incomplete at 6 weeks	<u>Alternative therapy regimens</u> Pyrimethamine (leucovorin)* plus clindamycin 600 mg IV or PO q6h; **or** TMP-SMX (5 mg/kg TMP and 25 mg/kg SMX) IV or PO BID; **or** Atovaquone 1,500 mg PO BID with food (or nutritional supplement) plus pyrimethamine (leucovorin)*; **or** Atovaquone 1,500 mg PO BID with food (or nutritional supplement) plus sulfadiazine 1,000–1,500 mg PO q6h; **or** Atovaquone 1,500 mg PO BID with food; **or** Pyrimethamine (leucovorin)* plus azithromycin 900–1200 mg PO daily	Adjunctive corticosteroids (e.g., dexamethasone) should be administered when clinically indicated only for treatment of mass effect attributed to focal lesions or associated edema; discontinue as soon as clinically feasible Anticonvulsants should be administered to patients with a history of seizures and continued through the acute treatment; but should not be used prophylactically
<u>Preferred chronic maintenance therapy</u> Pyrimethamine 25–50 mg PO daily plus sulfadiazine 2,000–4,000 mg PO daily (in two to four divided doses) plus leucovorin 10–25 mg PO daily	<u>Alternative chronic maintenance therapy/secondary prophylaxis</u> Clindamycin 600 mg PO every 8 hours plus pyrimethamine 25–50 mg PO daily plus leucovorin 10–25 PO daily [should add additional agent to prevent PCP]; **or** Atovaquone 750 mg PO every 6–12 hours +/- [(pyrimethamine 25 mg PO daily plus leucovorin 10 mg PO daily) or sulfadiazine 2,000–4,000 mg PO] daily	

* Pyrimethemine and leucovorin doses—same as in "Preferred therapy" for toxoplasmosis

Clinical Presentation: Wide spectrum of neurologic symptoms, including sensorimotor deficits, seizures, confusion, ataxia. Fever/headache are common.

Diagnostic Considerations: Diagnosis by characteristic radiographic appearance and response to empiric therapy in a for *T. gondii* seropositive patient.

Pitfalls: Use leucovorin (folinic acid) 10 mg (PO) daily with pyrimethamine-containing regimens, not folate/folic acid. Radiographic improvement may lag behind clinical response.

Therapeutic Considerations: Alternate agents include atovaquone, azithromycin, clarithromycin, minocycline (all with pyrimethamine if possible). Decadron 4 mg (PO or IV) q6h is useful for edema/mass effect. Intravenous TMP-SMX useful for critically ill or neurologically compromised patients who cannot take oral therapy. Chronic suppressive therapy can be discontinued if patients are free from signs and symptoms of disease and have a CD4 cell count > 200/mm^3 for > 6 months due to ART.

Prognosis: Usually responds to treatment if able to tolerate drugs. Clinical response is evident by 1 week in 70%, by 2 weeks in 90%. Radiographic improvement is usually apparent by 2 weeks. Neurologic recovery is variable.

Treponema pallidum (Syphilis)

Preferred Therapy, Duration of Therapy, Chronic Maintenance	Alternate Therapy	Other Options/Issues
Preferred therapy early stage (primary, secondary, and early latent syphilis) Benzathine penicillin G 2.4 million units IM for 1 dose	Alternative therapy early stage (primary, secondary, and early latent syphilis) *For penicillin-allergic patients:* Doxycycline 100 mg PO BID for 14 days; **or** Ceftriaxone 1 g IM or IV daily for 8–10 days; **or** Azithromycin 2 g PO for 1 dose	The efficacy of non-penicillin alternatives has not been evaluated in HIV-infected patients and should be undertaken only with close clinical and serologic monitoring Combination of procaine penicillin and probenecid is not recommended for patients with history of sulfa allergy
Preferred therapy late-latent disease (> 1 year or of unknown duration, CSF examination ruled out neurosyphilis) Benzathine penicillin G 2.4 million units IM weekly for 3 doses	Alternative therapy late-latent disease (without CNS involvement) *For penicillin-allergic patients:* Doxycycline 100 mg PO BID for 28 days	The Jarisch-Herxheimer reaction is an acute febrile reaction accompanied by headache and myalgias that might occur within the first 24 hours after therapy for syphilis
Preferred therapy late-stage (tertiary–cardiovascular or gummatous disease)	Alternative therapy neurosyphilis	

Treponema pallidum (Syphilis) (cont'd)

Preferred Therapy, Duration of Therapy, Chronic Maintenance	Alternate Therapy	Other Options/Issues
Rule out neurosyphilis before therapy with 3 doses of benzathine penicillin and obtain infectious diseases consultation to guide management Preferred therapy neurosyphilis (including otic and ocular disease) Aqueous crystalline penicillin G, 18–24 million units per day, administered as 3–4 million units IV q4h or by continuous IV infusion for 10–14 days +/- benzathine penicillin G 2.4 million units IM weekly for 3 doses after completion of IV therapy	Procaine penicillin 2.4 million units IM daily plus probenecid 500 mg PO QID for 10–14 days +/- benzathine penicillin G 2.4 million units IM weekly for 3 doses after completion of above; **or** *For penicillin-allergic patients:* Desensitization to penicillin is the preferred approach; if not feasible, Ceftriaxone 2 grams IM or IV daily for 10–14 days	

Epidemiology: Syphilis is highly prevalent among some groups with high rates of HIV, notably gay men. Studies have shown that syphilis facilitates HIV transmission, and case reports/series suggest that syphilis in HIV-infected patients is associated with multiple and slower resolving primary chancres, higher titer RPR, slower decline of RPR titers, higher rate of serologic failure, increased frequency of CSF abnormalities and CSF-VDRL positivity, higher incidence of ocular disease, and higher rates of relapse after treatment (Sex Transm Dis 2001;28:158–65; N Engl J Med 1997 Jul;337:307–14; Ann Intern Med 1990;113:872).

Clinical Presentation: The causative organism of syphilis is *Treponema pallidum*, which cannot be cultured in routine clinical laboratories. As a result, the diagnosis of syphilis depends on recognizing the clinical stages and use of serologic tests:

- Primary syphilis: Following an incubation period of 2–6 weeks, primary syphilis presents as a papule that later ulcerates to form a syphilitic chancre. These are generally painless and may occur on any mucosal surface. Non-tender regional adenopathy may also be present. Serologic tests for syphilis (RPR or VDRL) can be negative early in primary syphilis, so empiric treatment is indicated in suspected cases, with follow-up testing necessary to confirm the disease.
- Secondary syphilis: Approximately 60–90% of patients with untreated primary syphilis will develop secondary syphilis as a manifestation of *T. pallidum* dissemination. The time course is typically within 6 months of infection acquisition, and the clinical manifestations are highly variable. The most common manifestation of secondary syphilis is a non-pruritic macular-papular rash over the entire body, including the palms and soles. Other symptoms

and laboratory abnormalities can include condyloma lata (white genital lesions similar in appearance to condyloma acuminata), mucous patches (shallow ulcerations on the oral or genital mucosa), fever, malaise, lymphadenopathy, anorexia, hepatitis, and diminished vision secondary to uveitis.

- Latent syphilis: Defined by a reactive serologic test in the absence of active symptoms, latent syphilis is divided into "early-latent" (< 1 year after exposure) and "late-latent" (> 1 year after exposure). Patients who are unable to give an accurate exposure date are classified as "latent syphilis of unknown duration" and treated as late-latent disease.

- Tertiary (late) syphilis: This develops in 25–40% of patients untreated for earlier disease, usually months to years later. Tertiary syphilis can cause CNS disease, cardiovascular disorders, and gummatous lesions involving the skin and bones. Cardiovascular and gummatous syphilis have become extremely rare, but CNS syphilis still occurs with some frequency and can present in various ways. *Acute syphilitic meningitis* and *meningovascular syphilis* occur relatively early after exposure (typically within the first 1–5 years), sometimes during dissemination of the organism with secondary syphilis. By contrast, *parenchymatous syphilis* usually occurs decades later, and includes general paresis, tabes dorsalis, and focal lesions due to CNS gummas.

Diagnostic Considerations: Diagnostic strategies for syphilis are the same as in HIV-negative patients, and rely mostly on serologic studies since the organism cannot be cultured. Darkfield microscopy on fluid obtained from chancres or condyloma lata may demonstrate the characteristic spiral-shaped organism; however, this technique is of limited utility since it cannot be used in the absence of obvious lesions, and most clinicians do not have access to a darkfield microscope. As a result, a positive serologic test for syphilis (RPR or VDRL) followed by a positive confirmatory test (MHA-TP, FTA-ABS, or TP-PA) is the most common way to diagnose syphilis in patients with (or without) HIV. Although case reports have cited unusually high titers, false negative results, and delayed onset of seropositivity in patients with HIV infection, no alternative testing strategy is routinely recommended. Neurosyphilis is diagnosed via clinical presentation and CSF examination. In symptomatic neurosyphilis, presenting complaints may include cognitive dysfunction, motor or sensory deficits, cranial nerve palsies, ophthalmic or auditory symptoms, and symptoms or signs of meningitis. Diagnostic criteria for neurosyphilis by CSF examination vary, but one commonly used definition is a CSF white blood cell count > 20 cells/mcL or a reactive CSF VDRL. (Although considered highly sensitive, the FTA-ABS test of the spinal fluid is not specific and can be used only to rule out disease.) The diagnosis of neurosyphilis is challenging since the CSF VDRL (the most specific test) is positive in only 30–70%, even in HIV-negative-patients. Furthermore, HIV itself may induce cellular responses independent of syphilis, and clinical manifestations are extremely varied. As a result, there is some debate about which patients with HIV and syphilis should undergo lumbar puncture (LP). One study of 326 HIV-infected patients with syphilis who underwent LP found that 65 (20%) met criteria for neurosyphilis by CSF exam; the risk was substantially higher if the CD4 cell count was ≤ 350 or the RPR was ≥ 1:32 (J Infect Dis 2004;189:369–76). Based on this study, the diagnostic approach shown in Table 5.5 is reasonable.

Therapeutic Considerations: The treatment of syphilis is generally the same as for HIV-negative patients, with penicillin as the mainstay of therapy. The criteria for treatment response are the same in HIV-infected and HIV-negative individuals. Specifically, the RPR or VDRL titer should decline ≥ 4-fold by one year after treatment for early syphilis and by 2–3 years after treatment for latent syphilis. (For HIV patients with early syphilis, there is an increased rate of treatment failure when using serologic criteria; therefore, our practice is to include an RPR as part of monitoring labs performed every 3–4 months unless the titer has reverted to negative.) Failure to achieve ≥ 4-fold decline in titer should prompt investigation of reinfection or a CSF examination to exclude neurosyphilis. For patients with neurosyphilis, follow-up CSF examinations are performed every 6 months until CSF pleocytosis has normalized; if still abnormal 2 years after treatment, consider retreatment with intravenous penicillin. In general, non-penicillin therapies for syphilis have had limited evaluation in HIV patients; hence these cases warrant close clinical and laboratory follow-up. Procaine penicillin/probenecid options may not be used in patients with sulfa allergy.

Table 5.5. Need for Lumbar Puncture (LP) in HIV-Infected Patients with Syphilis

Stage of Syphilis	Recommendation
Primary, secondary, or early latent	No LP; if RPR > 1:32 or CD4 < 350, be especially vigilant for lack of response
Late-latent or syphilis of unknown duration	Perform LP (some clinicians only LP for RPR > 1:32 or CD4 < 350)
Positive RPR and confirmatory test with neurologic, ophthalmic, or auditory symptoms/signs	Perform LP

Varicella-Zoster Virus (VZV) Disease

Preferred Therapy, Duration of Therapy, Chronic Maintenance	Alternate Therapy	Other Options/Issues
Varicella (chickenpox) *Uncomplicated cases* Acyclovir (20 mg/kg body weight up to a maximum of 800 mg PO 5x daily), valacyclovir 1,000 mg PO TID, or famciclovir 500 mg PO TID × 5–7 days *Severe or complicated cases* Acyclovir 10–15 mg/kg IV q8h × 7–10 days May switch to oral acyclovir, famciclovir, or valacyclovir after defervescence if no evidence of visceral involvement is evident Herpes zoster (shingles) *Acute localized dermatomal*	Infection caused by acyclovir-resistant VZV Foscarnet 90 mg/kg IV q12h	Involvement of an experienced ophthalmologist with management of VZV retinitis is strongly recommended Corticosteroid therapy for herpes zoster is not recommended

Varicella-Zoster Virus (VZV) Disease (cont'd)

Preferred Therapy, Duration of Therapy, Chronic Maintenance	Alternate Therapy	Other Options/Issues
Valacyclovir 1g TID or famciclovir 500 mg TID, or acyclovir 800 mg PO 5x daily × 7–10 days, longer duration should be considered if lesions are slow to resolve *Extensive cutaneous lesion or visceral involvement* Acyclovir 10–15 mg/kg IV q8h until clinical improvement is evident Switch to oral therapy (valacyclovir 1,000 mg TID or famciclovir 500 mg TID, or acyclovir 800 mg PO 5x daily) after clinical improvement is evident, to complete a 10–14 day course Progressive outer retinal necrosis (PORN) Ganciclovir 5 mg/kg IV q12h, plus foscarnet 90 mg/kg IV q12h, plus ganciclovir 2 mg/0.05mL intravitreal twice weekly, and/or foscarnet 1.2 mg/0.05mL intravitreal twice weekly Optimization of ART Acute retinal necrosis (ARN) Acyclovir 10 mg/kg IV q8h × 10–14 days, followed by valacyclovir 1,000 mg PO TID × 6 weeks		

Clinical Presentation: Primary varicella (chickenpox) presents as widely disseminated clear vesicles on an erythematous base that heal with crusting and sometimes scarring. Zoster usually presents as painful tense vesicles on an erythematous base in a dermatomal distribution. In patients with HIV, primary varicella is more severe/prolonged, and zoster is more likely to involve multiple dermatomes/disseminate. VZV can rarely cause acute retinal necrosis, which requires close consultation with ophthalmology.

Diagnostic Considerations: Diagnosis is usually clinical. In atypical cases, immunofluorescence can be used to distinguish herpes zoster from herpes simplex.

Pitfalls: Extend treatment beyond 7–10 days if new vesicles are still forming after initial treatment period. Corticosteroids for dermatomal zoster are not recommended in HIV-positive patients.

Therapeutic Considerations: IV therapy is generally indicated for severe disease/cranial nerve zoster.

Prognosis: Usually responds slowly to treatment.

Chapter 6

Complications of HIV Infection*

*   Also see Chapter 5 for Opportunistic Infections and Chapters 3 and 9 for Drug-Induced
    Adverse Effects

HEMATOLOGIC COMPLICATIONS

A. **Thrombocytopenia.** May be the first and only sign of HIV infection. Treatment is only required for platelet count < 20,000/mm^3, active bleeding, or planned procedures. Causes include medications, alcohol, idiopathic thrombocytopenic purpura (ITP), thrombotic thrombocytopenic purpura (TTP), and advanced HIV disease ± marrow infiltration with secondary opportunistic infections (usually accompanied by pancytopenia).

1. **Idiopathic Thrombocytopenic Purpura (ITP).** Can occur at any stage of HIV disease and sometimes emerges as antiretroviral therapy induces an immune response. Consultation with a hematologist is advised for platelet count < 20,000 or if rapid recovery of platelet count is required.

   a. **Preferred therapy.** Combination antiretroviral therapy. Although ZDV is the best studied agent for ITP treatment, alternative combination regimens may be effective as well.

   b. **If rapid control of platelet count is needed.** IVIG 1–2 gm/kg total dose, over 2–5 days. Duration of response is typically 3–4 weeks. <u>Alternative</u>: Anti-RH D globulin (WinRho) 50–75 mcg/kg IV (effective only in RH-positive, non-splenectomized patients). Causes mild hemolysis. Duration of response is similar to IVIG, and may work in some patients who do not respond to IVIG.

   c. **Miscellaneous alternative therapies.** Prednisone 1 mg/kg daily, with taper as tolerated; danazol 400–800 mg (PO) QD; dapsone 100 mg (PO) QD (if not G6PD-deficient); alpha-interferon 3 million units 3×/week; splenectomy. Some anecdotal evidence for use of vincristine, splenic irradiation, anti-cd20 antibody (Rituximab).

2. **Thrombotic Thrombocytopenic Purpura (TTP).** Manifests as microangiopathic hemolytic anemia associated with renal insufficiency and neurologic symptoms. TTP is a **medical emergency**—if it is suspected based on clinical grounds and examination of blood smear, consult hematologist immediately. Standard treatment is prednisone 60–100 mg (PO) QD (or IV equivalent) plus plasmapheresis.

B. **Anemia.** Anemia is associated with a lower quality of life; several studies also suggest it is independently associated with reduced survival (Clin Infect Dis 1999;29:44–9).

1. **Etiology**

   a. **Decreased RBC production (low reticulocyte count)**

   - **Direct effect of HIV** (usually CD4 < 100/mm^3); responds well to initiation of antiretroviral therapy.
   - **Infiltration of bone marrow:** in particular MAC—suspect in a patient with advanced AIDS who has fever, weight loss, and anemia out of proportion to drop in other cell lines; can also be due to lymphoma.

- **Iron deficiency (women)**
- **B12 or folate deficiency:** a high MCV is usually related to a side effect of NRTIs (especially ZDV), but need to rule out B12 and folate deficiency, which appears to be more common among patients with HIV.
- **Certain infections:** Parvovirus B19: infects and inhibits early RBC precursors, with characteristic bone marrow showing giant pronormoblasts; diagnosed by viral DNA by PCR of blood (not by serology); treated with IVIG. MAC: diagnosed by isolator blood cultures or bone marrow biopsy; treated as described on p. 123.
- **Drugs:** ZDV (most common in advanced HIV disease, but can occur at any stage; other antiretroviral agents rarely cause anemia); ganciclovir and valganciclovir (lower WBC also); TMP-SMX; amphotericin; interferon.

    b. **Increased RBC destruction (high reticulocyte count)**

- **Drug-induced:** Dapsone and primaquine if patient is G6PD deficient; ribavirin as part of HCV therapy (causes dose-related hemolytic anemia), which may further compromise fatigue associated with HCV therapy.
- **TTP** (described on p. 139)

2. **Evaluation.** As a minimum work-up, evaluate clinical status, stage of HIV disease, stool for occult blood, CBC/differential, RBC indices, reticulocyte count, iron, TIBC, creatinine, LFTs, B12, folate. Bone marrow aspiration is indicated when above work-up and history fail to identify a cause.

3. **Treatment.** If no reversible cause of anemia is identified, or if the cause cannot be removed (for example, ribavirin-associated anemia during HCV treatment), consider erythropoietin (EPO) for patients with Hgb < 10 gm/dL or HCT < 30. Start with 40,000 units (SQ) once weekly with iron supplementation; if at 4 weeks, Hgb has increased by > 1 gm/dL, continue same dose until Hgb reaches 11–12 gm/dL. Dose can then be reduced to 10,000 units (SQ) once weekly to maintain Hgb at this level. Higher levels have been associated with increased risk of thromboembolic events in non-HIV populations. For non-responders, 60,000 units (SQ) once weekly may be effective. Supplemental iron should also be given.

C. **Neutropenia.** As with anemia, neutropenia is much more common in advanced HIV disease. The risk of infection is increased with lower absolute neutrophil counts (ANC), especially when < 500/mm^3.

1. **Etiology**

    a. **Direct effect of HIV.** Responds well to initiation of antiretroviral therapy.

    b. **Drugs.** ZDV, ganciclovir and valganciclovir (ZDV and ganciclovir given together can cause particularly severe neutropenia), pyrimethamine, TMP-SMX at PCP treatment doses, interferon (pegylated interferon more likely to cause neutropenia than standard interferon), flucytosine. Uncommon causes include other NRTIs, ribavirin, amphotericin, TMP-SMX at dose used for PCP prophylaxis, pentamidine, rifabutin. TMP-SMX given at doses used for PCP prophylaxis rarely is the sole cause of neutropenia; if neutropenia does not improve after a trial of an alternative prophylactic regimen, TMP-SMX can be restarted.

c. **Infections.** MAC, CMV, disseminated fungal diseases (e.g., histoplasmosis).

2. **Treatment.** Only indicated if ANC is consistently < 750/mm^3 (some experts cite 500/mm^3). After underlying causes are corrected, consider G-CSF (Neupogen) 150–300 mcg (SQ) every 1–7 days. Start with 3x/week dosing, then titrate dose to maintain ANC > 1000/mm^3.

D. Eosinophilia

1. **Etiology**

   a. **Direct effect of HIV.** Sometimes seen with no apparent cause, especially in advanced HIV disease.

   b. **Drug allergy.** Most commonly to TMP-SMX and other sulfonamides.

   c. **Parasitic infection (rare).** Most HIV-related parasitic infections (e.g., toxoplasmosis, cryptosporidiosis) do not cause eosinophilia. Rare exceptions include *Isospora belli* and strongyloidiasis (if patient from endemic area).

2. **Treatment.** Consider withdrawal of offending agent if associated with other allergic phenomena. Check stool for ova and parasites, strongyloides serology.

ONCOLOGIC COMPLICATIONS

Malignancies definitely associated with HIV infection include Kaposi's sarcoma, non-Hodgkin's lymphoma, Hodgkin's disease, lung cancer, squamous cell carcinomas (cervical, anal, head and neck), and soft tissue sarcoma (in children). Possible associated malignancies include seminoma, lung cancer, and multiple myeloma. Prolonged survival due to ART has led to a greater appreciation of the increased incidence of non-AIDS malignancies in HIV patients (Ann Intern Med 2008 May 20;148:728);risk appears strongly related to CD4 cell count (AIDS 2008 Oct 18;22:2143).

A. Kaposi's Sarcoma. Infection with HHV-8 is a critical viral cofactor; interaction between host immunosuppression, genetic factors, and this virus determine a patient's risk. In North America, Australia, and Western Europe, Kaposi's sarcoma occurs most commonly in gay/bisexual men. The incidence has diminished markedly since the introduction of potent antiretroviral therapy. In developing countries (especially in certain parts of Africa), Kaposi's sarcoma is more evenly distributed among men and women.

1. **Presentation.** Usually presents as violaceous nodules and plaques on the skin; oral cavity and other mucosal surfaces may be involved. With more advanced immunosuppression, visceral involvement (lungs, gastrointestinal tract) can be life-threatening. Invasion of local lymphatics can lead to chronic edema of the limbs, face, and genitals, with increased risk of bacterial superinfection.

   2. **Treatment.** Initiation of antiretroviral therapy is often sufficient to cause regression of disease. For disease that progresses despite antivirals, options include local measures (intralesional chemotherapy, radiation therapy) and systemic chemotherapy (liposomal anthracyclines are especially effective). Occasionally clinical disease may temporarily worsen soon after starting ART as a manifestation of the immune reconstitution inflammatory syndrome (IRIS); in these cases, ART should be continued and systemic chemotherapy considered or intensified.

B. **Non-Hodgkin's Lymphoma (NHL).** In patients with HIV infection, NHL is most commonly a manifestation of advanced immunosuppression (CD4 < 100/mm³).

   1. **Presentation.** Clinical presentation reflects extranodal involvement of the disease: typically, gastrointestinal tract (45%), bone marrow (20%), and CNS (20–30%). Often multiple sites are involved simultaneously. Of note, the patient with AIDS who has diffuse adenopathy and fever will more likely have a systemic infection (most commonly *M. avium* complex, histoplasmosis, cryptococcus) rather than lymphoma. Although the incidence of NHL has declined since the introduction of potent antiretroviral therapy, it has done so to a lesser degree than other opportunistic infections. As a result, NHL in some centers is responsible for a higher proportion of AIDS-related complications compared with the pre-antiretroviral era.

   2. **Treatment.** Generally involves full-dose chemotherapy (e.g., CHOP), with use of recombinant growth factors (G-CSF, erythropoietin) as needed to support cell lines. Initiation of antiretroviral therapy concurrently with chemotherapy may improve outcome by reducing infectious complications and improving recovery time of bone marrow function. It is important to avoid the use of antiviral agents that may have overlapping toxicities with the prescribed chemotherapy (e.g., avoid d4T or ddI when patients are receiving systemic vincristine therapy, as this increases the risk of peripheral neuropathy; avoid ZDV since this may further suppress the bone marrow).

C. **Primary CNS Lymphoma.** Usually a manifestation of advanced HIV disease, with the vast majority of patients having a CD4 cell count < 50/mm³.

   1. **Presentation.** The typical presentation is one of focal neurologic deficits or seizures, reflecting focal lesion(s) in the brain. MRI findings typically show lesions with irregular enhancement, sometimes involving the corpus callosum and crossing the midline; mass effect is generally evident. Appearance of primary CNS lymphoma is similar to that of CNS toxoplasmosis; in the latter, lesions are often greater in number, but radiographic abnormalities overlap significantly.

   2. **Diagnosis.** If a patient with advanced AIDS presents with focal enhancing lesion(s) on MRI or CT scan and is either toxoplasmosis seronegative or taking TMP-SMX for toxoplasmosis prophylaxis, then primary CNS lymphoma is the most likely diagnosis. While noninvasive testing such as thallium SPECT scan, PET scan, and CSF studies for cytology and Epstein-Barr virus DNA (by PCR) can sometimes be helpful, the definitive

diagnosis is generally made through stereotactic brain biopsy. Of note, Epstein-Barr virus PCR of the CSF in HIV patients without characteristic CNS mass lesions has a very low specificity for CNS lymphoma; the test should not be routinely ordered (Clin Infect Dis 2004 Jun 1;38[11]:1629–32).

3. **Treatment.** The prognosis of primary CNS lymphoma remains quite poor, especially for patients who fail antiretroviral therapy. Treatment with steroids and radiation therapy is palliative. Rare patients have experienced sustained remissions after initiating antiretroviral therapy and achieving a significant improvement in immune function.

D. Cervical Cancer. Compared to HIV-negative women, the incidence of cervical cancer in HIV-infected women is higher and the disease may be more aggressive. Cervical cancer is strongly associated with HPV infection and progressive immunosuppression. A diagnosis of cervical cancer along with a positive HIV serology is considered AIDS defining. Recommendations for screening include a Pap smear twice the first year after HIV diagnosis, and yearly thereafter if normal. This strategy is associated with a low risk of invasive cervical cancer, comparable to HIV-negative women.

E. Anal Cancer. The incidence of anal cancer in gay men is approximately 80 times that of the general population. As with cervical cancer, anal cancer is strongly associated with HPV infection. Although screening for anal cancer using anal Pap smears could identify precancerous lesions much as with cervical cancer, guidelines for screening have not been incorporated into formal recommendations. Pending these recommendations, a reasonable strategy is as follows:

1. At a minimum, perform annual periodic visual inspection and a digital rectal exam.

2. Perform anal Pap smear for any anorectal complaints; some recommend annual testing on all HIV-positive gay men.

3. For atypical cells of uncertain significance, repeat anal Pap smear in 6–12 months.

4. For squamous intraepithelial lesion (SIL), refer to a colorectal surgeon for anoscopy and/or anal colposcopy with biopsy.

ENDOCRINE COMPLICATIONS

A. Disorders of Adrenal Function. Although adrenal gland involvement has been documented in up to two-thirds of patients with AIDS on postmortem examination, clinically relevant adrenal insufficiency is rare (~ 3% of patients with AIDS) and is generally a manifestation of late-stage AIDS.

1. **Etiology.** Potential causes of primary adrenal dysfunction include destruction of the adrenal gland from opportunistic infections (especially CMV), neoplasms (Kaposi's sarcoma, lymphoma), hemorrhage, and infarction. More commonly, adrenal

insufficiency results from the adverse effect of medications, including ketoconazole (decreased steroidogenesis), rifampin/rifabutin (enhanced cortisol metabolism), and corticosteroids/megestrol acetate (suppressed pituitary secretion of corticotropin due to intrinsic glucocorticoid activity; latter may actually induce Cushing's syndrome with prolonged use). An cause of cortisol excess is the use of inhaled (especially fluticasone) or intramuscular steroids with ritonavir. Ritonavir blocks the metabolism of many corticosteroids, leading to increased exposure and iatrogenic Cushing's syndrome. Conversely, stopping the inhaled steroid can cause adrenal insufficiency (J Clin Endocrinol Metab 2005;90:4394–8).

2. **Diagnosis.** Adrenal insufficiency should be suspected in a patient with advanced HIV disease or recent therapy with steroid-interfering medications who presents with hypotension, profound weakness, or electrolyte abnormalities (hyponatremia, hyperkalemia). Evaluation consists of measurement of a.m. cortisol; if normal and the diagnosis is still suspected, perform a corticotropin stimulation test. If the diagnosis is still suspected despite a normal corticotropin stimulation test, referral to an endocrinologist is warranted since some patients with AIDS have peripheral resistance to glucocorticoid action.

3. **Treatment.** Patients with basal low cortisol levels, even if asymptomatic, require lifelong replacement therapy (prednisone 5 mg [PO] at bedtime). For corticotropin hyporesponsiveness, steroid supplementation for stressing conditions (e.g., surgery, intercurrent illness) is indicated. For life-threatening situations, immediate treatment with dexamethasone 4 mg (IV) is indicated; this will not impair the diagnostic utility of the corticotropin stimulation test.

B. **Hypogonadism.** Men with HIV infection are more likely to be hypogonadal than HIV-negative controls. The frequency of this abnormality increases with progressive immunodeficiency and may reach 50% in patients with AIDS. In general, there is no detectable underlying etiology. HIV-related hypogonadism is associated with weakness, weight loss, decreased libido, and impaired quality of life. Replacement therapy can improve many of these symptoms, especially when combined with a resistance exercise program. While low testosterone levels have also been observed in HIV-infected women, replacement therapy is experimental. Treatment for men consists of testosterone gel (Androgel) 5 mg QD, testosterone transdermal patch, or injectable testosterone cypionate/enanthate 200 mg every other week. Potential side effects include acne, gynecomastia, and testicular atrophy. Monitor prostate specific antigen annually for patients on replacement therapy.

C. **Thyroid Disease.** The thyroid gland is rarely involved in disseminated opportunistic infections (e.g., extrapulmonary pneumocystis). Chronically ill patients with HIV may have low T3, but TSH is generally normal. Immune response to antiretroviral therapy may unmask subclinical Grave's disease, leading to clinical hyperthyroidism. Treatment of Grave's disease consists of radioactive thyroid ablation or an anti-thyroid medication (e.g., methimazole) as directed by an endocrinologist. Beta-blockers can be used to ameliorate the symptoms of hyperthyroidism.

D. Pancreatitis. Clinical presentation is similar to HIV-negative patients, with nausea, vomiting, abdominal pain.

  1. Etiology

   a. Medications: <u>Common</u>: ddI (increased risk with higher doses, hydroxyurea, alcohol use), d4T (risk especially high when d4T and ddI are prescribed together), pentamidine, corticosteroids. <u>Less common</u>: other NRTIs, TMP-SMX, protease inhibitors (when accompanied by very high triglyceride levels), INH, erythromycin.

   b. Opportunistic infections. Most commonly identified opportunistic infection to cause pancreatitis is CMV. Can rarely be caused by TB, MAC, intestinal protozoa (cryptosporidia, microsporidia), widely disseminated toxoplasmosis.

   c. Non-HIV–related. Alcohol, obesity, gallstones.

  2. Treatment. Discontinue potentially offending drug; treat identified cause.

E. Hyperglycemia. Patients with HIV appear to be at higher risk of developing insulin resistance and diabetes mellitus than HIV-negative controls. Potential contributing factors include lipodystrophy syndrome (especially subcutaneous fat loss) and medications (most notably indinavir and the NRTI stavudine).

  1. Diagnosis. For patients on antiretroviral therapy, monitor serum glucose every 3–6 months as part of safety labs. If elevated or abnormal, consider a fasting glucose, insulin level, and hemoglobin A1C. A fasting blood glucose > 126 mg/dL or a glucose level > 200 mg/dL two hours after administration of 75 gm of glucose is diagnostic of diabetes mellitus.

  2. Treatment. If the patient is on a protease inhibitor and has an undetectable HIV RNA and no history of extensive NRTI resistance, consider substituting an NNRTI (e.g., efavirenz, nevirapine) for the protease inhibitor. Alternatively, there is evidence that atazanavir may be least likely to lead to insulin resistance, and hence can be substituted for other protease inhibitors. If the patient is not on a protease inhibitor and fasting hyperglycemia persists, follow established guidelines for treatment of diabetes mellitus in the general population, including weight loss, dietary modification, and exercise. When medical therapy is required, consider the use of insulin-sensitizing agents such as metformin 500 mg (PO) q12h or pioglitazone 15–30 mg (PO) QD. In small studies, metformin therapy in patients with HIV has led to improvements in insulin sensitivity, reduction in waist circumference, and decreased blood pressure; potential adverse effects include diarrhea, progression of lipoatrophy, and (rarely) lactic acidosis. Pioglitazone in one study improved insulin sensitivity and subcutaneous fat stores, and appears to be safer in HIV patients than rosiglitazone, which has been associated with hyperlipidemia.

F. Hypoglycemia. Pentamidine induces hypoglycemia by lysing pancreatic islet cells. Monitor fingerstick glucose levels daily while patients receive this therapy. Prolonged, repeated use of pentamidine may result in diabetes mellitus from irreversible damage to islet cells, leading to insulin deficiency.

G. Ovarian Complications. Amenorrhea is common in women with advanced AIDS who have significant weight loss. Menses may resume with weight gain and improvement in clinical status accompanying antiretroviral therapy.

H. Bone Disease

1. **Osteonecrosis.** This complication has been reported in association with HIV infection since the late 1980s, but it appears to be more common since the introduction of effective antiretroviral therapy (J AIDS 2006;42:286–92). It is not clear if the increased incidence is due simply to prolonged survival, or to a direct toxic effect of antiretroviral medications. The most commonly involved sites are the femoral heads, followed by the humeral heads, femoral condyles, proximal tibia, and small bones of the hands and wrists. Most patients will have traditional underlying risk factors, such as a history of corticosteroid use, hyperlipidemia, alcohol abuse, or a hypercoagulable state. The relationship to any specific form of antiretroviral therapy has not been conclusively demonstrated (HIV Med 2004 Nov;5[6]:421–6).

   a. **Diagnosis.** Consider osteonecrosis in a patient with refractory hip pain, especially if there are underlying risk factors (see above). If plain film imaging is negative, proceed to MRI, which is more sensitive. Bilateral imaging is indicated since the disease is often bilateral.

   b. **Treatment.** Conservative management with physical therapy is recommended initially. If pain persists, refer to an orthopedic surgeon for consideration of hip stabilization/hip replacement.

2. **Osteoporosis.** Osteopenia and osteoporosis have been reported in 22–50% and 3–21% of patients receiving chronic antiretroviral therapy, respectively. Low bone mineral density appears to be substantially more common in patients with HIV than those who are HIV negative (AIDS 2006 Nov 14;20[17]:2165–74). Spontaneous fractures have also been reported, although the risk is low. As with osteonecrosis, the relationship between bone demineralization and a specific antiretroviral drug class has not been established. As part of initial therapy, the use of tenofovir (in combination with other agents) leads to a modest decline in bone density that then stabilizes. For example, in a randomized trial of either tenofovir or stavudine in combination with lamivudine and efavirenz, those receiving tenofovir had a significant decline from baseline in lumbar spine bone density at 48 weeks compared to those in the stavudine arm. No further decrement was seen at 144 weeks of follow-up, and there was no significant difference in the incidence of fractures (JAMA 2004 Jul 14;292[2]:191–201).

   a. **Diagnosis.** Routine screening is not indicated. If other risk factors for loss of bone density are present, the appropriate screening test is regional DEXA scanning. Secondary causes of osteopenia and osteoporosis should be evaluated, including thyrotoxicosis, hyperparathyroidism, hypogonadism, weight loss, alcohol intake, and certain medications (especially corticosteroids).

   b. **Treatment.** All patients should receive adequate diet, and if needed, supplements of calcium and vitamin D. If osteoporosis is demonstrated on DEXA scan (t-score of –2.5 or lower), consider biphosphonate therapy. Both alendronate and zoledronate have been tested in prospective clinical studies (J Acquir Immune Defic Syndr 2005 Apr 1;38[4]:426–31; J Clin Endocrinol Metab 2007 Apr;92[4]: 1283–8).

GASTROINTESTINAL TRACT COMPLICATIONS

A. Anorexia

1. **Etiology.** Commonly associated with advanced HIV disease, possibly due to high cytokine (especially TNF) levels that correlate with high titer HIV RNA. Other causes include depression, medications, opportunistic infections (especially MAC), and lactic acidosis (related to mitochondrial toxicity).

2. **Treatment.** <u>Megecetrol acetate</u> (Megace) liquid suspension 400–800 mg (PO) QD improves appetite, quality of life (Ann Intern Med 1994 Sep 15;121[6]:400–8). Weight gain that results is generally fat, not lean body mass. Side effects include hypogonadism, DVT, gynecomastia. Megecetrol has corticosteroid properties, and therefore can lead to Cushings-like state (prolonged use) or adrenal insufficiency (when drug is withdrawn). Prolonged use should be avoided; if required, dose should be tapered gradually. <u>Dronabinol</u> (Marinol) 2.5 mg q12h stimulates appetite and reduces nausea. Dronabinol is a synthetic delta-9-tetrahydrocannabinol (THC), the active ingredient in marijuana. The main side effect is oversedation. Patients should start with a dose at bedtime and then increase to q12h as tolerated.

B. Nausea/Vomiting

1. **Etiology**

   a. **Medications.** Direct effect of antiretroviral medications (especially PIs, ZDV, abacavir hypersensitivity), medication-related pancreatitis (see above), or lactic acidosis from NRTIs.

   b. **Opportunistic infections.** Intestinal protozoa (e.g., cryptosporidiosis, isospora, giardiasis—all usually accompanied by diarrhea), CMV esophagitis/gastritis, GI tract involvement of MAC.

   c. **Others.** Gastric lymphoma, CNS process producing mass effect (toxoplasmosis or lymphoma) or raised intracerebral pressure (cryptococcal meningitis).

2. **Treatment.** Address underlying etiology. If felt to be due to the direct effect of antiretrovirals, choose an alternate regimen if safe from the virologic perspective (e.g., substitute tenofovir for ZDV, efavirenz for PI). If underlying cause cannot be treated or removed, or for temporary relief of symptoms, therapeutic options include: prochlorperazine (Compazine) 10 mg (PO) or 25 mg (PR) q12h prn; metoclopramide (Reglan) 10 mg (PO) q6h prn; trimethobenzamide (Tigan) 250 mg (PO) q6h prn; lorazepam 0.5–1.0 mg (PO or IV) q6h prn; ondansetron (Zofran) 4–8 mg (PO) q8h prn or 32 mg (IV or IM) as a single dose; dronabinol (Marinol) 2.5–5.0 mg (PO) q12h.

Patients with HIV are at increased risk for phenothiazine-related dystonia, which may occur with prochlorperazine, metoclopramide, and trimethobenzamide. Treat dystonia with diphenhydramine (Benadryl) 50 mg (PO or IV) × 1 dose.

C. Diarrhea

1. Etiology

a. **Infection.** <u>Acute diarrhea</u>: salmonella, shigella, campylobacter, *C. difficile*, giardiasis, cyclospora; <u>subacute/chronic diarrhea</u>: giardiasis, cryptosporidia, microsporidia, isospora, CMV.

b. **Medication-related.** Especially nelfinavir, all ritonavir-boosted PIs, full-dose ritonavir (rarely used), buffered version of ddl; can be part of abacavir hypersensitivity syndrome. Medication-related diarrhea is rarely associated with weight loss or fever (abacavir excluded). Risk of ritonavir-related diarrhea appears to be dose related—several comparative studies have shown lower rates of diarrhea when the total daily dose is 100 mg rather than 200 mg.

2. Treatment.
Treat underlying cause (see Chapter 5). If PI-related, consider changing to an alternative PI that is less likely to cause diarrhea (e.g., nelfinavir or lopinavir/ritonavir to atazanavir/ritonavir or darunavir/ritonavir), or to an NNRTI (efavirenz or nevirapine). To avoid resistance, NNRTI replacement should only be considered when the HIV RNA is < 50 copies/mL, and preferably when there is no history of treatment failure that would lead to NRTI resistance. If diarrhea persists or if medication changes are not possible, offer symptomatic therapy with psyllium 1 tsp q12h–24h, loperamide 2 mg q6h prn, calcium 500 mg q12h; pancreatic enzymes 1–2 tabs with each meal, Lomotil 1–2 tabs q8h prn, or octreotide 100–500 mcg (SQ) q12h.

D. Oral or Esophageal Ulcers

1. Presentation.
Intensely painful ulcers of various size; esophageal ulcers cause severe dysphagia. May occur at any stage of HIV disease (including primary infection), but more common with progressive immunosuppression (CD4 < 100, associated neutropenia). Most common diagnosis is idiopathic aphthous ulcers; other causes include CMV, HSV, histoplasmosis, lymphoma. For first-time presentation, culture for HSV and refer for biopsy to exclude other causes.

2. Treatment.
For idiopathic aphthous ulcers, start with symptom relief, followed by application of local steroids, followed by either systemic steroids or thalidomide. Lesions sometimes respond to immune reconstitution from antiretroviral therapy along with resolution of neutropenia (adjunctive therapy with G-CSF may hasten healing). Therapeutic modalities include:

a. Symptom reduction with viscous lidocaine (2%).

b. Topical fluocinonide (Lidex) 0.05% ointment mixed 1:1 with Orobase; apply q6h as needed.

c. Dexamethasone 0.5/5M elixir mouth rinse q8h–12h.

d. Local corticosteroid injections by oral surgeon.

e. Prednisone 40–60 mg/day × 1–2 weeks, tapered as tolerated over 1–2 weeks or longer as needed.

f. Thalidomide 200 mg (PO) at bedtime × 4–6 weeks, followed by 100 mg (PO) at bedtime twice weekly. Side effects include sedation, constipation, peripheral neuropathy. Severe teratogenicity of thalidomide requires that physicians register with company-sponsored monitoring program before prescribing (see http://www.thalomid.com/steps_program.aspx). Women of childbearing age must use at least two forms of contraception and have regular pregnancy tests while receiving thalidomide. Informed consent in package insert must be signed before therapy is initiated.

E. HIV Cholangiopathy
1. **Presentation.** Presents with right upper quadrant pain, fever, and sometimes jaundice. Laboratory evaluation invariably demonstrates increased alkaline phosphatase. Generally occurs with severe immunosuppression (CD4 < 100/mm³). Imaging with ultrasound or ERCP shows dilated or prominent intrahepatic and extrahepatic ducts. Papillary stenosis may also be present.

2. **Etiology.** Differential diagnosis include cholelithiasis, acalculous cholecystitis, infiltrative infectious or neoplastic diseases of the liver. Screen for infectious etiology, including stool for ova/parasites and/or ERCP aspirates for cryptosporidia, microsporidia, cyclospora, CMV.

3. **Treatment.** Symptomatic improvement is sometimes seen with endoscopic-guided sphincterotomy or stenting. Treat underlying infectious process, if identified.

RENAL COMPLICATIONS

A. HIV-Associated Nephropathy. A form of progressive glomerulosclerosis, leading to massive proteinuria and progressive renal dysfunction. Over 80% of cases occur in Africans–Americans. Renal biopsy shows extensive collapsing glomerulosclerosis, tubular ectasia, and tubulo-interstitial disease. Occurs most commonly with low CD4 cell counts (< 100/mm³), but may occur at any level of immunosuppression. Very uncommon with undetectable HIV RNA (Clin Infect Dis 2006;43:377–80).
1. **Presentation.** Clinical presentation varies from asymptomatic to symptoms of hypoalbuminemia and renal failure (edema, fatigue, anemia). Hypertension generally is absent. Renal ultrasound demonstrates enlarged or normal-sized kidneys. The cardinal laboratory feature is proteinuria > 1 gm/day, usually with rapidly progressive renal failure evolving over weeks to months to end-stage renal disease requiring dialysis.

2. **Diagnostic Considerations.** Biopsy should be considered to rule out other causes of progressive renal disease, such as HCV-associated renal disease, medication-associated toxicity (see below), or a non-HIV-related cause.

3. **Treatment.** Effective options include antiretroviral therapy (case reports suggest PI-based therapy may lead to resolution of disease), ACE inhibitors, and high-dose corticosteroids (60 mg prednisone QD × 1 month followed by gradual taper) (Kidney International 2000;58:1253). Since high-dose steroids are associated with further immune suppression and other complications, a reasonable approach is to begin with antiretroviral therapy plus an ACE inhibitor (e.g., captopril 6.25 mg q8h).

B. **Medication-Related Renal Disease.** HIV-related medications most likely to cause nephrotoxicity are listed below. (See antiretroviral drug summaries in Chapter 9 for dosing in renal insufficiency.)

1. **Tenofovir.** Can rarely cause tubular injury, leading to increased creatinine. Sometimes accompanied by Fanconi's syndrome, with phosphate wasting and acidosis. Renal toxicity is more likely to occur in those with underlying renal disease or advanced HIV infection (Clin Infect Dis 2005;15:1194–8; J Infect Dis 2008;197:102). Use calculated creatinine clearance (Cockgroft-Gault equation) to assess renal function, and reduce dose based on degree of renal insufficiency as recommended in the package insert.

2. **Indinavir.** Can crystalize in urine, leading to a variety of renal conditions, including nephrolithiasis, crystal-related nephropathy, and sterile pyuria. Risk may be dose-related and is more common when indinavir is dosed with ritonavir as a PK booster. Risk can be reduced by ingestion of at least 1.5 liters of water daily. For acute renal colic, a trial of increasing oral hydration is warranted, after which IV hydration and cessation of indinavir and other antiretroviral medications is recommended until the condition resolves. For severe nephrolithiasis or other renal complication of indinavir, strongly consider changing the patient to an alternative PI. As atazanavir may also cause nephrolithiasis, best options would be lopinavir/ritonavir, darunavir/ritonavir, or fosamprenavir/ritonavir.

3. **Pentamidine.** Can cause renal failure in up to 50% of patients; other adverse effects include electrolyte/mineral wasting and hypoglycemia. Risk is related to cumulative dose; monitor creatinine, electrolytes, glucose, calcium, and phosphate during therapy.

4. **Foscarnet.** Induces dose-related renal failure as well as wasting of potassium, calcium, and phosphate. Dose adjustment is necessary for reduced creatinine clearance. Supplement potassium, calcium, and phosphorus as needed.

5. **Cidofovir.** Associated with dose-related renal toxicity, which can be reduced by concomitant administration of probenecid and hydration. Check serum creatinine and urine for protein prior to each dose; if creatinine is > 2 gm/dL or there is more than 2+ proteinuria, do not administer further cidofovir as renal toxicity may be irreversible.

6. **Amphotericin B.** Dose-dependent renal toxicity is common. Liposomal preparations are less nephrotoxic.

7. **Trimethoprim-sulfamethoxazole (TMP-SMX).** May cause hyperkalemia through amiloride-like effect from trimethoprim, especially when used at high doses for PCP treatment. Sulfonamide component can rarely cause crystal nephropathy (reversible with hydration).

8. **Acyclovir.** High-dose IV administration can crystalize in kidney and cause acute renal failure. Risk can be reduced with adequate hydration, and renal dysfunction usually responds to hydration and cessation of drug.

C. **HCV-Associated Renal Disease.** Often a manifestation of HCV-associated mixed cryoglobulinemia.

1. **Presentation.** Patients may present with palpable purpura or other dermatologic signs, along with hematuria, proteinuria, and sometimes renal failure. Other related laboratory findings include HCV RNA in plasma, cryoglobulins in blood, and low complement; renal biopsy shows HCV-related immune complexes.

2. **Treatment.** Therapy directed at hepatitis C (PEG-interferon plus ribavirin) can lead to improvement in renal disease and other manifestations of cryoglobulinemia.

D. **Heroin Nephropathy.** Can coexist with other forms of renal failure listed above. Results from glomerular injury, presumably from toxic effects of heroin or other contaminants. Distinguished from HIV-associated nephropathy by a slower rate of progression, small (as opposed to large) kidneys on ultrasound, and less proteinuria. Treatment consists of cessation of drug use.

CARDIAC COMPLICATIONS

A. **HIV-Related Cardiomyopathy** (JAMA 2008;299:324–31). Biventricular reduction in ejection fraction, with pathologic features typical of myocarditis and/or immune-mediated cardiomyopathy. Prevalence varies widely depending on definition; echocardiogram may show reduced ejection fraction in up to 50% of patients with AIDS, but symptomatic cardiomyopathy occurs in only 1–3%. More common with progressive immunodeficiency, especially when CD4 cell count < 100.

1. **Etiology.** Usually idiopathic. Differential diagnosis includes several causes, not mutually exclusive: HIV itself, secondary infection (CMV, toxoplasmosis, coxsackie, adenovirus, Chagas), disordered immune response leading to autoimmune myocarditis, nutritional deficiencies (selenium, carnitine), drug toxicity (NRTI-associated mitochondrial toxicity, alcohol, doxorubicin).

2. **Presentation.** Presents as left ventricular failure, with dyspnea, congestive heart failure, elevated jugular venous pressure, a prominent S_3 on exam. Chest x-ray typically demonstrates an enlarged heart, and echocardiogram shows marked biventricular dysfunction with reduced ejection fraction. Diagnosis is made after exclusion of other common causes of low EF (alcohol, poor nutrition, myocardial ischemia). Cardiac biopsy is rarely useful.

3. Treatment. Patients should receive antiretroviral therapy plus usual therapies for heart failure (diuretics, beta-blockers, ACE inhibitors are often quite effective in reducing symptoms). For manifestations of disseminated CMV disease or a positive blood CMV viral load, empiric CMV treatment with valganciclovir 900 mg (PO) q12h × 3 weeks. Although case reports have shown improvement in ejection fraction after cessation of NRTIs, this is a much less common cause of cardiomyopathy than HIV itself.

B. Pericarditis/Pericardial Effusion

1. Etiology. Pericardial fluid may be due to HIV itself or a complicating malignancy/opportunistic infection. The most common malignancy is lymphoma, where an effusion may be the first manifestation of an extranodal high-grade B-cell lymphoma; Kaposi's sarcoma causes effusions generally only when the disease is widespread elsewhere. In addition, numerous common and opportunistic infections have been reported to cause pericarditis in HIV patients, including pyogenic bacteria (especially *S. aureus* and *S. pneumoniae*), TB, atypical mycobacteria, cryptococcal disease, disseminated histoplasmosis, and CMV.

2. Presentation and Diagnosis. Often diagnosed incidentally through enlarged cardiac silhouette and subsequent echocardiogram. May be asymptomatic or cause chest pain, dyspnea, cardiac tamponade, pericardial friction rub. Pericardiocentesis is indicated for large or symptomatic effusions, with fluid sent for cultures (routine, fungal, mycobacterial) and cytology.

3. Treatment. Directed at underlying condition. If idiopathic pericarditis, consider starting antiretroviral therapy, and manage symptoms with NSAIDs and corticosteroids (as in HIV-negative patients).

C. Tricuspid Valve Endocarditis

1. Etiology. Injection drug users (IDUs) with HIV, particularly those with lower CD4 cell counts, are at substantially higher risk for endocarditis than HIV-negative IDUs (J Infect Dis 2002;185:1761–6). *Staphylococcus aureus* is the most common pathogen. In one series, rates of infection included *S. aureus* (73%), coagulase-negative *Staphylococcus* species (1%), *Staphylococcus* species not otherwise classified (7%), *Streptococcus* species (13%), *Pseudomonas* species (2%), *Bacillus* species (2%), and other organisms (2%). Most urban centers are experiencing an increasing rate of MRSA.

2. Presentation and Diagnosis. Patients typically present with fever, weight loss, and sometimes pulmonary symptoms (dyspnea, chest pain) reflective of septic emboli arising from an infected tricuspid valve. Physical examination usually reveals a heart murmur ± evidence of peripheral septic emboli. Chest x-ray may show multiple septic emboli, some with cavitation. An echocardiogram should be performed to assess for valvular vegetations. Diagnosis is confirmed when a patient with the above clinical presentation has positive blood cultures for an organism known to be associated with endocarditis.

3. Treatment. While a short course (2 weeks) of therapy has been effective in HIV-negative IDUs with tricuspid endocarditis, this regimen cannot be recommended in HIV-positive patients. Recommended regimens include:

- <u>Methicillin-sensitive *S. aureus*</u>: Nafcillin 2 gm (IV) q4h × 28 days plus gentamicin 1 mg/kg (IV) q8h × 3–5 days or until blood cultures clear.
- <u>Methicillin-resistant *S. aureus* or beta-lactam allergy</u>: Vancomycin 1 gm (IV) q12h × 28 days plus gentamicin 1 mg/kg (IV) q8h × 3–5 days or until blood cultures clear. Alternative to vancomycin is daptomycin (IV) 6 mg/kg QD × 4 weeks.
- <u>Unable or unwilling to receive IV therapy</u>: Ciprofloxacin 750 mg (PO) q12h plus rifampin 300 mg (PO) q12h × 4 weeks. This regimen cannot be used with PIs due to rifampin-PI interaction. Linezolid 600 mg (PO) q12h × 4 weeks can be used as an alternative (limited data).

PULMONARY COMPLICATIONS

A. Pulmonary Hypertension (see also JAMA 2008;299:324–31). Idiopathic elevation of pulmonary pressures is sometimes seen in HIV infection. The pathological process is similar to primary pulmonary hypertension (i.e., hypertrophy of vascular endothelium). Pulmonary hypertension is more common in women and can occur at any CD4 cell count.

    1. Presentation. Dyspnea on exertion, palpitations, chest pain. Exam may reveal elevated JVP and precordial heave. Diagnosis is supported by echocardiogram and doppler studies showing right ventricular hypertrophy and elevated PA pressures. Most sensitive test is right heart catheterization, where pressures will exceed 30 mmHg. Recurrent pulmonary emboli should be excluded as a possible cause.

    2. Treatment. Epoprostenol (FloLan) by continuous infusion. Requires placement of a permanent central venous catheter. Diuretics also help relieve symptoms. Anticoagulation is generally indicated. Sildenafil is also used as an adjunct to therapy. There are mixed reports on whether antiretroviral therapy improves hemodynamics or outcome.

B. Lymphocytic Interstitial Pneumonitis (LIP). An idiopathic form of diffuse lung disease that is more common in children. Tends to occur with moderate immunosuppression (CD4 cell count 200–400/mm^3) and mimics PCP.

    1. Presentation and Diagnosis. Cough, dyspnea on exertion, exercise oxygen desaturation. Usually afebrile. Chest x-ray and chest CT show diffuse bilateral reticulonodular infiltrates. Differentiated from PCP by generally higher CD4 cell counts and lower LDH. Diagnosed by bronchioalveolar lavage (BAL) with biopsy, which will exclude PCP and yield the characteristic histopathology of LIP (patchy lymphocytic infiltration and no microorganisms on special stains).

    2. Treatment. Antiretroviral therapy can either improve LIP or worsen it through enhanced immune activity. Prednisone usually achieves rapid reduction in dyspnea, but tapering dose may be accompanied by a relapse of symptoms.

C. Emphysema. Cigarette smoking is associated with a more rapid progression to bullous emphysema in patients with HIV compared to HIV-negative controls. Clinical presentation and treatment are the same as for the general population.

D. Pulmonary Kaposi's Sarcoma. Generally occurs only in patients with advanced HIV disease and extensive Kaposi's sarcoma elsewhere.

    1. Presentation and Diagnosis. Chest x-ray demonstrates nodules, masses, and/or pleural effusions. Diagnosed by visual inspection of the airway during bronchoscopy, where typical violaceous plaques may be observed.

    2. Treatment. Antiretroviral therapy may lead to dramatic improvement in even severe Kaposi's sarcoma, although temporary flares due to immune reconstitution have been reported. Concomitant systemic chemotherapy is also generally required.

HEENT COMPLICATIONS

A. Aphthous Ulcers. See p. 148.

B. Oral Hairy Leukoplakia

    1. Presentation. Presents as ribbed, "corduroy"-like white patches on the side of the tongue. More common with increased immunosuppression (CD4 < 200/mm^3). Usually painless. Distinguished from oral thrush in that oral hairy leukoplakia does not rub off with tongue depressor. Caused by Epstein-Barr virus.

    2. Treatment. No treatment is needed unless the patient is symptomatic. If treatment is desired, antiretroviral therapy often leads to resolution. Other treatment options include acyclovir 800 mg (PO) 5×/day or famciclovir 500 mg (PO) q12h or valacyclovir 1000 mg (PO) q8h until resolution. Topical application of podophyllin is sometimes effective.

C. Salivary Gland Enlargement

    1. Presentation. Can occur at any stage of HIV infection and usually worsens with disease progression. Often accompanied by xerostomia. Biopsy shows lymphoid infiltration, possibly due to HIV itself; may be part of diffuse infiltrative lymphocytosis syndrome (DILS), which can be accompanied by involvement of the lungs, kidneys, and peripheral nerves. For progressive parotid enlargement, a CT scan is recommended to differentiate solid from cystic enlargement. Differential diagnosis includes infectious parotitis, which presents more acutely with fever and local pain.

    2. Treatment. Antiretroviral therapy is the preferred approach. Other forms of treatment include repeated aspiration of fluid-filled cysts when symptomatic, local measures for dry mouth (sugarless gum, artificial saliva), and prednisone 40 mg (PO) QD × 1 week followed by gradual taper over 1–2 weeks.

D. Lymphoepithelial Cysts

    1. Presentation. Presents as enlarged cervical cysts that can mimic lymphadenopathy. Can occur at any CD4 cell count. A biopsy is needed to rule out lymphoma, other malignancies (notably squamous cell carcinoma), opportunistic infections. Cause is unknown.

2. **Treatment.** Antiretroviral therapy often causes dramatic reduction in size of cysts.

E. **Gingivitis/Periodontitis**
   1. **Presentation.** Presents as painful gums with easy bleeding, along with erythematous and receding gingiva. May be the initial manifestation of underlying HIV disease. Severity correlates with stage of immunosuppression. Caused by oral anaerobic bacteria (usually polymicrobial), and exacerbated by poor local oral hygiene, smoking, alcoholism.

   2. **Treatment.** Improve local hygiene, (brush, floss, antibacterial mouth rinse). Curettage by dentist/periodontist may be helpful. For severe cases, treat for 7–10 days with metronidazole 500 mg (PO) q8h or clindamycin 300 mg (PO) q6h or amoxicillin-clavulanate 850 mg (PO) q12h.

MUSCULOSKELETAL COMPLICATIONS

A. **HIV Arthropathy**
   1. **Presentation.** Presents as painful arthropathy, often involving multiple joints. Pain out of proportion to physical findings. Cause is unknown.

   2. **Treatment.** NSAIDs, other pain relievers.

B. **Reiter's Syndrome**
   1. **Presentation.** Asymmetrical polyarthritis involving the large joints of lower extremities. Arthritis is seen in conjunction with urethritis, skin lesions (circinate balanitis, keratoderma blennorrhagica), ocular disease. May also occur after gastroenteritis. Appears to occur with greater frequency among HIV patients, usually in association with HLA-B27.

   2. **Diagnosis.** Differential diagnosis includes septic arthritis; if joint effusions are present, arthrocentesis with cultures/gram stain is indicated. Urethral swab for chlamydia and gonorrhea is also recommended.

   3. **Treatment.** Consider treatment of urethritis with empiric chlamydia therapy with azithromycin 1 gm (PO) × 1 dose. Other measures include NSAIDs and referral to rheumatology for possible immunosuppressive therapy (prednisone, methotrexate, TNF antagonists).

C. **Pyomyositis.** Focal infection of muscle often occurring at site of injections, trauma.
   1. **Presentation.** Presents as localized pain, swelling, fever. Usually caused by *Staphylococcus aureus* including MRA, less commonly other pyogenic bacteria, e.g., streptococci, gram-negative rods. More common with advanced HIV immunosuppression (CD4 cell count < 100).

   2. **Diagnosis.** Imaging of suspected area with CT followed by diagnostic aspiration for gram stain/culture.

   3. **Treatment.** Antibiotics directed at causative pathogen (usually an anti-staphylococcal penicillin or vancomycin). May also require surgical incision/drainage.

D. **HIV Myopathy and NRTI-Related Myopathy.** These two conditions may present similarly.

    1. **Presentation.** Patients present with myalgias, muscle tenderness, weakness, and elevated CPK levels. Proximal leg muscles are most commonly involved. Condition can occur at any stage of HIV disease.

    2. **Diagnosis.** Some experts recommend a biopsy to distinguish between HIV and NRTI-related myopathy. In the former, there is a more prominent inflammatory infiltrate; the latter usually shows evidence of mitochondrial myopathy. NRTI-related myopathy is most commonly associated with zidovudine.

    3. **Treatment.** For symptomatic HIV-related myopathy, corticosteroids at high doses (prednisone 1 mg/kg/day) are recommended. Once improvement occurs, this should be tapered over several weeks. For NRTI-related myopathy, change to a regimen that either avoids NRTIs entirely or switches to those NRTIs with lower mitochondrial toxicity (abacavir, emtricitabine, lamivudine, tenofovir).

E. **Rhabdomyolysis.** Extensive muscle necrosis with myoglobinuria and acute renal failure. May occur as part of medication toxicity (again, to NRTIs most commonly) or to HIV itself. Management is by withdrawal of possibly offending agents and hydration—hemodialysis if necessary.

NEUROLOGIC COMPLICATIONS

A. **Distal Sensory Neuropathy.** Caused by HIV itself and/or neurotoxic effects of medications, in particular the di-deoxy NRTIs (d4T, ddI, ddC).

    1. **Presentation.** Typically presents as pain, aching, burning, or tingling of the distal extremities (toes/feet more commonly than fingers/hands). Pain is often worse at night. Principal risk factors include the stage of HIV disease and exposure to the above listed drugs, especially when used in combination.

    2. **Diagnosis and Evaluation.** Usually clinical, based on patient history. Reduced pin-prick and vibration sense in the involved extremities support the diagnosis, but symptoms often precede objective physical findings. Attempt to identify contributing/other causes, including B_{12} deficiency, syphilis, CMV, multiple myeloma, other neurotoxic agents (dapsone, INH, vincristine; avoid using these drugs if possible with d4T or ddI). If presentation is confusing, refer for EMG and nerve conduction studies, which will show an axonal neuropathy.

    3. **Treatment.** Withdraw offending agents, in particular d4T and ddI; symptoms may persist or even worsen for several weeks after cessation of these drugs, and severe neuropathy may be irreversible. Antiretroviral therapy should be continued and one of several therapies used for neuropathic symptoms can be administered:

    • NSAIDs or acetaminophen for mild pain
    • Avoid tight-fitting shoes, extremes of temperature

- Gabapentin 300 mg at bedtime; increase up to 1200 mg divided q6–8h as needed
- Nortriptyline 10 mg at bedtime; increase up to 75 mg at bedtime as tolerated
- Lamictal 25 mg q12h; increase up to 150 mg q12h as tolerated
- Topical therapy: capsaicin (may make symptoms worse), lidocaine patches
- Acupuncture
- Severe pain may require chronic long-acting narcotic pain relievers (e.g., methadone, MS-Contin, transdermal fentanyl).

B. Other Forms of Neuropathy

1. Types

a. **Acute inflammatory demyelinating neuropathy (AIDP, Guillain-Barré syndrome).** Ascending motor weakness usually without sensory involvement. Reported in early and late stage HIV. May evolve into a chronic form with waxing and waning symptoms. Treatment consists of steroids, plasmapheresis, IVIG. Prognosis is variable for all—tends to be best for mononeuritis especially if due to acute HIV infection.

b. **Mononeuritis multiplex.** Scattered, asymmetrical, motor and sensory deficits (e.g., facial weakness, foot drop). Reported in acute and chronic HIV. Some cases ascribed to CMV in advanced HIV (CD4 < 50/mm^3). Treatment consists of steroids, IVIG. If caused by CMV, treat with valganciclovir at standard doses.

c. **HIV-associated neuromuscular weakness syndrome.** Rare complication of NRTI-therapy (especially d4T), presenting as progressive ascending paralysis in association with lactic acidosis. When severe, mechanical ventilation may be required. Treatment consists of withdrawal of NRTIs, especially d4T. Residual neurologic impairment is common after recovery.

d. **Progressive polyradiculopathy.** Complication of advanced HIV disease that typically presents with lower extremity weakness, anaesthesia in a "saddle" distribution (perineal area), and/or bowel and bladder dysfunction. Most common causes include CMV polyradiculitis (p. 105) and lymphoma. Diagnostically, obtain an MRI of the lumbosacral spine to exclude a mass lesion, then proceed to CSF exam. If due to CMV, the usual CSF finding is increased WBC (predominantly polys), increased protein, and positive CMV PCR. If due to lymphoma, the CSF shows increased protein and lymphoma cells on cytology. For CMV polyradiculitis, treat × 3–4 weeks or until improvement with either ganciclovir 5 mg/kg (IV) q12h or valganciclovir 900 mg (PO) q12h or foscarnet 90 mg/kg (IV) q12h; for severe cases, some advocate ganciclovir plus foscarnet. For lymphoma, treat with chemotherapy plus radiation.

2. Prognosis. Prognosis is variable for all forms of neuropathy but tends to be best for mononeuritis, especially if due to acute HIV infection.

C. HIV-Associated Dementia (AIDS dementia, HIV encephalitis/encephalopathy). Typical presentation at onset consists of short-term memory loss, often with apathy or withdrawal from usual activities. As the disease progresses, cognitive impairment worsens, and speech, motor, and gait disturbances develop. Seizures and akinetic mutism are late-stage manifestations. The incidence of this complication has decreased dramatically since the widespread introduction of combination antiretroviral therapy in 1996. Progression of dementia is gradual (usually over months) and can be arrested/reversed with potent antiretroviral therapy. A more rapidly progressive form has also been reported. HIV dementia almost always occurs in the late stages of HIV disease (CD4 < 100/mm³, HIV RNA > 100,000 copies/mL), but on rare occasions occurs with relatively preserved immune function and low plasma HIV RNA. In the latter case, relatively high HIV RNA levels are often present in the CSF.

1. **Diagnosis.** Diagnosis is based on a combination of clinical, laboratory, and imaging criteria, as well as exclusion of alternative causes (depression, adverse drug effects, neurosyphilis, CMV encephalitis). HIV-associated dementia should be suspected in a patient with advanced HIV disease and subacute to chronic cognitive impairment, especially short-term memory loss. Administration of the four-step HIV-dementia scale (AIDS Reader 2002;12:29) may help quantify the extent of deficits. MRI shows cerebral atrophy and often non-enhancing white matter abnormalities that can be indistinguishable from progressive multifocal leukoencephalopathy (PML). CSF exam is usually abnormal, with elevated protein and low-level lymphocytic pleocytosis. When HIV RNA in the CSF is measured, it is usually detectable at 1000 copies/mL or higher; an undetectable CSF HIV RNA is unusual in HIV dementia and suggests an alternative diagnosis.

2. **Treatment.** Potent antiretroviral therapy is the mainstay of therapy and can lead to dramatic improvement, especially in treatment-naïve individuals. Selection of drugs with higher penetration into the CNS is theoretically preferable (Arch Neurol 2008 Jan;65[1]:65–70), although there are no definitive clinical data to support this approach over choosing alternative agents. Antiretroviral agents with the best CSF penetration are ZDV, ABC, d4T, NVP, IDV, LPV, FTC; somewhat lower penetration occurs with ddI, 3TC, EFV, ATV, FPV. In a patient who has failed antiretroviral therapy, treatment is based on blood resistance testing to maximize antiviral potency.

PSYCHIATRIC COMPLICATIONS

Psychiatric illness is more common in patients with HIV than in those with other medical illnesses of comparable severity. Potential explanations include pre-existing psychiatric illness which predisposes to high-risk behavior for HIV acquisition (substance abuse, sexual addiction), extreme grief reactions from having a stigmatized illness, or neurotoxic effects of HIV manifesting as psychiatric illness. For all psychiatric illnesses, consider starting antiretroviral therapy even if there are otherwise no indications, as therapy is associated with improved neuropsychiatric function. Carefully review package inserts and drug interaction tables at www.aidsinfo.nih.gov prior to prescribing any psychotropic agent.

A. Depression

1. **Presentation and Diagnosis.** Common symptoms include depressed mood, decreased interest in work/leisure activities, blunted affect, sleep disturbances, alterations in appetite, forgetfulness, and diminished concentration. Key differential is HIV dementia, but depressed mood is usually not a prominent feature of dementia. Be sure to exclude contribution of medications, particularly efavirenz, ZDV, corticosteroids.

2. **Treatment.** SSRIs or tricyclic antidepressants are the mainstays of therapy, as for HIV-negative patients. In general, start with low-doses of all agents and titrate up as needed. Always check treatment guidelines for potential drug interactions with antiretroviral agents (aidsinfo.nih.gov). If rapid onset of response is needed, stimulants such as methylphenidate or dextroamphetamine may be tried. MAO inhibitors are contraindicated due to drug interactions.

B. Mania. HIV may produce an unusual form of mania as a manifestation of HIV encephalopathy.

1. **Presentation.** These patients usually have CD4 cell counts < 200/mm^3. It is distinguished from non-HIV-related bipolar disease in that there is no family history of bipolar illness and onset may occur at any age. Symptoms include expansive mood, grandiosity, and diminished sleep.

2. **Treatment.** Treatment should be undertaken with the assistance of a psychiatrist. Options include lithium 300 mg (PO) q8h or valproic acid 250 mg (PO) q12h or carbamazepine 200 mg (PO) q12h.

C. Insomnia

1. **Etiology.** Sleep disturbance may be a symptom of an underlying medical condition (hepatic encephalopathy, HIV dementia), a psychiatric illness (depression, mania, substance abuse, anxiety), or a medication side effect (efavirenz, corticosteroids).

2. **Treatment.** Attempt to identify/treat underlying causes, including "poor sleep hygiene" (excessive caffeine, alcohol, other stimulants). For patients with a history of substance abuse, avoid if possible the chronic use of benzodiazepines, which have addictive potential. As an alternative, trazodone 50–100 mg (PO) at bedtime can be very effective. Short-term insomnia due to anxiety or jet lag can be treated with benzodiazepines such as zolpidem (Ambien) 2.5–5.0 mg (PO) at bedtime or lorazepam 1.0 mg (PO) at bedtime.

DERMATOLOGIC COMPLICATIONS

A. Viral Infections

1. **Herpes Simplex Infection.** Oral/anogenital diseases occur more frequently and are more severe in patients with HIV. Infection may also occur on non-mucosal surfaces (e.g., skin), especially when the patient is severely immunocompromised.

a. **Diagnosis.** Characteristic vesicles on an erythematous base. Ulcerations may occur in primary disease and more advanced HIV-related immunosuppression. A viral culture for HSV is the diagnostic test of choice and is quite sensitive, especially early during the outbreak and prior to starting anti-herpes therapy.

b. **Treatment.** See p. 113.

2. **Varicella-Zoster Infection.** Herpes zoster is much more common (20- to 50-fold increased risk) in HIV patients than in age-matched HIV-negative controls and may be first sign of underlying HIV infection. AIDS patients are at increased risk for chronic non-healing zoster, which can last for several weeks. Appearance may also be atypical, with nodular rather than vesicular lesions.

a. **Diagnosis.** Diagnosed by clinical appearance. DFA test of a lesion can help distinguish zoster from HSV if the diagnosis is unclear.

b. **Treatment.** See p. 136.

3. **Molluscum Contagiosum**

a. **Presentation.** Manifests as clusters of white, umbilicated papules outside the groin/perineal area. Rarely seen except with severe immunosuppression (CD4 < $100/mm^3$); the number/size of lesions increase as immunosuppression progresses.

b. **Diagnosis.** Diagnosed by clinical appearance. Biopsy is rarely necessary, but when performed shows large inclusions known as "molluscum bodies." Etiologic virus (a pox virus) cannot be cultured in clinical practice.

c. **Treatment.** Effective antiretroviral therapy can often lead to dramatic, spontaneous improvement. If this is not possible, or for more immediate control, local cryosurgery, or other ablative methods can be effective.

4. **Oral Hairy Leukoplakia (OHL).** See p. 154.

5. **Warts.** Cutaneous and genital warts are extremely common in HIV disease, and in severe cases are disfiguring and difficult to treat. Although usually more severe with progressive HIV disease, in some patients they remain a debilitating problem even with good response to antiretroviral therapy.

a. **Diagnosis.** Generally a clinical diagnosis. In severe or refractory cases, biopsy is sometimes needed to exclude underlying squamous cell carcinoma.

b. **Treatment**

i. **Genital warts.** Imiquimod 5% cream 3x/week at bedtime, wash off in AM. Alternative: podofilox q12h application with cotton swab for 3 days followed by 4 days without treatment, then repeat. Local inflammation is common with both measures. Provider-applied therapies include cryotherapy, podophyllin resin (severe or bulky cases).

ii. **Cutaneous warts.** As in HIV-negative patients, spontaneous resolution may occur, especially in relatively immunocompetent patients. Therapy is otherwise similar as in HIV-negative patients, with multiple ablative therapies available (cryotherapy, liquid nitrogen, salicylic acid, bichloracetic acid, curettage). Refractory cases should be referred to a dermatologist for intra-lesional therapy or wide excision.

B. Bacterial Infections

1. Staphylococcal Infections. May cause staphylococcal folliculitis, a pruritic condition associated with small papules. Larger collections of soft tissue staph infection can cause furunculosis or subcutaneous abscesses (more common with advanced HIV-related immunosuppression.) In most parts of the United States, MRSA is the most common cause of purulent soft tissue infection.

a. Diagnosis. Clinical appearance. Culture to exclude MRSA.

b. Treatment. For furunculosis, which is usually due to MRSA, treat according to sensitivities; doxycycline or TMP-SMX 1–2 DS (PO) q12h are often effective; linezolid 600 mg (PO) q12h is recommended for severe cases. Clindamycin can be used if erythromycin sensitivity is documented. If organism is MSSA, dicloxacillin 500 mg QID or cephalexin 500 mg QID are options. Large furuncles or soft tissue collections must be surgically drained (Antimicrob Agents Chemother 2007 Nov;51[11]:4044–8). For multiple recurrences, consider decontamination strategies:

 i. Antibacterials: Mupirocin nasal ointment anterior nares BID, Bactrim 1 DS BID, ± rifampin 300 mg PO BID—all for 7–10 days (do not use rifampin with protease inhibitors).

 ii. Household contacts (including pets) cultured/treated.

 iii. Local measures

  — Keep cuts/abrasions covered.

  — Bathe for 10 minutes; 1 tsp bleach/gallon of water.

  — Using a bath sponge, lather armpits, groin, anus, and under the breasts with chlorhexidine topical antiseptic (Hibiclens scrub) after draining bath water.

  — Shower Hibiclens off.

 iv. Frequent laundering of towels, sheets, clothing.

2. Bacillary Angiomatosis. A cutaneous manifestation of *Bartonella quintanna* and *Bartonella henselae* infection (cat scratch bacillus). Presents as a dome-shaped and often pedunculated papule or papules in a patient with severe immunosuppression. Appearance can mimic Kaposi's sarcoma. Organism can also cause hepatic disease (peliosis hepatitis), fever, encephalopathy, endocarditis. Clinical syndromes due to bartonella infection have become extremely rare since the availability of potent antiretroviral therapy.

a. Diagnosis. Characteristic appearance and biopsy, with pathology showing the characteristic bacillus on Warthin-Starry and Dieterle stains. Organism can be cultured, but laboratory needs to be alerted so special media can be used. Serologies also may be helpful.

    b. Treatment. Azithromycin 250–500 mg (PO) QD or clarithromycin 500 mg (PO) q12h or doxycycline 100 mg (PO) q12h. Treatment duration is determined by recovery of immune system in response to antiretroviral therapy.

  3. Syphilis. See p. 133.

C. Fungal Infections

  1. Disseminated and Invasive Fungal Infections. All disseminated fungal infections can cause skin lesions. Most characteristic are molluscum-like lesions with cryptococcal disease, erythema nodosum with coccidioides, and nodular skin lesions with blastomycosis.

  2. Tinea Corporis, Cruris, or Pedis (jock itch, athlete's foot). Extensive erythematous plaques with severe pruritus.

    a. Diagnosis. Characteristic appearance, with KOH slide preparation showing branched, septated hyphae.

    b. Treatment. Topical therapy with over-the-counter preparations, or by prescription with one of several topical antifungals, including clotrimazole, ciclopirox, or butenafine q12h. For severe disease, use fluconazole 100–200 mg (PO) QD × 7–14 days or terbinafine 250 mg (PO) QD × 14 days.

  3. Candidiasis. In addition to mucosal infections, candida can cause disease in the skin and nails. In the skin, it is often seen in intertriginous areas (groin, under breasts), where it causes a pruritic papular eruption that can coalesce to form large plaques. Web spaces of the fingers and toes may also be involved. Heat and moisture in these areas encourage candidal growth.

    a. Diagnosis. Clinically suspected with papular, sometimes pustular eruption in intertriginous areas. A KOH slide shows yeast and pseudohyphae of candida.

    b. Treatment. Topical therapy with antifungals, such as clotrimazole q12h × 14 days. More severe cases may require systemic therapy with fluconazole 100–200 mg (PO) QD × 7–14 days. It is also important to maintain good hygiene, attempt to aerate and dry involved areas, and avoid tight clothing.

D. Miscellaneous Skin Conditions. All can be the first sign of underlying HIV infection.

  1. Seborrheic Dermatitis. Presents as waxy erythematous and sometimes flakey plaques with scale, usually on face and scalp. Usually worsens with progressive immunodeficiency. May be caused by the yeast *Pityrosporum ovale*. Antiretroviral therapy usually leads to improvement. Symptomatic treatment consists of ketoconazole cream q12h × 7–14 days or a low-potency topical steroid (e.g., hydrocortisone cream 2.5% q12h × 7–14 days). For refractory cases where higher-potency steroids may be indicated, referral to a dermatologist is recommended.

  2. Psoriasis. Severity of psoriasis correlates with the degree of immunosuppression. HIV can sometimes unmask a prior history of mild disease. May be accompanied by arthritis. Antiretroviral therapy is often useful. Other treatments as per HIV-negative patients.

3. **Eosinophilic Folliculitis.** An erythematous, papular, severely pruritic eruption, usually on the upper trunk and face. Appearance is similar to bacterial folliculitis, but the rash is unresponsive to antibacterials and biopsy demonstrates an eosinophilic infiltrate. The process becomes more difficult to treat as HIV disease progresses; rubbing/scratching can lead to ulcerations, prurigo nodularis, secondary staph infections. In darker-skinned individuals, this can ultimately lead to disfiguring post-inflammatory hyperpigmentation.

   a. **Diagnosis.** Skin biopsy is required.

   b. **Treatment.** The disease is characterized by its refractory nature and frequent relapses. Individual treatments may work well in some individuals but not in others. Options include ART, oral/topical corticosteroids, isotretinoin, and phototherapy. Antiretroviral therapy will ultimately lead to improvement in most patients. However, some individuals go through a paradoxical worsening due to a heightened inflammatory response, which can be difficult to distinguish from an adverse drug reaction and can sometimes last for weeks to months. Prednisone 70 mg (PO) QD, tapered by 5–10 mg/d, is also helpful. Intermittent therapy of 60 mg (PO) QD × 2–3 days may be useful to control flares after discontinuation. Potent topical corticosteroids q12h–q8h × 10–14 days can be effective but should not be used on the face. Isotretinoin (Accutane) 1 mg/kg/d or 40 mg (PO) q12h is also of value, with duration determined by response to therapy (associated with skin dryness). Ultraviolet B phototherapy may be used 3×/week until improvement, then maintenance as needed.

4. **Xerosis/Ichthyosis.** Manifests as dry, flakey, and extremely pruritic skin. Worsens as HIV disease progresses, and exacerbated by some antiretrovirals, particularly indinavir. Treatment consists of antiretroviral therapy (avoid indinavir) and emollients (e.g., Aquaphor, Eucerin, Cetaphil). Short-duration (7–14 days) topical steroids may also be considered for dry/inflamed skin.

Chapter 7

HIV Infection and Pregnancy

HIV AND PREGNANCY

Antiretroviral therapy reduces the risk of perinatal transmission by lowering maternal HIV RNA and by providing pre- and post-exposure prophylaxis for the infant. The risk of perinatal infection has dropped from 25–30% without intervention to 2% or lower with combination antiretroviral therapy (MMWR Morb Mortal Wkly Rep 2005;55:592-7), especially when ART reduces HIV RNA to below the levels of detection. Although the risk of vertical transmission correlates with maternal viral load, there is no maternal viral load below which the risk of transmission is zero (J Infect Dis 2001; 183:539-45). As a result, combination therapy is indicated for all pregnant women, regardless of baseline HIV RNA or CD4 cell count.

Treatment recommendations for pregnant women are updated frequently based on clinical studies and data collected by the Antiretroviral Pregnancy Registry (www.apregistry.com/index.htm). The most recent version of the US Public Health Service Task Force treatment guidelines was updated May 2010 and is available at aidsinfo.nih.gov. The National Perinatal HIV Hotline (1-888-448-8765) provides free clinical consultation on all aspects of perinatal HIV care. This service is particularly useful in settings where clinicians may not see a large volume of HIV-infected pregnant women.

In settings where safe, affordable and feasible alternatives are available and culturally acceptable, breastfeeding is not recommended for HIV-infected women. By contrast, in many resource-limited settings, breastfeeding is preferred, with data now strongly supporting the benefits of ongoing ART to the mother in preventing HIV transmission to the newborn during the breastfeeding period (Shapiro N Engl J Med. 2010 Jun 17;362(24):2282-94).

INITIAL EVALUATION

Initial evaluation of the HIV-infected pregnant woman requires assessment of the considerations shown in Table 7.1.

Table 7.1. Initial Evaluation of HIV-Infected Pregnant Women

- Degree of immunodeficiency (defined by current and past CD4 cell counts)
- Risk for disease progression and perinatal transmission (determined by HIV RNA)
- If HIV RNA is detectable, whether an antiretroviral resistance is present (determined by resistance testing; previous tests should also be reviewed)
- Need for opportunistic infection prophylaxis
- Baseline hematologic, metabolic, renal, and hepatic parameters
- Complete history of past and current antiretroviral therapy regimens
- Presence of co-infections that might require treatment or special care of the newborn (syphilis, gonorrhea, chlamydia, genital herpes simplex, hepatitis B, hepatitis C)
- Assessment of supportive care needs

INITIATION OF ANTIRETROVIRAL THERAPY IN PREGNANCY

Decisions regarding when to start treatment and what regimen to use depends on several factors, including; (1) gestational age of the pregnancy; (2) results of the laboratory testing (Table 7.2); and (3) known, suspected, or unknown effects of individual drugs on the fetus and newborn. An overview of antiretroviral therapy in pregnancy is shown in Tables 7.3 and 7.4.

HIV-infected women in their first trimester of pregnancy who are not on antiretroviral therapy may consider delaying initiation of treatment until after 10–12 weeks gestation, unless they require therapy for their own health, in which case treatment should be started as soon as indicated. For women already on ART who become pregnant, treatment should be continued, with modifications as indicated to avoid possible teratogenic agents (e.g., efavirenz) and to achieve virologic suppression (see following discussion). For pregnant women with acute HIV infection, treatment should be started immediately given the high HIV RNA levels associated with this condition. Before starting treatment, it is important to emphasize the need for adherence to medical therapy. Patients should also be instructed to have a low threshold for reporting any potential side effects early, especially those that may reduce medication compliance, so that treatment can be altered and/or symptomatic relief for the side effect can be provided.

GOALS OF THERAPY AND MONITORING

The goal of treatment is the same as for non-pregnant individuals: to ensure an undetectable HIV RNA using the most sensitive available assay. Once antiretroviral therapy is initiated, monitoring of HIV RNA is recommended at 1–2 weeks, then monthly thereafter until the HIV RNA is undetectable, then every 2 months after that. The CD4 cell count should be obtained every 3 months as for non-pregnant adults. Laboratory monitoring for toxicity can be performed at the same time as HIV RNA testing. A general overview of antiretroviral therapy during pregnancy and labor and to the newborn is summarized in Table 7.2.

In the case of virologic failure—i.e., inability to achieve an undetectable HIV RNA or viral rebound occurs—repeat resistance testing is indicated. Subsequent management will depend on assessment of medication adherence and the degree of resistance detected on testing, as described in Chapter 4. For women who have not achieved virologic suppression near the time of delivery, especially if the HIV RNA exceeds 1000 copies/mL, a scheduled cesarean delivery is recommended at 38 weeks gestation. In addition, an elective admission to the hospital for directly observed antiretroviral therapy might enable a greater decline in HIV RNA, further reducing risk of transmission.

Table 7.2. Overview of Antiretroviral Therapy (ART) During Pregnancy, Labor, and to the Infant Postpartum

Setting	Regimen
Antepartum	Combination ART should be started with a goal of HIV RNA suppression. Women who require ART solely to prevent perinatal HIV transmission may wish to delay starting therapy until after week 10–12 of gestation. If treatment is needed for maternal health based on standard adult treatment guidelines, it should be started when indicated, even during the first trimester. ZDV should be included in the regimen unless there is severe toxicity or resistance. Commonly used regimens include ZDV/3TC (co-formulated) plus a boosted PI such as LPV/r (preferred), ATV/r, or SQV/r. EFV should not be used (especially in the first trimester) due to animal data showing increased risk of CNS defects. Nevirapine may be considered only if the maternal CD4 cell count is < 250 cells/mm³. Tenofovir, a commonly-used and preferred NRTI in nonpregnant women, should be used only in certain circumstances (e.g., intolerance or resistance to zidovudine or chronic hepatitis B infection) because of concerns regarding the potential for fetal toxicity. In animal studies, this toxicity is decreased fetal growth and reduction in bone porosity. However, in many women already on tenofovir when they become pregant, our practice is to continue it rather than replacing it with zidovudine.
Intrapartum	ZDV is administered intravenously, with a loading dose of 2 mg/kg over 1 hour, followed by continuous infusion of 1 mg/kg/hr until delivery. Other components of the antiretroviral regimen are continued through delivery, with the exception of d4T (potential antagonism between ZDV and d4T). HIV-infected women who present in active labor without having received prepartum combination ART should receive intravenous ZDV as described above. Some clinicians also will give the mother a single dose of NVP, which further reduces the HIV transmission rate but also carries the risk of inducing NNRTI resistance. As a result, if such a strategy is chosen, strong consideration should be given to initiating a dual ART regimen (e.g., ZDV/3TC) and continuing it for at least 7 days postpartum to reduce risk of selecting for NVP or other resistance.
Postpartum	Combination ART is continued if indicated based on maternal clinical and immunological status. For women taking ART solely to prevent vertical transmission, the risks and benefits of continuing vs. discontinuing therapy should be discussed. Infants should receive oral ZDV syrup at a dose of 2 mg/kg q6h for the first 6 weeks of life. Infants born to women with known ZDV resistance should have their postpartum regimen selected in consultation with a pediatric infectious diseases/HIV specialist.

MANAGEMENT OF HIV-INFECTED PREGNANT WOMEN CURRENTLY RECEIVING ANTIRETROVIRAL THERAPY

Women currently receiving a <u>suppressive</u> antiretroviral regimen at the onset of pregnancy should continue the successful regimen, even in the first trimester. Discontinuation of therapy will lead to virologic rebound, potentially increasing the risk of disease progression, viral resistance, and vertical transmission. In general, the same suppressive regimen should be continued unless the regimen includes agents that might have an adverse effect on fetal or maternal outcomes. EFV should be avoided during pregnancy (especially in the first trimester) because of reports of malformations in monkeys and case reports of fetal open neural tube defects in infants exposed early in pregnancy (Arch Intern Med 2002;162:355). Similarly, women who are trying to conceive or who are sexually active without using effective or consistent contraception should not receive EFV-containing regimens. Regimens containing stavudine and didanosine should not be used during pregnancy due to an increased risk of lactic acidosis and hepatic steatosis in women on these agents; even using these drugs singly should be done with caution.

Women receiving a <u>non-suppressive</u> antiretroviral regimen at the onset of pregnancy should undergo assessment for virologic failure as described in Chapter 3. Selection of the optimal regimen is based on medication adherence, results of resistance testing, and understanding the known and unknown safety issues associated with antiretroviral agents in pregnancy.

In general, if antiretroviral therapy is given solely for prevention of perinatal HIV transmission—sometimes termed ART prophylaxis—the continuation of therapy after delivery is currently considered option, much as treatment in non-pregnant patients with CD4 cell counts > 500. Based on current treatment guidelines for non-pregnant adults, this option would be limited to asymptomatic pregnant women with a CD4 cell count > 500 cells/mm³. Depending on the pretreatment CD4 cell count and tolerability of the regimen, some women may elect to continue treatment given the possible benefits of early therapy and hence should be given this option. During pregnancy, if treatment must be stopped for severe toxicity or pregnancy-induced hyperemesis, all drugs should generally be stopped at the same time and then reinitiated together. The exception to this practice is for NNRTI-based treatment; if possible, the NRTI backbone should be continued for 7 days after stopping the NRTI to avoid selecting for NNRTI resistance.

OTHER MANAGEMENT AND MONITORING MEASURES

A. **Other Management Considerations.** Pregnant HIV-infected women should be instructed to discontinue cigarettes, illicit drugs, and unprotected sex, and to avoid breastfeeding. Prophylaxis against opportunistic infections is indicated as for nonpregnant HIV-infected women (Chapter 5). Because of concern over antiretroviral therapy and an increase in pregnancy-induced hyperglycemia, standard glucose-loading tests should be performed earlier in pregnancy than typical, and then repeated in the third trimester.

B. **Fetal Monitoring.** Specific adverse obstetrical outcomes have not been ascribed to antiretroviral therapy. Nevertheless, many providers monitor fetal anatomy, growth, and well-being with regular frequency using ultrasound, non-stress testing, and biophysical profiles. Specifically, first trimester ultrasound is recommended to confirm gestational age and to guide the timing of scheduled cesarean delivery (recommended at 38 weeks gestation for women who have not achieved virologic suppression). For patients not seen until later in gestation, second trimester ultrasound can be used to assess fetal anatomy and determine gestational age. Second trimester ultrasound assessment of fetal anatomy is also recommended for women receiving combination antiretroviral therapy during the first trimester, especially if the regimen included EFV. Third trimester ultrasound assessment of fetal growth and well-being should also be considered for woman receiving a combination drug regimen for which there is limited experience with use in pregnancy. The need for non-stress testing and other assessments is based on ultrasound findings and the presence of maternal comorbidities.

POSTPARTUM MANAGEMENT

Children born to HIV-infected women need to be assessed for the possibility of HIV infection and for short- and long-term toxicities due to in-utero exposure to antiretroviral agents. Exposure to antiretroviral agents should become a part of the child's permanent medical record. Further arrangements are needed for long-term care of the woman, including primary and HIV-specialty care appointments, made prior to hospital discharge, and family planning counseling. Mental health status and the possibility of postpartum depression also need to be assessed, and appropriate supports need to be put into place. The importance of adherence to antiretroviral therapy postpartum should be stressed at every patient visit. Case management services best assure adequate support and compliance with healthcare needs.

Table 7.3. Antiretroviral Drug Classes Used in Pregnant HIV-Infected Women (also see Table 7.4 for information on individual drugs)

Drug Class	Concerns in Pregnancy	Use in Pregnancy
NRTIs	Potential maternal and infant mitochondrial toxicity	NRTIs are recommended for use as part of combination regimens, usually including 2 NRTIs with either an NNRTI or one or more PIs. While single and dual NRTI therapy were used in the past for prevention of perinatal transmission, these strategies are no longer recommended and women should receive fully-suppressive regimens.

Table 7.3. Antiretroviral Drug Classes Used in Pregnant HIV-Infected Women (also see Table 7.4 for information on individual drugs) (cont'd)

Drug Class	Concerns in Pregnancy	Use in Pregnancy
NNRTIs	Hypersensitivity reactions to NVP, including hepatic toxicity and rash, more common in women; unclear if increased in pregnancy.	NNRTIs are recommended for use in combination regimens with 2 NRTI drugs.
Protease Inhibitors (PIs)	Hyperglycemia, new onset or exacerbation of diabetes mellitus, and diabetic ketoacidosis reported with PI use; unclear if pregnancy increases risk. Conflicting data regarding preterm delivery in women receiving PIs.	PIs are recommended for use in combination regimens with 2 NRTI drugs.
Entry Inhibitors (fusion inhibitors, CCR5 antagonists)	Little experience in human pregnancy.	Safety and pharmacokinetics data in pregnancy are insufficient to recommend use during pregnancy.
Integrase Inhibitors	Little experience in human pregnancy.	Safety and pharmacokinetics data in pregnancy are insufficient to recommend use during pregnancy.

From: Public Health Service Recommendation for Use of Antiretroviral Drugs in Pregnant HIV-Infected Women for Maternal Health and Interventions to Reduce Perinatal HIV Transmission in the United States. May 2010. aidsinfo.nih.gov.

Table 7.4. Antiretroviral Drug Use in Pregnant HIV-Infected Women: Pharmacokinetic and Toxicity Data in Human Pregnancy and Recommendations for Use in Pregnancy

Antiretroviral Drug	Pharmacokinetics in Pregnancy	Concerns in Pregnancy	Recommendations for Use in Pregnancy
NRTIs/NtRTIs		See text for discussion of potential maternal and infant mitochondrial toxicity.	NRTIs are recommended for use as part of combination regimens, usually including two NRTIs with either an NNRTI or one or more PIs. Use of single or dual NRTIs alone is not recommended for treatment of HIV infection.
		RECOMMENDED AGENTS	
Lamivudine*	Pharmacokinetics not significantly altered in pregnancy; no change in dose indicated.	No evidence of human teratogenicity (can rule out 1.5-fold increase in overall birth defects). Well-tolerated, short-term safety demonstrated for mother and infant. If hepatitis B coinfected, possible hepatitis B flare if drug stopped postpartum.	Because of extensive experience with lamivudine in pregnancy in combination with zidovudine, lamivudine plus zidovudine is the recommended dual NRTI backbone for pregnant women.
Zidovudine*	Pharmacokinetics not significantly altered in pregnancy; no change in dose indicated.	No evidence of human teratogenicity (can rule out 1.5-fold increase in overall birth defects). Well-tolerated, short-term safety demonstrated for mother and infant.	Preferred NRTI for use in combination antiretroviral regimens in pregnancy based on efficacy studies and extensive experience. Zidovudine should be included in the antenatal antiretroviral regimen unless there is severe toxicity, stavudine use, documented resistance, or the woman is already on a fully suppressive regimen.

Table 7.4. Antiretroviral Drug Use in Pregnant HIV-Infected Women: Pharmacokinetic and Toxicity Data in Human Pregnancy and Recommendations for Use in Pregnancy (cont'd)

Antiretroviral Drug	Pharmacokinetics in Pregnancy	Concerns in Pregnancy	Recommendations for Use in Pregnancy
ALTERNATE AGENTS			
Abacavir*	Pharmacokinetics not significantly altered in pregnancy; no change in dose indicated.	No evidence of human teratogenicity (can rule out 2-fold increase in overall birth defects). Hypersensitivity reactions occur in ~5%–8% of nonpregnant persons; fatal reactions occur in a much smaller percentage of persons and are usually associated with rechallenge. Rate of hypersensitivity reactions in pregnancy is unknown. Testing for HLA-B*5701 identifies patients at risk of reactions and should be done and documented as negative before starting abacavir. Patient should be educated regarding symptoms of hypersensitivity reaction.	Alternate NRTI for dual nucleoside backbone of combination regimens. See footnote regarding use in triple NRTI regimen.#
Didanosine	Pharmacokinetics not significantly altered in pregnancy; no change in dose indicated.	Cases of lactic acidosis, some fatal, have been reported in pregnant women receiving didanosine and stavudine together.	Alternate NRTI for dual nucleoside backbone of combination regimens. Didanosine should be used with stavudine only if no other alternatives are available.
Emtricitabine†	Pharmacokinetic study shows slightly lower levels in third trimester compared	No evidence of human teratogenicity (can rule out 2-fold increase in overall birth defects).	Alternate NRTI for dual nucleoside backbone of combination regimens.

Stavudine	to postpartum. No clear need to increase dose. Pharmacokinetics not significantly altered in pregnancy; no change in dose indicated.	No evidence of human teratogenicity (can rule out 2-fold increase in overall birth defects). Cases of lactic acidosis, some fatal, have been reported in pregnant women receiving didanosine and stavudine together.	Alternate NRTI for dual nucleoside backbone of combination regimens. Stavudine should be used with didanosine only if no other alternatives are available. Do not use with zidovudine due to potential for antagonism.

USE IN SPECIAL CIRCUMSTANCES

Tenofovir†	Limited studies in human pregnancy; data indicate AUC lower in third trimester than postpartum but trough levels similar.	No evidence of human teratogenicity (can rule out 2-fold increase in overall birth defects). Studies in monkeys at doses approximately 2-fold higher than dosage for human therapeutic use show decreased fetal growth and reduction in fetal bone porosity within 2 months of starting maternal therapy. Clinical studies in humans (particularly children) show bone demineralization with chronic use; clinical significance unknown. Significant placental passage in humans (cord:maternal blood ratio 0.6–0.99). If hepatitis B coinfected, possible hepatitis B flare if drug stopped postpartum.	Because of limited data on use in human pregnancy and concern regarding potential fetal bone effects, tenofovir should be used as a component of a maternal combination regimen only after careful consideration of other alternatives. Because of potential for renal toxicity, renal function should be monitored.

Table 7.4. Antiretroviral Drug Use in Pregnant HIV-Infected Women: Pharmacokinetic and Toxicity Data in Human Pregnancy and Recommendations for Use in Pregnancy (cont'd)

Antiretroviral Drug	Pharmacokinetics in Pregnancy	Concerns in Pregnancy	Recommendations for Use in Pregnancy
		USE IN SPECIAL CIRCUMSTANCES (cont'd)	
NNRTIs		Hypersensitivity reactions, including hepatic toxicity, and rash more common in women; unclear if increased in pregnancy.	NNRTIs are recommended for use in combination regimens with 2 NRTI drugs.
		RECOMMENDED AGENTS	
Nevirapine	Pharmacokinetics not significantly altered in pregnancy; no change in dose indicated.	No evidence of human teratogenicity (can rule out 2-fold increase in overall birth defects). Increased risk of symptomatic, often rash-associated, and potentially fatal liver toxicity among women with CD4 counts > 250/mm³ when first initiating therapy; unclear if pregnancy increases risk.	Nevirapine should be initiated in pregnant women with CD4 counts > 250 cells/mm³ only if benefit clearly outweighs risk, due to the increased risk of potentially life-threatening hepatotoxicity in women with high CD4 counts. Women who enter pregnancy on nevirapine regimens and are tolerating them well may continue therapy, regardless of CD4 count.
		USE IN SPECIAL CIRCUMSTANCES	
Efavirenz†	Small study in 13 breastfeeding women in Rwanda of 600 mg once daily; postpartum peak levels during lactation were 61% higher than previously reported in	FDA Pregnancy Class D; significant malformations (anencephaly, anophthalmia, cleft palate) were observed in 3 (15%) of 20 infants born to cynomolgus monkeys receiving efavirenz during the first trimester at a dose giving plasma levels	Use of efavirenz should be avoided in the first trimester. Use after the first trimester can be considered if, after consideration of other alternatives, this is the best choice for a specific woman. If efavirenz is to be continued postpartum, adequate contraception must be assured.

	HIV-infected nonpregnant individuals at that dose.	comparable to systemic human therapeutic exposure. There are 6 retrospective case reports and 1 prospective case report of neural tube defects in humans with first-trimester exposure; relative risk unclear.	Women of childbearing potential must be counseled regarding the teratogenic potential of efavirenz and avoidance of pregnancy while on the drug. Because of the known failure rates even with contraception, alternate antiretroviral regimens should be strongly considered in women of childbearing potential.
INSUFFICIENT DATA TO RECOMMEND USE			
Etravirine	No pharmacokinetic studies in human pregnancy.	No experience in human pregnancy.	Safety and pharmacokinetics in pregnancy data are insufficient to recommend use during pregnancy.
Protease Inhibitors (PIs)		Hyperglycemia, new onset or exacerbation of diabetes mellitus, and diabetic ketoacidosis reported with PI use; unclear if pregnancy increases risk. Conflicting data regarding preterm delivery in women receiving PIs (see text).	PIs are recommended for use in combination regimens with 2 NRTI drugs.
RECOMMENDED AGENTS			
Lopinavir/ritonavir	Pharmacokinetic studies of the new lopinavir/ritonavir tablet formulation are under way, but data are not yet available.	No evidence of human teratogenicity (can rule out 2-fold increase in overall birth defects). Well-tolerated, short-term safety demonstrated in Phase I/II studies.	Pharmacokinetic studies of the tablet formulation are under way but are not yet conclusive as to the optimal dose in pregnancy. Some experts would administer standard dosing (2 tablets twice daily) throughout pregnancy and monitor virologic response and lopinavir drug levels, if available. Other experts, extrapolating from the capsule formulation pharmacokinetic data, would increase the dose of the tablet formulation during the third trimester (from 2 tablets to

Table 7.4. Antiretroviral Drug Use in Pregnant HIV-Infected Women: Pharmacokinetic and Toxicity Data in Human Pregnancy and Recommendations for Use in Pregnancy (cont'd)

Antiretroviral Drug	Pharmacokinetics in Pregnancy	Concerns in Pregnancy	Recommendations for Use in Pregnancy
		RECOMMENDED AGENTS (cont'd)	
			3 tablets twice daily), returning to standard dosing postpartum. Once-daily lopinavir/ritonavir dosing is not recommended during pregnancy because there are no data to address whether drug levels are adequate with such administration.
		ALTERNATE AGENTS	
Atazanavir (recommended to be combined with low-dose ritonavir boosting)	Two of three intensive pharmacokinetic studies of atazanavir with ritonavir boosting during pregnancy suggest that standard dosing results in decreased plasma concentrations compared to nonpregnant adults. Atazanavir concentrations further reduced ~25% with concomitant tenofovir use.	No evidence of human teratogenicity (can rule out 2-fold increase in overall birth defects). Transplacental passage is low, with cord blood concentration averaging 10%–16% of the maternal delivery atazanavir concentration. Theoretical concern re: increased indirect bilirubin levels exacerbating physiologic hyperbilirubinemia in the neonate not observed in clinical trials to date.	Alternative PI for use in combination regimens in pregnancy. Should give as low-dose ritonavir-boosted regimen, may use once-daily dosing. In treatment-naïve patients unable to tolerate ritonavir, 400 mg once-daily dosing without ritonavir boosting may be considered, although there are no data describing atazanavir concentrations or efficacy under these circumstances. If coadministered with tenofovir, atazanavir must be given with low-dose ritonavir boosting.
Indinavir (combined with low-dose ritonavir boosting)	Two studies including 18 women receiving indinavir 800 mg three times daily showed markedly lower	No evidence of human teratogenicity (can rule out 2-fold increase in overall birth defects). Theoretical concern re: increased	Alternate PI for use in combination regimens in pregnancy. Must give as low-dose ritonavir-boosted regimen.

	levels during pregnancy compared to postpartum, although suppression of HIV RNA was seen. In a study of ritonavir-boosted indinavir (400 mg indinavir/100 mg ritonavir twice daily), 82% of women met the target trough level.	indirect bilirubin levels, which may exacerbate physiologic hyperbilirubinemia in the neonate, but minimal placental passage. Use of unboosted indinavir during pregnancy is not recommended.	
Nelfinavir	Adequate drug levels are achieved in pregnant women with nelfinavir 1,250 mg given twice daily, although levels are variable in late pregnancy. In a study of pregnant women in their second and third trimester dosed at 1,250 mg given twice daily, women in the third trimester had lower concentration of nelfinavir than women in the second trimester. In a study of the new 625-mg tablet formulation dosed at 1, 250 mg twice daily, lower AUC and peak levels were observed during the third trimester of pregnancy than postpartum.	No evidence of human teratogenicity (can rule out 2-fold increase in overall birth defects). Well-tolerated, short-term safety demonstrated for mother and infant.	Given pharmacokinetic data and extensive experience with use in pregnancy, nelfinavir is an alternative PI for combination regimens in pregnant women receiving combination antiretroviral drugs only for perinatal prophylaxis. In clinical trials of initial therapy in nonpregnant adults, nelfinavir-based regimens had a lower rate of viral response compared to lopinavir-ritonavir or efavirenz-based regimens but similar viral response to atazanavir- or nevirapine-based regimens.

Table 7.4. Antiretroviral Drug Use in Pregnant HIV-Infected Women: Pharmacokinetic and Toxicity Data in Human Pregnancy and Recommendations for Use in Pregnancy (cont'd)

Antiretroviral Drug	Pharmacokinetics in Pregnancy	Concerns in Pregnancy	Recommendations for Use in Pregnancy
		ALTERNATE AGENTS (cont'd)	
Ritonavir	Phase I/II study in pregnancy showed lower levels during pregnancy compared to postpartum.	Limited experience at full dose in human pregnancy; has been used as low-dose ritonavir boosting with other PIs.	Given low levels in pregnant women when used alone, recommended for use in combination with second PI as low-dose ritonavir "boost" to increase levels of second PI.
Saquinavir HGC (combined with low-dose ritonavir boosting)	Limited pharmacokinetic data on saquinavir HGC and the new 500-mg tablet formulation suggest that 1,000 mg saquinavir HGC/100 mg ritonavir given twice daily achieves adequate saquinavir drug levels in pregnant women.	Well-tolerated, short-term safety demonstrated for mother and infant for saquinavir in combination with low-dose ritonavir.	There are only limited pharmacokinetic data on saquinavir HGC and the new tablet formulation in pregnancy. Ritonavir-boosted saquinavir HGC or saquinavir tablets are alternative PIs for combination regimens in pregnancy and are alternative initial antiretroviral recommendations for nonpregnant adults. Must give as low-dose ritonavir-boosted regimen.
		INSUFFICIENT DATA TO RECOMMEND USE	
Darunavir (combined with low-dose ritonavir boosting)	No pharmacokinetic studies in human pregnancy.	No experience in human pregnancy.	Safety and pharmacokinetics in pregnancy data are insufficient to recommend use during pregnancy. Must give as low-dose ritonavir-boosted regimen.
Fosamprenavir (recommended to be combined with low-dose ritonavir boosting)	No pharmacokinetic studies in human pregnancy.	Limited experience in human pregnancy.	Safety and pharmacokinetics in pregnancy data are insufficient to recommend use during pregnancy. Recommended to be given as low-dose ritonavir-boosted regimen.

Tipranavir (combined with low-dose ritonavir boosting)	No pharmacokinetic studies in human pregnancy.	No experience in human pregnancy.	Safety and pharmacokinetics in pregnancy data are insufficient to recommend use during pregnancy. Must give as low-dose ritonavir-boosted regimen.
ENTRY INHIBITORS			
INSUFFICIENT DATA TO RECOMMEND USE			
Enfuvirtide	No pharmacokinetic studies in human pregnancy.	Minimal data in human pregnancy.	Safety and pharmacokinetics in pregnancy data are insufficient to recommend use during pregnancy.
Maraviroc	No pharmacokinetic studies in human pregnancy.	No experience in human pregnancy.	Safety and pharmacokinetics in pregnancy data are insufficient to recommend use during pregnancy.
INTEGRASE INHIBITORS			
INSUFFICIENT DATA TO RECOMMEND USE			
Raltegravir	No pharmacokinetic studies in human pregnancy.	No experience in human pregnancy.	Safety and pharmacokinetics in pregnancy data are insufficient to recommend use during pregnancy.

Abbreviations: AUC: area under the curve; HGC: hard gel capsule; NRTI: nucleoside reverse transcriptase inhibitor; NtRTI: nucleotide reverse transcriptase inhibitor; NNRTI: non-nucleoside reverse transcriptase inhibitor; PI: protease inhibitor.

* Zidovudine and lamivudine are included as a fixed-dose combination in Combivir; zidovudine, lamivudine, and abacavir are included as a fixed-dose combination in Trizivir; lamivudine and abacavir are included as a fixed-dose combination in Epzicom.

† Emtricitabine and tenofovir are included as a fixed-dose combination in Truvada; emtricitabine, tenofovir, and efavirenz are included as a fixed-dose combination in Atripla.

\# Triple NRTI regimens including abacavir have been less potent virologically compared to PI-based combination antiretroviral drug regimens. Triple NRTI regimens should be used only when an NNRTI- or PI-based combination regimen cannot be used (e.g., due to significant drug interactions).

From: Public Health Service Recommendation for Use of Antiretroviral Drugs in Pregnant HIV-Infected Women for Maternal Health and Interventions to Reduce Perinatal HIV Transmission in the United States. May 2010. aidsinfo.nih.gov.

Chapter 8

Post-Exposure Prophylaxis

OCCUPATIONAL POST-EXPOSURE PROPHYLAXIS (PEP)

The CDC estimates > 600,000 significant exposures to blood-borne pathogens occur yearly. Of 56 confirmed cases of HIV acquisition in healthcare workers, more than 90% involved percutaneous exposure, with the remaining cases due to mucous membrane/non-intact skin exposure. Estimates of HIV seroconversion rates after percutaneous and mucous membrane exposure to HIV-infected blood are 0.3% and 0.09%, respectively; lower rates of transmission occur after nonintact skin exposure, and no transmission has thus far been reported to occur through intact skin. (By comparison, the risks of seroconversion after percutaneous exposure to Hepatitis B and Hepatitis C viruses are 30% and 3%, respectively.) Risk factors for increased risk of HIV transmission after percutaneous exposure include deep injury (odds ratio 16.1), visible blood on device (odds ratio 5.2), source patient is terminally ill (odds ratio 6.4), or needle was in source patient's artery/vein (odds ratio 5.1); ZDV prophylaxis reduces the risk of transmission (odds ratio 0.2). All guidelines suggest PEP should be administered as soon as possible after exposure, but there is no absolute window (e.g., within 1–2 weeks) after which PEP should be withheld following serious exposure. Because clear-cut efficacy data for patient selection and PEP regimens are lacking, most experts rely on CDC guidelines, which emphasize the type of exposure and potential infectivity of the source patient (Tables 8.1 and 8.2). The latest US Public Health Service (USPHS) guidelines for the management of occupational exposure to HIV and post-exposure prophylaxis are summarized below and are detailed in *Morbidity Mortality Weekly Review* 54(RR9):1–17, Sept 30, 2005, or at www.aidsinfo.nih.gov/guidelines. Additional information can be found at the National Clinicians' Post-exposure Prophylaxis Hotline (www.ucsf.edu/hivcntr). Occupationally acquired HIV infections and PEP failures should be reported to the CDC at (800) 893-0485.

Recommendations from the updated 2005 USPHS guidelines include:

* Initiate PEP as soon as possible after exposure (preferably within hours), and continue PEP for 4 weeks if tolerated (Tables 8.1 and 8.2)

* Seek expert consultation if viral resistance is suspected

* Offer pregnancy testing to all women of childbearing age not known to be pregnant

* Advise exposed persons to seek medical evaluation for any acute illness during follow-up

* Perform HIV-antibody testing and HIV RNA testing for any illness compatible with an acute retroviral syndrome (e.g., pharyngitis, fever, rash, myalgia, fatigue, malaise, lymphadenopathy)

* Perform HIV-antibody testing for at least 6 months post-exposure (at baseline, 6 weeks, 3 months, and 6 months)

* Advise exposed persons to use precautions to prevent secondary transmission during follow-up, especially during the first 6–12 weeks, when most HIV-infected patients will seroconvert. Precautions include sexual abstinence or use of condoms, refrain from donating blood, plasma, organs, tissue or semen, and discontinuation of breast-feeding after high-risk exposures

- Evaluate exposed persons taking PEP within 72 hours after exposure, and monitor for drug toxicity for at least 2 weeks. Approximately 50% will experience nausea, malaise, headache, or anorexia, and about one-third will discontinue PEP due to drug toxicity. Lab monitoring should include (at a minimum) a CBC, serum creatinine, liver function tests, serum glucose (if receiving a protease inhibitor to detect hyperglycemia), and monitoring for HBV and HCV. Serious adverse events should be reported to the FDA's MedWatch Program

- If available, employees with workplace exposure should follow up in their designated occupational health sites according to employer policies. This will help retain rights and/ or benefits defined by the job in case of infection

Table 8.1. Recommendations for Occupational HIV Post-Exposure Prophylaxis (see Table 8.2 for basic and expanded PEP regimens)

Exposure Type	Infection Status of Source Patient				
	HIV (+) Class 1*	HIV (+) Class 2*	HIV status unknown†	Unknown source††	HIV (−)
Percutaneous injuries *Less severe*+	Recommend basic 2-drug PEP	Recommend expanded 3-drug PEP	Generally no PEP warranted; consider basic 2-drug PEP††† for source with HIV risk factors**	Generally no PEP warranted; consider basic 2-drug PEP††† if exposure to HIV-infected persons is likely	No PEP warranted
More severe+	Recommend expanded 3-drug PEP	Recommend expanded ≥ 3-drug PEP			
Mucous membrane/ nonintact skin exposure *Small volume*++	Consider basic 2-drug PEP	Recommend basic 2-drug PEP			
Large volume++	Recommend basic 2-drug PEP	Recommend expanded ≥ 3-drug PEP			

HIV (+) = HIV-positive; HIV (−) = HIV-negative; PEP = post-exposure prophylaxis

*   Class 1: Asymptomatic HIV infection or known low HIV RNA (e.g., < 1500 RNA copies/mL)
    Class 2: Symptomatic HIV infection, AIDS, acute seroconversion, or known high HIV RNA. If drug resistance is a concern, obtain expert consultation; do not delay PEP pending consultation

**   Source with HIV risk factors: If PEP is administered and the source patient is later determined to be HIV-negative, PEP should be discontinued

†   HIV status unknown: for example, source patient is deceased with no samples available for HIV testing

††   Unknown source: for example, a needle from a sharps disposal container (percutaneous injury)

††† PEP is optional; discuss with patient and individualize decision

+   Less severe: for example, a solid needle and superficial injury. More severe: for example, a large-bore hollow needle, deep puncture, visible blood on device, or needle used in patient's artery/vein

++   Small volume: a few drops. Large volume: major blood splash

From: Updated US Public Health Service Guidelines for the Management of Occupational Exposures to HBV, HCV, and HIV and Recommendations for Post-exposure Prophylaxis, MMWR;50 (RR-9):1–17, September 30, 2005 (www.aidsinfo.nih.gov)

Table 8.2. Basic and Expanded Occupational HIV Post-Exposure Prophylaxis Regimens (see Table 8.1 for patient selection guidelines)

Regimen	Dosage	Comments
Basic regimen *Preferred*	Zidovudine 300 mg BID or 200 mg TID with food + lamivudine 300 mg QD or 150 mg BID. Available as Combivir tablet: dose = 1 tablet BID	<u>Advantages</u>: ZDV associated with decreased risk for HIV transmission; ZDV used more often than other drugs for PEP for healthcare personnel (HCP); serious toxicity rare when used for PEP; side effects predictable and manageable with antimotility and antiemetic agents; can be used by pregnant HCP; can be given as a single tablet (Combivir™) twice daily <u>Disadvantages</u>: side effects (especially nausea and fatigue) common and might result in low adherence; source-patient virus resistance to this regimen possible; potential for delayed toxicity (oncogenic/teratogenic) unknown
	Zidovudine 300 mg BID or 200 mg TID with food + emtricitabine 200 mg (one capsule) QD	<u>Advantages</u>: ZDV: see above; convenient (once daily); well tolerated; long intracellular half-life (~ 40 hours) <u>Disadvantages</u>: ZDV: see above; FTC: rash perhaps more frequent than with 3TC; no long-term experience with this drug; cross resistance to 3TC; hyperpigmentation among non-Caucasians with long-term use: 3%
	Tenofovir 300 mg QD + lamivudine 300 mg QD or 150 mg BID	<u>Advantages</u>: 3TC: see above; TDF: convenient dosing (single pill once daily); resistance profile activity against certain thymidine analogue mutations; well tolerated <u>Disadvantages</u>: TDF: same class warnings as nucleoside reverse transcriptase inhibitors (NRTIs); drug interactions; increased TDF concentrations among persons taking atazanavir and lopinavir/ritonavir; need to monitor patients for TDF-associated toxicities; preferred dosage of atazanavir if used with TDF: ATV 300 mg + ritonavir 100 mg once daily + TDF 300 mg once daily

Table 8.2. Basic and Expanded Occupational HIV Post-Exposure Prophylaxis Regimens (see Table 8.1 for patient selection guidelines) (cont'd)

Regimen	Dosage	Comments
Basic regimen *Preferred* (cont'd)	Tenofovir 300 mg QD + emtricitabine 200 mg QD. Available as Truvada tablet: dose = 1 tablet QD	<u>Advantages</u>: FTC: see above; TDF: convenient dosing (single pill once daily Truvada); resistance profile activity against certain thymidine analogue mutations; well tolerated; <u>this is our preferred NRTI pair for most exposures due to lower GI and hematologic toxicity compared to ZDV/3TC.</u> <u>Disadvantages</u>: TDF: same class warnings as (NRTIs); drug interactions; increased TDF concentrations among persons taking atazanavir and lopinavir/ritonavir; need to monitor patients for TDF-associated toxicities; preferred dosage of atazanavir if used with TDF: ATV 300 mg + ritonavir 100 mg once daily + TDF 300 mg once daily
Basic regimen *Alternate*	Lamivudine 300 mg QD or 150 mg BID + stavudine 40 mg BID (can use lower doses of 20–30 mg BID if toxicity occurs) or 30 mg BID for body weight < 60 kg	<u>Advantages</u>: 3TC: see above; d4T: gastrointestinal (GI) side effects rare <u>Disadvantages</u>: possibility that source-patient virus is resistant to this regimen; potential for delayed toxicity (oncogenic/teratogenic) unknown
	Emtricitabine 200 mg QD + stavudine 40 mg BID (can use lower doses of 20–30 mg BID if toxicity occurs) or 30 mg BID for body weight < 60 kg	<u>Advantages</u>: 3TC: see above; d4T's GI side effects rare <u>Disadvantages</u>: potential that source-patient virus is resistant to this regimen; unknown potential for delayed toxicity (oncogenic/teratogenic) unknown
Expanded regimen *Preferred*	<u>Basic regimen plus:</u> Lopinavir/ritonavir (Kaletra) 400/100 mg = 2 tablets BID with or without food	<u>Advantages</u>: potent HIV protease inhibitor; generally well-tolerated; <u>this is our preferred 3rd drug for expanded regimens due to convenient formulation and low likelihood of broad PI resistance in most sources of occupational exposures</u> <u>Disadvantages</u>: potential for serious or life-threatening drug interactions (Chapter 3); might accelerate clearance of certain drugs, including

Table 8.2. Basic and Expanded Occupational HIV Post-Exposure Prophylaxis Regimens (see Table 8.1 for patient selection guidelines) (cont'd)

Regimen	Dosage	Comments
Expanded regimen _Preferred_ (cont'd)		oral contraceptives (requiring alternative or additional contraceptive measures for women taking these drugs); can cause severe hyperlipidemia, especially hypertriglyceridemia; GI (e.g., diarrhea) events common
Alternate (basic regimen plus one of the following drugs)	Atazanavir 400 mg QD, or atazanavir 300 mg QD + ritonavir 100 mg QD	<u>Advantages</u>: potent HIV protease inhibitor; convenient dosing—once daily; generally well-tolerated <u>Disadvantages</u>: hyperbilirubinemia and jaundice common; potential for serious or life-threatening drug interactions (Chapter 3); avoid coadministration with proton pump inhibitors; separate antacids and buffered medications by 2 hours and H2-receptor antagonists by 12 hours to avoid decreasing ATV levels; caution should be used with ATV and products known to induce PR prolongation (e.g., diltiazem)
	Fosamprenavir 1400 mg BID (without ritonavir), or fosamprenavir 1400 mg QD + ritonavir 200 mg QD, or fosamprenavir 700 mg BID + ritonavir 100 mg BID	<u>Advantages</u>: once daily dosing when given with ritonavir <u>Disadvantages</u>: tolerability: GI side effects common; multiple drug interactions. Oral contraceptives decrease fosamprenavir concentrations; incidence of rash in healthy volunteers, especially when used with low doses of ritonavir. Differentiating between early drug-associated rash and acute seroconversion can be difficult and cause extraordinary concern for the exposed person
	Indinavir 800 mg BID + ritonavir 100 mg BID without regard to food, or indinavir 800 mg TID on empty stomach	<u>Advantages</u>: potent HIV inhibitor <u>Disadvantages</u>: potential for serious or life-threatening drug interactions; serious toxicity (e.g., nephrolithiasis) possible; consumption of 8 glasses of fluid/day required; hyperbilirubinemia common; must avoid this drug during late pregnancy; requires acid for absorption and cannot be taken

Table 8.2. Basic and Expanded Occupational HIV Post-Exposure Prophylaxis Regimens (see Table 8.1 for patient selection guidelines) (cont'd)

Regimen	Dosage	Comments
Expanded regimen _Alternate_ (basic regimen plus one of the following drugs) (cont'd)		simultaneously with ddI, chewable/dispersible buffered tablet formulation (doses must be separated by ≥ 1 hour)
	Saquinavir 1000 mg (given as Invirase) BID + ritonavir 100 mg BID	<u>Advantages</u>: generally well-tolerated, although GI events common <u>Disadvantages</u>: potential for serious or life-threatening drug interactions (Chapter 3)
	Nelfinavir 1250 mg (2 × 625-mg tablets or 5 × 250-mg tablets) BID with a meal	<u>Advantages</u>: generally well-tolerated, although diarrhea common <u>Disadvantages</u>: potential for serious or life-threatening drug interactions (Chapter 3); diarrhea
	Efavirenz 600 mg once daily at bedtime	<u>Advantages</u>: does not require phosphorylation before activation and might be active earlier than other antiretroviral agents (a theoretic advantage of no demonstrated clinical benefit); once daily dosing <u>Disadvantages</u>: drug associated with rash (early onset) that can be severe and might rarely progress to Stevens-Johnson syndrome; differentiating between early drug-associated rash and acute seroconversion can be difficult and cause extraordinary concern for the exposed person; CNS side effects (e.g., dizziness, somnolence, insomnia, or abnormal dreaming) common; severe psychiatric symptoms possible (dosing before bedtime might minimize these side effects); teratogen; should not be used during pregnancy; potential for serious or life-threatening drug interactions (Chapter 3)

Adapted from: US Public Health Service Guidelines. MMWR;54(RR-9):1–17, September 30, 2005

NONOCCUPATIONAL POST-EXPOSURE PROPHYLAXIS (NPEP)

In January, 2005, the US Department of Health and Human Services issued recommendations for antiretroviral PEP after sexual, injection-drug use, and other nonoccupational exposures to HIV (MMWR 2005;54[RR-2]:1–28).

A. **Evaluation.** The evaluation of person seeking nonoccupational PEP should include determination of the HIV status of the potentially exposed person, the timing and characteristics of the most recent exposure, the frequency of exposures to HIV, the HIV status of the source, and the likelihood of concomitant infection with other pathogens. Available data indicate that nonoccupational PEP is less likely to be effective if initiated > 72 hours after HIV exposure. Therefore, if initiation of nonoccupational PEP is delayed, the likelihood of benefit might not outweigh the risks associated with antiretroviral medications. Persons who engage in behaviors that result in frequent, recurrent exposures that would require sequential or near-continuous courses of antiretroviral medications (e.g., discordant sex partners who rarely use condoms or injection-drug users who often share injection equipment) should not take nonoccupational PEP. In these instances, exposed persons should instead be provided with intensive risk-reduction interventions. If the risk associated with the exposure is considered substantial, nonoccupational PEP can be started pending determination of the HIV status of the source and then stopped if the source is determined to be noninfected. The highest levels of estimated per-act risk for HIV transmission are associated with blood transfusion, needle sharing by injection-drug users, receptive anal intercourse, and percutaneous needlestick injuries. Insertive anal intercourse, penile-vaginal exposures, and oral sex represent substantially less per-act risk.

B. **Use of Antiretroviral Therapy (Tables 8.1 and 8.2).** A 28-day course of antiretroviral therapy is recommended for persons who have had nonoccupational exposure to blood, genital secretions, or other potentially infected body fluids of a persons known to be HIV infected when: (1) that exposure represents a substantial risk for HIV transmission (Figure 8.1); and (2) when the person seeks care within 72 hours of exposure. When indicated, antiretroviral nonoccupational PEP should be initiated promptly for the best chance of success. If there is concern about potential adherence and toxicity issues associated with a 3-drug regimen, a 2-drug regimen may be considered (i.e., a combination of two reverse transcriptase inhibitors). When the source-person is available for interview, their history of antiretroviral medication use and most recent viral load measurement might help avoid prescribing antiretroviral medications to which the source-virus is likely to be resistant. If the source-person is willing, it may be useful to draw blood for viral load and resistance testing if the results can be obtained promptly.

C. Follow-up Testing. All patients seeking care after HIV exposure should be tested for the presence of HIV antibodies at baseline and at 4–6 weeks, 3 months, and 6 months after exposure to determine whether HIV infection has occurred. In addition, testing for sexually transmitted diseases, hepatitis B and C, and pregnancy should be offered (Table 8.3). Patients should be instructed about the signs and symptoms associated with acute retroviral infection especially fever and rash, and asked to return for evaluation if these occur during or after nonoccupational PEP.

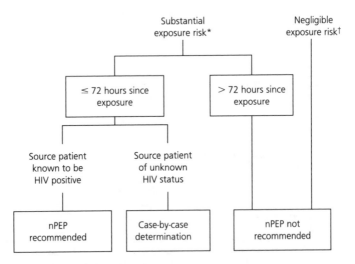

Figure 8.1. Evaluation and Treatment of Possible Nonoccupational HIV Exposures

nPEP = nonoccupational post-exposure prophylaxis

* Substantial risk for HIV exposure = exposure of vagina, rectum, eye, mouth, or other mucous membrane, nonintact skin, or percutaneous contact with blood, semen, vaginal secretions, rectal secretions, breast milk, or any body fluid that is visibly contaminated with blood when the source is know to be HIV-infected

† Negligible risk for HIV exposure = exposure of vagina, rectum, eye, mouth, or other mucous membrane, intact or nonintact skin, or percutaneous contact with urine, nasal secretions, saliva, sweat, or tears if not visibly contaminated with blood regardless of the known or suspected HIV status of the source

Table 8.3. Recommended Laboratory Evaluation for Nonoccupational Post-Exposure Prophylaxis (nPEP) of HIV Infection

Test	Baseline	During nPEP*	Time After Exposure 4–6 Weeks	Time After Exposure 3 Months	Time After Exposure 6 Months
HIV antibody testing	E, S		E	E	E
Complete blood count with differential	E	E			
Serum liver enzymes	E	E			
Sexually transmitted diseases screen (gonorrhea, chlamydia, syphilis)	E, S	E¶	E¶		
Hepatitis B serology	E, S		E¶	E¶	
Hepatitis C serology	E, S			E	E
Pregnancy test (women of reproductive age)	E	E¶	E¶		
HIV viral load	S		E**	E**	E**
HIV resistance testing	S		E**	E**	E**
CD4+ T lymphocyte count	S		E**	E**	E**

E = exposed patient, S = source

*   Other specific tests might be indicated depending on antiretrovirals prescribed. Literature pertaining to individual agents should be consulted.

§   HIV antibody testing of the source patient is indicated for sources of unknown serostatus.

¶   Additional testing for pregnancy, sexually transmitted diseases, and hepatitis B should be performed as clinically indicated.

** If determined to be HIV infected on follow-up testing; perform as clinically indicated once diagnosed.

From: Antiretroviral Post-exposure Prophylaxis after Sexual, Injection-drug Use, or Other Nonoccupational Exposure to HIV in the United States. MMWR January 21, 2005;54 (No. RR-2):1–16

Chapter 9

Antiretroviral Drug Summaries

David W. Kubiak, PharmD, BCPS
Demary Torres, PharmD

This section contains prescribing information pertinent to the clinical use of antiretroviral agents in adults, as compiled from a variety of sources, including MICROMEDEX®, Up to Date on-line version 18.2®, Department of Health and Human Services Guidelines for the use of antiretroviral agents in HIV-1-infected adults and adolescents (www.aidsinfo.nih.gov/guidelines/), December 1, 2009, manufacturers' product information, among others. The information provided is not exhaustive, and the reader is referred to other drug information references and the manufacturer's product literature for further information. Clinical use of the information provided and any consequences that may arise from its use are the responsibilities of the prescribing physician. The authors, editors, and publisher do not warrant or guarantee the information contained in this section, and do not assume and expressly disclaim any liability for errors or omissions or any consequences that may occur from such. **The use of any drug should be preceded by careful review of the package insert, which provides indications and dosing approved by the U.S. Food and Drug Administration. This information can be obtained on the website provided at the end of the reference list for each drug summary.**

Drugs are listed alphabetically by generic name; trade names follow in parentheses. To search by trade name, consult the index. Each drug summary contains the following information:

Usual Dose. Represents the usual dose to treat HIV infection in adult patients with normal hepatic and renal function. Additional information can be found in the manufacturer's package insert and product literature.

Bioavailability. Refers to the percentage of the dose reaching the systemic circulation from the site of administration (PO or IM). For PO antibiotics, bioavailability refers to the percentage of dose adsorbed from the GI tract.

Excreted Unchanged. Refers to the percentage of drug excreted unchanged, and provides an indirect measure of drug concentration in the urine/feces.

Serum Half-Life (normal/ESRD). The serum half-life ($T_{1/2}$) is the time (in hours) in which serum concentration falls by 50%. Serum half-life is useful in determining dosing interval. If the half-life of drugs eliminated by the kidneys is prolonged in end-stage renal disease (ESRD), then the total daily dose is reduced in proportion to the degree of renal dysfunction. If the half-life in ESRD is similar to the normal half-life, then the total daily dose does not change.

Plasma Protein Binding. Expressed as the percentage of drug reversibly bound to serum albumin. It is the unbound (free) portion of a drug that equilibrates with tissues and imparts antiviral activity. Plasma protein binding is not typically a factor in antimicrobial effectiveness unless binding exceeds 95%. Decreases in serum albumin (nephrotic syndrome, liver disease) or competition for protein binding from other drugs or endogenously produced substances (uremia, hyperbilirubinemia) will increase the percentage of free drug available for antimicrobial activity, and may require a decrease in dosage. Increases in serum binding proteins (trauma, surgery, critical illness) will decrease the percentage of free drug available for antimicrobial activity, and may require an increase in dosage.

Volume of Distribution (V_d). Represents the apparent volume into which the drug is distributed, and is calculated as the amount of drug in the body divided by the serum concentration (in liters/kilogram). V_d is related to total body water distribution (V_d H_2O = 0.7 L/kg). Hydrophilic (water soluble) drugs are restricted to extracellular fluid and have a $V_d \leq 0.7$ L/kg. In contrast, hydrophobic (highly lipid soluble) drugs penetrate most fluids/tissues of the body and have a large V_d. Drugs that are concentrated in certain tissues (e.g., liver) can have a V_d greatly exceeding total body water. V_d is affected by organ profusion, membrane diffusion/permeability, lipid solubility, protein binding, and state of equilibrium between body compartments. For hydrophilic drugs, increases in V_d may occur with burns, heart failure, dialysis, sepsis, cirrhosis, or mechanical ventilation; decreases in V_d may occur with trauma, hemorrhage, pancreatitis (early), or GI fluid losses. Increases in V_d may require an increase in total daily drug dose for antimicrobial effectiveness; decreases in V_d may require a decrease in drug dose. In addition to drug distribution, V_d reflects binding avidity to cholesterol membranes and concentration within organ tissues (e.g., liver).

Mode of Elimination. Refers to the primary route of inactivation/excretion of the drug, which impacts dosing adjustments in renal/hepatic failure.

Dosage Adjustments. Each grid provides dosing adjustments based on renal and hepatic function. Antimicrobial dosing for hemodialysis (HD)/peritoneal dialysis (PD) patients is the same as indicated for patients with a CrCl < 10 mL/min. Some antimicrobial agents require a supplemental dose immediately after hemodialysis (post-HD)/peritoneal dialysis (post-PD); following the supplemental dose, antimicrobial dosing should once again resume as indicated for a CrCl < 10 mL/min. "No change" indicates no change from the usual dose. "Avoid" indicates the drug should be avoided in the setting described. "None" indicates no supplemental dose is required. "No information" indicates there are insufficient data from which to make a dosing recommendation. Dosing recommendations are based on data, experience, or pharmacokinetic parameters. CVVH dosing recommendations represent general guidelines, since antibiotic removal is dependent on area/type of filter, ultrafiltration rates, and sieving coefficients; replacement dosing should be individualized and guided by serum levels, if possible. Creatinine clearance (CrCl) is used to gauge the degree of renal insufficiency, and can be estimated by the following calculation: CrCl (mL/min) = [(140 − age) × weight (kg)] / [72 × serum creatinine (mg/dL)]. The calculated value is multiplied by 0.85 for females. It is important to recognize that due to age-dependent decline in renal function, elderly patients with "normal" serum creatinines may have low CrCls requiring dosage adjustments. (For example, a 70-year-old, 50-kg female with a serum creatinine of 1.2 mg/dL has an estimated CrCl of 34 mL/min.) "Antiretroviral Dosage Adjustment" grids indicate recommended dosage adjustments when protease inhibitors (PIs) and non-nucleoside reverse transcriptase inhibitor (NNRTIs) are combined or used in conjunction with rifampin or rifabutin. These grids were compiled, in part, from "Guidelines for the Use of Antiretroviral Agents in HIV-Infected Adults and Adolescents," Panel on Clinical Practices for Treatment of HIV Infection, Department of Health and Human Services , www.aidsinfo.nih.gov/guidelines/. December 1, 2009.

Drug Interactions. Refers to common/important drug interactions, as compiled from various sources. If a specific drug interaction is well-documented, then other drugs from the same drug class (e.g., atorvastatin) may also be listed, based on theoretical considerations. Drug interactions may occur as a consequence of altered absorption (e.g., metal ion chelation of tetracycline), altered distribution (e.g., sulfonamide displacement of barbiturates from serum albumin), altered metabolism (e.g., rifampin–induced hepatic P-450 metabolism of theophylline/warfarin; chloramphenicol inhibition of phenytoin metabolism), or altered excretion (e.g., probenecid competition with penicillin for active transport in the kidney).

Adverse Side Effects. Common/important side effects are indicated.

Allergic Potential. Described as low or high. Refers to the likelihood of a hypersensitivity reaction to a particular antimicrobial.

Safety in Pregnancy. Designated by the U.S. Food and Drug Administration's (USFDA) use-in-pregnancy letter code (Table 9.1).

Antiretroviral Pregnancy Registry. To monitor maternal-fetal outcomes of pregnant women exposed to antiretroviral drugs, an Antiretroviral Pregnancy Registry has been established. Clinicians who are treating HIV-infected pregnant women are strongly encouraged to report cases of prenatal exposure to antiretroviral drugs (either administered alone or in combinations). The registry collects observational, non-experimental data regarding antiretroviral exposure during pregnancy for the purpose of assessing potential teratogenicity. Telephone: 910-251-9087 or 1-800-258-4263. Website: http://www.apregistry.com/who.htm; e-mail: registries@kendle.com

Comments. Includes various useful information for each antimicrobial agent.

Biliary Tract Penetration. Indicated as a percentage relative to peak serum concentrations. Percentages > 100% reflect concentration within the biliary system. This information is useful for the treatment of biliary tract infections.

Selected References. These references are classic, important, or recent. When available, the website containing the manufacturer's prescribing information/package insert is provided.

Table 9.1. USFDA Use-in-Pregnancy Letter Code

Category	Interpretation
A	**Controlled studies show no risk.** Adequate, well-controlled studies in pregnant women have not shown a risk to the fetus in any trimester of pregnancy
B	**No evidence of risk in humans.** Adequate, well-controlled studies in pregnant women have not shown increased risk of fetal abnormalities despite adverse findings in animals, or, in the absence of adequate human studies, animal studies show no fetal risk. The chance of fetal harm is remote, but remains a possibility
C	**Risk cannot be ruled out.** Adequate, well-controlled human studies are lacking, and animal studies have shown a risk to the fetus or are lacking. There is a chance of fetal harm if the drug is administered during pregnancy, but potential benefit from use of the drug may outweigh potential risk
D	**Positive evidence of risk.** Studies in humans or investigational or post-marketing data have demonstrated fetal risk. Nevertheless, potential benefit from use of the drug may outweigh potential risk. For example, the drug may be acceptable if needed in a life-threatening situation or serious disease for which safer drugs cannot be used or are ineffective
X	**Contraindicated in pregnancy.** Studies in animals or humans or investigational or post-marketing reports have demonstrated positive evidence of fetal abnormalities or risk which clearly outweigh any possible benefit to the patient

Abacavir (Ziagen) ABC

Drug Class: Antiretroviral NRTI (nucleoside reverse transcriptase inhibitor)
Usual Dose: HLA-B*5701 negative patients—300 mg (PO) BID
How Supplied: Oral Solution: 20 mg/mL, Oral Tablet: 300 mg
Pharmacokinetic Parameters:
Peak serum level: 3 mcg/mL
Bioavailability: 83%
Excreted unchanged (urine): 1.2%
Serum half-life (normal/ESRD): 1.5/8 hrs
Plasma protein binding: 50%
Volume of distribution (V_d): 0.86 L/kg
Primary Mode of Elimination: Hepatic
Dosage Adjustments*

CrCl 50–80 mL/min	No change
CrCl 10–50 mL/min	No change
CrCl < 10 mL/min	No change
Post-HD dose	None
Post-PD dose	None
CVVH dose	No change
Mild hepatic insufficiency	200 mg (PO) QD
Moderate or severe hepatic insufficiency	Avoid

Drug Interactions: Methadone (↑ methadone clearance with abacavir 600 mg BID); ethanol (↑ abacavir serum levels/half-life and may ↑ toxicity).
Adverse Effects: *Abacavir may cause severe hypersensitivity reactions (see comments), usually during the first 4–6 weeks of therapy,* **which may be fatal;** report cases of hypersensitivity syndrome to Abacavir

Hypersensitivity Registry at 1-800-270-0425. Drug fever/rash, abdominal pain/diarrhea, nausea, vomiting, anorexia, insomnia, weakness, headache, ↑ SGOT/SGPT, hyperglycemia, hypertriglyceridemia, lactic acidosis with hepatic steatosis (rare, but potentially life-threatening toxicity with use of NRTIs). Potential for increased cardiovascular events, especially in patients with cardiovascular risk factors.
Allergic Potential: High (~ 5%)
Safety in Pregnancy: C
Comments: May be taken with or without foods. **HLA-B*5701 testing should precede the use of abacavir or an abacavir-containing regimen to reduce the risk of hypersensitivity reaction. Immediately and permanently discontinue if a hypersensitivity reaction occurs; never restart abacavir sulfate/lamivudine following a hypersensitivity reaction** or if hypersensitivity cannot be ruled out, which may include fever, rash, fatigue, nausea, vomiting, diarrhea, abdominal pain, anorexia, respiratory symptoms., which may include fever, rash, fatigue, nausea, vomiting, diarrhea, abdominal pain, anorexia, respiratory symptoms. Ethanol increases abacavir levels by 41%.
Cerebrospinal Fluid Penetration: 27–33%

REFERENCES:
Carr A, Workman C, Smith DE, et al. Abacavir substitution for nucleoside analogs in patients with HIV lipoatrophy. A randomized trial. JAMA 288:207–15, 2002.

Cutrell A, Brothers C, Yeo J, et al. Abacavir and the potential risk of myocardial infarction. Lancet 2008 April 1, e-pub.

Katalama C, Clotet B, Plettenberg A, et al. The role of abacavir (AVC, 1592) in antiretroviral therapy-experiences patients: results from randomized, double-blind, trial. CNA3002 European Study Team. AIDS 14:781–9, 2000.

Keating MR. Antiviral agents. Mayo Clin Proc 67:160–78, 1992.

"Usual dose" assumes normal renal/hepatic function. * For renal insufficiency, give usual dose × 1 followed by maintenance dose per CrCl. For dialysis patients, dose the same as for CrCl < 10 mL/min and give supplemental (post-HD/PD dose) immediately after dialysis. CrCl = creatinine clearance; CVVH = continuous veno-venous hemo-filtration; HD/PD = hemodialysis/peritoneal dialysis. See pp. 190–193 for explanations, p. x for abbreviations

Mallal S, Phillips E, Carosi G, et al. HLA-B*5701 screening for hypersensitivity to abacavir. N Engl J Med 358:568–79, 2008.

McDowell JA, Lou Y, Symonds WS, et al. Multiple-dose pharmacokinetics and pharmacodynamics of abacavir alone and in combination with zidovudine in human immunodeficiency virus-infected adults. Antimicrob Agents Chemother 44:2061–7, 2000.

Panel on Antiretroviral Guidelines for Adults and Adolescents. Guidelines for the use of antiretroviral agents in HIV-1-infected adults and adolescents. Department of Health and Human Services. December 1, 2009; 1–161. Available at http://www.aidsinfo.nih.gov/ContentFiles/AdultandAdolescentGL.pdf.

Staszewski S, Keiser P, Mantaner J, et al. Abacavir-lamivudine-zidovudine vs. indinavir-lamivudine-zidovudine in antiretroviral-naïve HIV-infected adults: a randomized equivalence trial. JAMA 285:1155–63, 2001.

Abacavir + Lamivudine (Epzicom)

Drug Class: Antiretroviral NRTI combination
Usual Dose: HLA-B*5701 negative patients—
Epzicom tablet = abacavir 600 mg + lamivudine 300 mg. Usual dose: 1 tablet QD
How supplied: Oral Tablet: Contains 300 mg Abacavir Sulfate + 600 mg Lamivudine
Pharmacokinetic Parameters:
Peak serum level: 3/1.5 mcg/L
Bioavailability: 83/86%
Excreted unchanged (urine): 1.2/71%
Serum half-life (normal/ESRD): (1.5/8)/(5–7/20) hrs
Plasma protein binding: 50/36%
Volume of distribution (V_d): 0.86/1.3 L/kg
Primary Mode of Elimination: Hepatic/Renal
Dosage Adjustments*

CrCl < 50 mL/min	Not recommended
Post-HD dose	Not recommended
Post-PD dose	Not recommended

CVVH dose	Not recommended
Mild hepatic insufficiency	Contraindicated
Moderate or severe hepatic insufficiency	Contraindicated

Drug Interactions: Methadone (↑ methadone clearance with abacavir 600 mg BID); ethanol (↑ abacavir serum levels/half-life; may ↑ toxicity); didanosine, zalcitabine (↑ risk of pancreatitis); TMP-SMX (↑ lamivudine levels); zidovudine (↑ zidovudine levels).
Adverse Effects: Abacavir may cause severe hypersensitivity reactions that may be fatal (see comments), usually during the first 4–6 weeks of therapy; report cases of hypersensitivity reactions to Abacavir Hypersensitivity Registry at 1-800-270-0425. Drug fever, rash, abdominal pain, diarrhea, nausea, vomiting, anorexia, anemia, leukopenia, photophobia, depression, insomnia, weakness, headache, cough, nasal complaints, dizziness, peripheral neuropathy, myalgias, ↑ AST/ALT, hyperglycemia, hypertriglyceridemia, pancreatitis, lactic acidosis with hepatic steatosis (rare, but potentially life-threatening toxicity with the NRTIs).
Allergic Potential: High (~ 5%)/Low
Safety in Pregnancy: C
Comments: May be taken with or without food. **HLA-B*5701 testing should precede the use of abacavir or an abacavir-containing regimen to reduce the risk of hypersensitivity reaction. Immediately and permanently discontinue if a hypersensitivity reaction occurs; never restart abacavir sulfate/lamivudine following a hypersensitivity reaction** or if hypersensitivity cannot be ruled out, which may include fever, rash, fatigue, nausea, vomiting, diarrhea, abdominal pain, anorexia, respiratory symptoms. Potential cross-resistance with didanosine.

"Usual dose" assumes normal renal/hepatic function. * For renal insufficiency, give usual dose × 1 followed by maintenance dose per CrCl. For dialysis patients, dose the same as for CrCl < 10 mL/min and give supplemental (post-HD/PD dose) immediately after dialysis. CrCl = creatinine clearance; CVVH = continuous veno-venous hemo-filtration; HD/PD = hemodialysis/peritoneal dialysis. See pp. 190–193 for explanations, p. x for abbreviations

Lamivudine prevents development of ZDV resistance and restores ZDV susceptibility. For patients co-infected with HIV and HBV, monitor hepatic function closely during therapy and for several months afterward.

Cerebrospinal Fluid Penetration: 27–33/15%

REFERENCES:

Mallal S, Phillips E, Carosi G, et al. HLA-B*5701 screening for hypersensitivity to abacavir. N Engl J Med 358:568–79, 2008.

No authors listed. Two once-daily fixed-dose NRTI combination for HIV. Med Lett Drugs Ther. 47: 19–20, 2005.

Panel on Antiretroviral Guidelines for Adults and Adolescents. Guidelines for the use of antiretroviral agents in HIV-1-infected adults and adolescents. Department of Health and Human Services. December 1, 2009; 1–161. Available at http://www.aidsinfo.nih.gov/ContentFiles/AdultandAdolescentGL.pdf.

Sosa N, Hill-Zabala C, Dejesus E, et al. Abacavir and lamivudine fixed-dose combination tablet once daily compared with abacavir and lamivudine twice daily in HIV-infected patients over 48 weeks. J Acquir Immune Defic Syndr 40:422–7, 2005.

Abacavir + Lamivudine + Zidovudine (Trizivir)

Drug Class: Antiretroviral NRTI combination
Usual Dose: HLA-B*5701 negative patients—Trizivir tablet = abacavir 300 mg + lamivudine 150 mg + zidovudine 300 mg. Usual dose = 1 tablet (PO) BID
How supplied: Oral Tablet: Contains 300 mg Abacavir Sulfate + 600 mg Lamivudine
Pharmacokinetic Parameters:
Peak serum level: 3/1.5/1.2 mcg/mL
Bioavailability: 86/86/64%
Excreted unchanged (urine): 1.2/90/16%
Serum half-life (normal/ESRD): [1.5/6/1.1]/8/20/2.2] hrs

Plasma protein binding: 30/36/20%
Volume of distribution (V_d): 0.86/1.3/1.6 L/kg
Primary Mode of Elimination: Hepatic/renal
Dosage Adjustments*

CrCl < 50 mL/min	Avoid
Post-HD or Post-PD	Avoid
CVVH dose	Avoid
Moderate or severe hepatic insufficiency	Not recommended

Drug Interactions: Amprenavir, atovaquone (↑ zidovudine levels); clarithromycin (↓ zidovudine levels); cidofovir (↑ zidovudine levels, flu-like symptoms); doxorubicin (neutropenia); stavudine (antagonistic to zidovudine; avoid combination); TMP-SMX (↑ lamivudine and zidovudine levels); zalcitabine (↓ lamivudine levels).
Adverse Effects: HLA-B*5701 testing should precede the use of abacavir or an abacavir-containing regimen to reduce the risk of hypersensitivity reaction. Immediately and permanently discontinue if a hypersensitivity reaction occurs; never restart abacavir sulfate/lamivudine/zidovudine following a hypersensitivity reaction or if hypersensitivity cannot be ruled out, which may include fever, rash, fatigue, nausea, vomiting, diarrhea, abdominal pain, anorexia, respiratory symptoms. Most common (> 5%): nausea, vomiting, diarrhea, anorexia, insomnia, fever/chills, headache, malaise/fatigue. Others (less common): peripheral neuropathy, myopathy, steatosis, pancreatitis. Lab abnormalities: mild hyperglycemia, anemia, LFT elevations, hypertriglyceridemia, leukopenia.
Allergic Potential: High (~ 5%)
Safety in Pregnancy: C
Comments: Avoid in patients with CrCl < 50 mL/min. May be taken with or without food. HBV hepatitis may relapse if lamivudine is discontinued.

"Usual dose" assumes normal renal/hepatic function. * For renal insufficiency, give usual dose × 1 followed by maintenance dose per CrCl. For dialysis patients, dose the same as for CrCl < 10 mL/min and give supplemental (post-HD/PD dose) immediately after dialysis. CrCl = creatinine clearance; CVVH = continuous veno-venous hemo-filtration; HD/PD = hemodialysis/peritoneal dialysis. See pp. 190–193 for explanations, p. x for abbreviations

REFERENCES:

Havlir DV, Lange JM. New antiretrovirals and new combinations. AIDS 12 (Suppl A):S165–74, 1998.

Mallal S, Phillips E, Carosi G, et al. HLA-B*5701 screening for hypersensitivity to abacavir. N Engl J Med 358:568–79, 2008.

McDowell JA, Lou Y, Symonds WS, et al. Multiple-dose pharmacokinetics and pharmacodynamics of abacavir alone and in combination with zidovudine in human immunodeficiency virus-infected adults. Antimicrob Agents Chemother 44:2061–7, 2000.

Panel on Antiretroviral Guidelines for Adults and Adolescents. Guidelines for the use of antiretroviral agents in HIV-1-infected adults and adolescents. Department of Health and Human Services. December 1, 2009; 1–161. Available at http://www.aidsinfo.nih.gov/ContentFiles/AdultandAdolescentGL.pdf.

Three new drugs for HIV infection. Med Lett Drugs Ther 40:114–6, 1998.

Weverling GJ, Lange JM, Jurriaans S, et al. Alternative multidrug regimen provides improved suppression of HIV-1 replication over triple therapy. AIDS 12:117–22, 1998.

CrCl 10–20 mL/min	10 mg (PO) q3d
Hemodialysis	10 mg (PO) q7d
Post-HD or PD dose	No information
CVVH dose	No information
Moderate or severe hepatic insufficiency	No change

Drug Interactions: No significant interaction with lamivudine, TMP-SMX, acetaminophen, ibuprofen.

Adverse Effects: Asthenia, headache, abdominal pain, nausea, flatulence, diarrhea, dyspepsia.

Allergic Potential: Low

Safety in Pregnancy: C

Comments: May be taken with or without food. Does not inhibit CP450 isoenzymes. Do not discontinue abruptly to avoid exacerbation of HBV hepatitis.

Cerebrospinal Fluid Penetration: No data

Adefovir dipivoxil (Hepsera)

Drug Class: Anti-Hepatitis B agent (Nucleotide Reverse Transcriptase Inhibitor)
Usual Dose: 10 mg (PO) QD
How supplied: Oral Tablet: 10 mg
Pharmacokinetic Parameters:
Peak serum level: 18 ng/mL
Bioavailability: 59%
Excreted unchanged (urine): 45%
Serum half-life (normal/ESRD): 7.5/9 hrs
Plasma protein binding: 4%
Volume of distribution (V_d): 0.4 L/kg
Primary Mode of Elimination: Renal
Dosage Adjustments*

| CrCl ≥ 50 mL/min | 10 mg (PO) QD |
| CrCl 20–50 mL/min | 10 mg (PO) q2d |

REFERENCES:

Buti M, Esteban R. Adefovir dipivoxil. Drugs of Today 39:127–35, 2003.

Cundy KC, Burditch-Crovo P, Walker RE, et al. Clinical pharmacokinetics of adefovir in human HIV-1 infected patients. Antimicrob Agents Chemother 35:2401–2405, 1995.

Davis GL. Update on the management of chronic hepatitis B. Rev Gastroenterol Disord 2: 106–15, 2002.

Hadziyannis SJ, Tassopoulos NC, Heathcote E, et al. Adefovir dipivoxil for the treatment of hepatitis B e antigen-negative chronic hepatitis B. N Engl J Med 348:800–7, 2003.

Perrillo R, Schiff E, Yoshida E, et al. Adefovir for the treatment of lamivudine-resistant hepatitis B mutants. Hepatology 32:129–34, 2000.

Peters MG, Hann Hw H, Martin P, et al. Adefovir dipivoxil alone or in combination with lamivudine in patients with lamivudine-resistant chronic hepatitis B. Gastroenterology 126:90–101, 2004.

"Usual dose" assumes normal renal/hepatic function. * For renal insufficiency, give usual dose × 1 followed by maintenance dose per CrCl. For dialysis patients, dose the same as for CrCl < 10 mL/min and give supplemental (post-HD/PD dose) immediately after dialysis. CrCl = creatinine clearance; CVVH = continuous veno-venous hemo-filtration; HD/PD = hemodialysis/peritoneal dialysis. See pp. 190–193 for explanations, p. x for abbreviations

Atazanavir (Reyataz) ATV

Drug Class: Antiretroviral protease inhibitor
Usual Dose: 400 mg (PO) QD; 300 mg (PO)
QD when given with ritonavir 100 mg (PO) QD
How Supplied: Oral Capsule: 100 mg,
150 mg, 200 mg, 300 mg
Pharmacokinetic Parameters:
Peak serum level: 3152 ng/mL
Bioavailability: No data
Excreted unchanged (urine) (urine/feces): 7%/20%
Serum half-life (normal/ESRD): 7 hrs/no data
Plasma protein binding: 86%
Volume of distribution (V_d): No data
Primary Mode of Elimination: Hepatic
Dosage Adjustments*

CrCl < 50 mL/min	No data
Post-HD or PD dose	No data
CVVH dose	No data
Moderate hepatic insufficiency	300 mg (PO) QD
Severe hepatic insufficiency	Avoid

Antiretroviral Dosage Adjustments

Delavirdine	No information
Didanosine	Give atazanavir 2 hrs before or 1 hr after didanosine buffered formulations
Efavirenz	Do not coadminister with unboosted ATV. In treatment-naïve patients (ATV 400 mg + RTV 100 mg) once daily. Do not coadminister in treatment-experienced patients.
Indinavir	Avoid combination

Lopinavir/ ritonavir	ATV 300 mg once daily + LPV/r 400/100 mg BID
Nelfinavir	No information
Nevirapine	Do not co-administer with atazanavir +/− ritonavir
Ritonavir	Atazanavir 300 mg/d + ritonavir 100 mg/d as single daily dose with food
Saquinavir	↑ saquinavir (soft-gel) levels; no information
Rifampin	Avoid combination
Rifabutin	150 mg q2d or 3x/week
Etravirine	Do not co-administer with atazanavir +/− ritonavir
Maraviroc	MVC 150 mg BID with ATV +/− RTV
Raltegravir	No change

Drug Interactions: Antacids or buffered
medications (↓ atazanavir levels; give atazanavir
2 hours before or 1 hour after); H₂-receptor
blockers (↓ atazanavir levels. In <u>treatment-naïve</u>
patients taking an H₂-receptor antagonist, give
either atazanavir 400 mg once daily with food
at least 2 hours before and at least 10 hours
after the H₂-receptor antagonist, or give
atazanavir 300 mg once daily with ritonavir
100 mg once daily with food, without the need
for separation from the H₂-receptor antagonist. In
<u>treatment-experienced</u> patients, give atazanavir
300 mg once daily with ritonavir 100 mg once
daily with food at least 2 hours before and at
least 10 hours after the H₂-receptor antagonist);
antiarrhythmics (↑ amiodarone, systemic lidocaine,
quinidine levels; prolongs PR interval; monitor
antiarrhythmic levels); antidepressants (↑ tricyclic

"Usual dose" assumes normal renal/hepatic function. * For renal insufficiency, give usual dose × 1 followed
by maintenance dose per CrCl. For dialysis patients, dose the same as for CrCl < 10 mL/min and give supplemental (post-HD/PD dose) immediately after dialysis. CrCl = creatinine clearance; CVVH = continuous
veno-venous hemo-filtration; HD/PD = hemodialysis/peritoneal dialysis. See pp. 190–193 for explanations,
p. x for abbreviations

antidepressant levels; monitor levels); calcium channel blockers ($\uparrow$ calcium channel blocker levels, $\uparrow$ PR interval; $\downarrow$ diltiazem dose by 50%; use with caution; consider ECG monitoring); clarithromycin ($\uparrow$ clarithromycin and atazanavir levels; consider 50% dose reduction; consider alternate agent for infections not caused by MAI); cyclosporine, sirolimus, tacrolimus ($\uparrow$ immunosuppressant levels; monitor levels); ethinyl estradiol, norethindrone ($\uparrow$ oral contraceptive levels; use lowest effective oral contraceptive dose); lovastatin, simvastatin ($\uparrow$ risk of myopathy, rhabdomyolysis; avoid combination); sildenafil ($\uparrow$ sildenafil levels; do not give more than 25 mg q2h); tadalafil (max. 10 mg/72 hours); vardenafil (max. 2.5 mg/72 hours); St. John's wort (avoid combination); warfarin ($\uparrow$ warfarin levels; monitor INR); tenofovir (tenofovir reduces systemic exposure to atazanavir. Whenever the two are coadministered, the recommended dose of atazanavir is 300 mg once daily with ritonavir 100 mg once daily). *Drugs that should not be coadministered with atazanavir* include beta-blockers, cisapride, pimozide, rifampin, irinotecan, midazolam, triazolam, lovastatin, simvastatin, bepridil, some ergot derivatives, indinavir, proton pump inhibitors, St. John's wort.

Adverse Effects: Reversible, asymptomatic $\uparrow$ in indirect (unconjugated) bilirubin may occur. Asymptomatic, dose-dependent $\uparrow$ PR interval (~ 24 msec). Use with caution with drugs that $\uparrow$ PR interval (e.g., beta-blockers, verapamil, digoxin). May $\uparrow$ risk of hyperglycemia/diabetes. May $\uparrow$ risk of bleeding in hemophilia (types A + B).

Allergic Potential: Low
Cerebrospinal Fluid Penetration: Intermediate
Safety in Pregnancy: B
Comments: Monitor LFTs in patients with HBV, HCV. Take 400 mg (two 200-mg capsules) once daily with food.

Cerebrospinal Fluid Penetration: Intermediate

REFERENCES:
Colonno RJ, Thiry A, Limoli K, Parkin N. Activities of atazanavir (BMS-232632) against a large panel of Human Immunodeficiency Virus Type 1 clinical isolates resistant to one or more approved protease inhibitors. *Antimicrob Agents Chemother* 47: 1324–33, 2003.

Haas DW, Zala C, Schrader S, et al. Therapy with atazanavir plus saquinavir in patients failing highly active antiretroviral therapy: a randomized comparative pilot trial. *AIDS* 17:1339–1349, 2003.

Havlir DV, O'Marro SD. Atazanavir: new option for treatment of HIV infection. *Clin Infect Dis* 38: 1599–604, 2004.

Jemsek JG, Arathoon E, Arlotti M, et al. Body fat and other metabolic effects of atazanavir and efavirenz, each administered in combination with zidovudine plus lamivudine, in antiretroviral-naïve HIV-infected patients. *Clin Infect Dis* 42:273–80, 2006.

Panel on Antiretroviral Guidelines for Adults and Adolescents. Guidelines for the use of antiretroviral agents in HIV-1-infected adults and adolescents. Department of Health and Human Services. December 1, 2009; 1–161. Available at http://www.aidsinfo.nih.gov/ContentFiles/AdultandAdolescentGL.pdf.

Piliero PJ. Atazanavir: a novel HIV-1 protease inhibitor. *Expert Opin Investig Drugs* 11:1295–301, 2002.

Sanne I, Piliero P, Squires K, et al. Results of a phase 2 clinical trial at 48 weeks (AI424-007): a dose-ranging, safety, and efficacy comparative trial of atazanavir at three doses in combination with didanosine and stavudine in antiretroviral-naïve subjects. *J Acquir Immune Defic Syndr* 32:18–29, 2003.

Wang F, Ross J. Atazanavir: a novel azapeptide inhibitor of HIV-1 protease. *Formulary* 38:691–702, 2003.

Darunavir Ethanolate (Prezista) DRV

Drug Class: Antiretroviral protease inhibitor
Usual Dose: Treatment-naïve patients: 800 mg (two 400 mg tablets) of darunavir (PO) QD + 100

"Usual dose" assumes normal renal/hepatic function. * For renal insufficiency, give usual dose × 1 followed by maintenance dose per CrCl. For dialysis patients, dose the same as for CrCl < 10 mL/min and give supplemental (post-HD/PD dose) immediately after dialysis. CrCl = creatinine clearance; CVVH = continuous veno-venous hemo-filtration; HD/PD = hemodialysis/peritoneal dialysis. See pp. 190–193 for explanations, p. x for abbreviations

mg of ritonavir (PO) QD. Treatment-experienced patients: 600 mg (one 600-mg tablet) of darunavir (PO) BID plus 100 mg of ritonavir (PO) BID

How Supplied: Oral Tablet: 75 mg, 150 mg, 400 mg, 600 mg

Pharmacokinetic Parameters:

Peak serum level: 3578 ng/mL
Bioavailability: 37% (alone) 82% (with ritonavir)
Excreted unchanged: 41.2% (feces), 7.7% (urine)
Serum half-life (normal/ESRD): 15/15 hrs
Plasma protein binding: 95%
Volume of distribution (V_d): not studied

Primary Mode of Elimination: Fecal/renal

Dosage Adjustments*

CrCl 50–80 mL/min	No change
CrCl 10–50 mL/min	No change
CrCl < 10 mL/min	No change
Post-HD dose	No change
Post-PD dose	No change
CVVH dose	No change
Mild hepatic insufficiency	Not studied
Moderate or severe hepatic insufficiency	Not studied

Antiretroviral Dosage Adjustments

Efavirenz	No change
Nevirapine	No change
Didanosine	1 hour before or 1 hour after darunavir
Tenofovir	No change
Fosamprenavir	No change
Indinavir	No information
Lopinavir/ritonavir	Avoid
Saquinavir	Avoid
Rifabutin	150 mg QOD
Etravirine	No change
Maraviroc	150 mg BID
Raltegravir	No change

Drug Interactions: Indinavir, ketoconazole, nevirapine, tenofovir (↑ darunavir levels); lopinavir/ritonavir, saquinavir, efavirenz (↓ darunavir levels); concomitant administration of darunavir/ritonavir with agents highly dependent on CYP3A for clearance, astemizole, cisapride, dihydroergotamine, ergonovine, ergotamine, methylergonovine, midazolam, pimozide, terfenadine, midazolam, triazolam (may ↓ darunavir levels and ↓ effectiveness); sildenafil, vardenafil, tadalafil (↑ PDE-5 inhibitors; sildenafil do not exceed 25 mg in 48 hrs, vardenafil do not exceed 2.5 mg in 72 hrs, or tadalafil do not exceed 10 mg in 72 hrs).

Adverse Effects: Diarrhea, nausea, headache, nasopharyngitis.

Allergic Potential: High (see comments)

Safety in Pregnancy: C

Comments: Always take with food (increases AUC, Cmax by approximately 30%). Must be given with ritonavir to boost bioavailability. Darunavir contains a sulfonamide moiety (as do fosamprenavir and tipranavir); use with caution in patients with sulfonamide allergies. A mild-to-moderate rash occurred in 7% of patients receiving the drug in clinical trial; it did not usually require drug cessation, but severe rashes (including Stevens-Johnson syndrome) have been reported.

Cerebrospinal Fluid Penetration: No data

"Usual dose" assumes normal renal/hepatic function. * For renal insufficiency, give usual dose × 1 followed by maintenance dose per CrCl. For dialysis patients, dose the same as for CrCl < 10 mL/min and give supplemental (post-HD/PD dose) immediately after dialysis. CrCl = creatinine clearance; CVVH = continuous veno-venous hemo-filtration; HD/PD = hemodialysis/peritoneal dialysis. See pp. 190–193 for explanations, p. x for abbreviations

REFERENCES:

Clotet B, Bellos N, Moloina JM, et al. Efficacy and safety of darunavir-ritonavir at week 48 in treatment-experienced patients with HIV-1 infection in POWER 1 and 2: a pooled subgroup analysis of data from two randomised trials. *Lancet* 369:1169–78, 2007.

De Meyer SM, Spinosa-Guzman S, Vangeneugden TJ, et al. Efficacy of once-daily darunavir/ritonavir 800/100 mg in HIV-infected, treatment-experienced patients with no baseline resistance-associated mutations to darunavir. *J Acquir Immune Defic Syndr* 49(2):179–82, 2008.

De Meyer S, Azijn H, Surleraux D, et al. TMC114, a novel human immunodeficiency virus type 1 protease inhibitor active against protease inhibitor-resistant viruses, including a broad range of clinical isolates. *Antimicrob Agents Chemother* 49:2314–21, 2005.

Dominique L.N.G, Surleraux T, Abdellah Tahri T, et al. Discovery and selection of TMC114, a next generation HIV-I protease inhibitor. *J Med Chem* 48:1813–22, 2005.

Grinsztejn, B. TMC114/r is well tolerated in 3-class-experienced patients: week 24 of POWER 1 (TMC114–C213). Tibotec Pharmaceuticals. Rio de Janerio, Brazil. Available from URL: www.tibotec.com

Katlama C. TMC114/r outperforms investigator-selected PI(s) in 3-class-experienced patients: week 24 primary efficacy analysis of POWER 1 (TMC114–C213). Tibotec Pharmaceuticals. Rio de Janerio, Brazil. Available from URL: www.tibotec.com

Madruga JV, Berger D, McMurchie M, et al. Efficacy and safety of darunavir-ritonavir compared with that of lopinavir-ritonavir at 48 weeks in treatment-experienced, HIV-infected patients in TITAN: a randomized controlled phase III trial. *Lancet* 370:3–5, 2007.

Ortiz R, Dejesus E, Khanlou H, et al. Efficacy and safety of once-daily darunavir/ritonavir versus lopinavir/ritonavir in treatment-naive HIV-1-infected patients at week 48 (ARTMIS). *AIDS* 2008;22(12):1389–97.

Panel on Antiretroviral Guidelines for Adults and Adolescents. Guidelines for the use of antiretroviral agents in HIV-1-infected adults and adolescents. Department of Health and Human Services. December 1, 2009; 1–161. Available at http://www.aidsinfo.nih.gov/ContentFiles/AdultandAdolescentGL.pdf.

Product Information: PREZISTA(TM) oral tablets, darunavir oral tablets. Tibotec Therapeutics, Inc, Raritan, NJ, 2006.

Sorbera LA, Castaner J, Bayes M. Darunavir: Anti-HIV agent HIV protease inhibitor. Drugs of the Future. 30:441–449, 2005.

Website: www.prezista.com

Delavirdine (Rescriptor)

Drug Class: Antiretroviral NNRTI (non-nucleoside reverse transcriptase inhibitor)
Usual Dose: 400 mg (PO) BID
How Supplied: Oral Tablet: 100 mg, 200 mg
Pharmacokinetic Parameters:
Peak serum level: 35 mcg/mL
Bioavailability: 85%
Excreted unchanged (urine): 5%
Serum half-life (normal/ESRD): 5.8 hrs/no data
Plasma protein binding: 98%
Volume of distribution (V_d): 0.5 L/kg
Primary Mode of Elimination: Hepatic
Dosage Adjustments*

CrCl 50–80 mL/min	No change
CrCl 10–50 mL/min	No change
CrCl < 10 mL/min	No change
Post-HD dose	None
Post-PD dose	None
CVVH dose	No change
Moderate hepatic insufficiency	No information
Severe hepatic insufficiency	No information/ use caution

Antiretroviral Dosage Adjustments

Efavirenz	No information
Indinavir	Indinavir 600 mg TID

"Usual dose" assumes normal renal/hepatic function. * For renal insufficiency, give usual dose × 1 followed by maintenance dose per CrCl. For dialysis patients, dose the same as for CrCl < 10 mL/min and give supplemental (post-HD/PD dose) immediately after dialysis. CrCl = creatinine clearance; CVVH = continuous veno-venous hemo-filtration; HD/PD = hemodialysis/peritoneal dialysis. See pp. 190–193 for explanations, p. x for abbreviations

Lopinavir/ritonavir	No information
Nelfinavir	No information (monitor for neutropenia)
Nevirapine	No information
Ritonavir	Delavirdine: no change; ritonavir: No information
Saquinavir soft-gel	Saquinavir soft-gel 800 mg TID (monitor transaminases)
Rifampin, rifabutin	Avoid combination
Statins	Not recommended

Drug Interactions: Antiretrovirals, rifabutin, rifampin (see dose adjustment grid, above); astemizole, terfenadine, benzodiazepines, cisapride, H_2 blockers, proton pump inhibitors, ergot alkaloids, quinidine, statins (avoid if possible); carbamazepine, phenobarbital, phenytoin (may ↓ delavirdine levels, monitor anticonvulsant levels); clarithromycin, dapsone, nifedipine, warfarin (↑ interacting drug levels); sildenafil (do not exceed 25 mg in 48 hrs); tadalafil (max. 10 mg/72 hrs); vardenafil (max. 2.5 mg/72 hrs).

Adverse Effects: Drug fever/rash, Stevens-Johnson syndrome (rare), headache, nausea/vomiting, diarrhea, ↑ SGOT/SGPT.

Allergic Potential: High

Safety in Pregnancy: C

Comments: May be taken with or without food, but food decreases absorption by 20%. May disperse four 100-mg tablets in > 3 oz. water to produce slurry; 200-mg tablets should be taken as intact tablets and not used to make an oral solution. Separate dosing with ddI or antacids by 1 hour.

Cerebrospinal Fluid Penetration: 0.4%

REFERENCES:

Been-Tiktak AM, Boucher CA, Brun-Vezinet F, et al. Efficacy and safety of combination therapy with delavirdine and zidovudine: A European/Australian phase II trial. *Intern J Antimicrob Agents* 11:13–21, 1999.

Conway B. Initial therapy with protease inhibitor-sparing regimens: Evaluation of nevirapine and delavirdine. *Clin Infect Dis* 2:130–4, 2000.

Demeter LM, Shafer RW, Meehan PM, et al. Delavirdine susceptibilities and associated reverse transcriptase mutations in human immunodeficiency virus type 1 isolates from patients in a phase I/II trial of delavirdine monotherapy (ACTG260). *Antimicrob Agents Chemother* 44:794–7, 2000.

Justesen US, Klitgaard NA, Brosen K, et al. Dose-dependent pharmacokinetics of delavirdine in combination with amprenavir in healthy volunteers. *J Antimicrob Chemother* 54:206–10, 2004.

Panel on Antiretroviral Guidelines for Adults and Adolescents. Guidelines for the use of antiretroviral agents in HIV-1-infected adults and adolescents. Department of Health and Human Services. December 1, 2009; 1–161. Available at http://www.aidsinfo.nih.gov/ContentFiles/AdultandAdolescentGL.pdf.

Didanosine (Videx) ddI

Drug Class: Antiretroviral NRTI (nucleoside reverse transcriptase inhibitor)

Usual Dose: 400 mg QD for weight > 60 kg; 250 QD for < 60 kg

How Supplied:

Generic—Oral Capsule, Delayed Release: 125 mg, 200 mg, 250 mg, 400 mg

Videx EC—Oral Capsule, Delayed Release: 125 mg, 200 mg, 250 mg, 400 mg

Videx—Oral Tablet, Chewable: 100 mg

Videx Pediatric—Oral Powder for Suspension: 10 mg/mL

Pharmacokinetic Parameters:

Peak serum level: 29 mcg/mL
Bioavailability: 42%
Excreted unchanged (urine): 60%

"Usual dose" assumes normal renal/hepatic function. * For renal insufficiency, give usual dose × 1 followed by maintenance dose per CrCl. For dialysis patients, dose the same as for CrCl < 10 mL/min and give supplemental (post-HD/PD dose) immediately after dialysis. CrCl = creatinine clearance; CVVH = continuous veno-venous hemo-filtration; HD/PD = hemodialysis/peritoneal dialysis. See pp. 190–193 for explanations, p. x for abbreviations

Serum half-life (normal/ESRD): 1.6/4.1 hrs
Plasma protein binding: ≤ 5%
Volume of distribution (V_d): 1.1 L/kg
Primary Mode of Elimination: Renal
Dosage Adjustments*: > 60 kg/[< 60 kg]:

CrCl 30–59 mL/min	200 mg (PO) QD (125 mg [PO] QD)
CrCl 10–29 mL/min	125 mg (PO) QD (125 mg [PO] QD)
CrCl < 10 mL/min	125 mg (PO) QD (not recommended)
Post-HD dose	No information
Post-PD dose	100 mg (PO)
CVVH dose	150 mg (PO) QD
Moderate hepatic insufficiency	No change
Severe hepatic insufficiency	No change

Drug Interactions: Alcohol, lamivudine, pentamidine, valproic acid (↑ risk of pancreatitis); dapsone, fluoroquinolones, ketoconazole, itraconazole, tetracyclines (↓ absorption of interacting drug; give 2 hours after didanosine); dapsone, INH, metronidazole, nitrofurantoin, stavudine, vincristine, zalcitabine, neurotoxic drugs or history of neuropathy (↑ risk of neuropathy); dapsone (↓ dapsone absorption, which increases risk of PCP); tenofovir (if possible, avoid concomitant tenofovir due to impaired CD4 response and increased risk of virologic failure). Avoid ribavirin in HIV patients.
Adverse Effects: Headache, depression, nausea, vomiting, GI upset/abdominal pain, diarrhea, drug fever/rash, anemia, leukopenia, thrombocytopenia, hepatotoxicity/

hepatic necrosis, pancreatitis (may be fatal; ↑ risk in patients on concomitant tenofovir), hypertriglyceridemia, hyperuricemia, lactic acidosis, lipoatrophy, wasting, dose-dependent (≥ 0.06 mg/kg/d) peripheral neuropathy, hyperglycemia, reports of noncirrhotic portal hypertension lactic acidosis with hepatic steatosis (rare, but potentially life-threatening toxicity with use of NRTIs; **_pregnant women taking didanosine + stavudine may be at increased risk_**).
Allergic Potential: Low
Safety in Pregnancy: B; should be avoided in pregnancy as it may cause fatal pancreatitis
Comments: Available as buffered powder for oral solution and enteric-coated extended-release capsules (Videx EC 400 mg PO QD). Take 30 minutes before or 2 hours after meal (food decreases serum concentrations by 49%). Avoid in patients with alcoholic cirrhosis/history of pancreatitis. Use with caution with ribavirin. Na^+ content = 11.5 mEq/g. Buffered tablets discontinued by US manufacturer in February 2006.
Cerebrospinal Fluid Penetration: 20%

REFERENCES:
Barreiro P, Corbaton A, Nunez M, et al. Tolerance of didanosine as enteric-coated capsules versus buffered tablets. *AIDS Patient Care STDS* 18:329–31, 2004.
Hirsch MS, D'Aquila RT. Therapy for human immunodeficiency virus infection. *N Engl J Med* 328:1686–95, 1993.
HIV Trialists' Collaborative Group. Zidovudine, didanosine, and zalcitabine in the treatment of HIV infection: Meta-analyses of the randomised evidence. *Lancet* 353:2014–2025, 1999.
Montaner JS, Reiss P, Cooper D, et al. A randomized, double-blind trial comparing combinations of nevirapine, didanosine, and zidovudine for HIV-infected patients: The INCAS trial. Italy, the Netherlands, Canada and Australia Study. *J Am Med Assoc* 279:930–937, 1998.

- -
"Usual dose" assumes normal renal/hepatic function. * For renal insufficiency, give usual dose × 1 followed by maintenance dose per CrCl. For dialysis patients, dose the same as for CrCl < 10 mL/min and give supplemental (post-HD/PD dose) immediately after dialysis. CrCl = creatinine clearance; CVVH = continuous veno-venous hemo-filtration; HD/PD = hemodialysis/peritoneal dialysis. See pp. 190–193 for explanations, p. x for abbreviations

Negredo E, Molto J, Munoz-Moreno JA, et al. Safety and efficacy of once-daily didanosine, tenofovir and nevirapine as a simplification antiretroviral approach. *Antivir Ther* 9:335–42, 2004.

Panel on Antiretroviral Guidelines for Adults and Adolescents. Guidelines for the use of antiretroviral agents in HIV-1-infected adults and adolescents. Department of Health and Human Services. December 1, 2009; 1–161. Available at http://www.aidsinfo.nih.gov/ ContentFiles/AdultandAdolescentGL.pdf.

Perry CM, Balfour JA. Didanosine: An update on its antiviral activity, pharmacokinetic properties, and therapeutic efficacy in the management of HIV disease. *Drugs* 52:928–62, 1996.

Rathbun RC, Martin ES 3rd. Didanosine therapy in patients intolerant of or failing zidovudine therapy. *Ann Pharmacother* 26:1347–51, 1992.

Efavirenz (Sustiva) EFV

Drug Class: Antiretroviral NNRTI (non-nucleoside reverse transcriptase inhibitor)
Usual Dose: 600 mg (PO) QD or QHS
How Supplied: Oral Capsule: 50 mg, 200 mg; Oral Tablet: 600 mg
Pharmacokinetic Parameters:
Peak serum level: 12.9 mcg/mL
Bioavailability: Increased with food
Excreted unchanged (urine): 14–34%
Serum half-life (normal/ESRD): 40–55 hrs/ no data
Plasma protein binding: 99%
Volume of distribution (V_d): No data
Primary Mode of Elimination: Hepatic
Dosage Adjustments*

CrCl < 60 mL/min	No change
Post-HD or PD dose	None
CVVH dose	No change
Moderate or severe hepatic insufficiency	No information

Antiretroviral Dosage Adjustments

Delavirdine	No information
Indinavir	Indinavir 1000 mg TID
Lopinavir/ ritonavir (l/r)	Consider l/r 533/133 mg BID in PI-experienced patients
Nelfinavir	No changes
Nevirapine	Do not coadminister
Ritonavir	Ritonavir 600 mg BID (500 mg BID for intolerance)
Saquinavir	Avoid use as sole PI
Rifampin	No changes
Rifabutin	Rifabutin 450–600 mg QD or 600 mg 2–3x/week if not on protease inhibitor
Etravirine	Do not coadminister
Maraviroc	600 mg BID
Raltegravir	No change

Drug Interactions: Antiretrovirals, rifabutin, rifampin (see dose adjustment grid, above); astemizole, terfenadine, cisapride, ergotamine, midazolam, triazolam (avoid); carbamazepine, phenobarbital, phenytoin (monitor anticonvulsant levels; use with caution); caspofungin (↓ caspofungin levels, may ↓ caspofungin effect); methadone, clarithromycin (↓ interacting drug levels; titrate methadone dose to effect; consider using azithromycin instead of clarithromycin).
Adverse Effects: Drug fever/rash, CNS symptoms (nightmares, dizziness, neuropsychiatric symptoms, difficulty concentrating, somnolence), ↑ SGOT/SGPT, E. multiforme/Stevens-Johnson syndrome (rare), false positive cannabinoid test.
Allergic Potential: High

"Usual dose" assumes normal renal/hepatic function. * For renal insufficiency, give usual dose × 1 followed by maintenance dose per CrCl. For dialysis patients, dose the same as for CrCl < 10 mL/min and give supplemental (post-HD/PD dose) immediately after dialysis. CrCl = creatinine clearance; CVVH = continuous veno-venous hemo-filtration; HD/PD = hemodialysis/peritoneal dialysis. See pp. 190–193 for explanations, p. x for abbreviations

Safety in Pregnancy: D
Comments: Rash/CNS symptoms usually resolve spontaneously over 2–4 weeks. Take at bedtime. Avoid taking after high fat meals (levels ↑ 50%). 600-mg dose available as single tablet.
Cerebrospinal Fluid Penetration: 0.26%–1.19%

REFERENCES:

Albrecht MA, Bosch RJ, Hammer SM, et al. Nelfinavir, efavirenz, or both after the failure of nucleoside treatment of HIV infection. *N Engl J Med* 345:398–407, 2001.

Gallant JE, DeJesus D, Arribas JR, et al. Tenofovir DF, emtricitabine, and efavirenz vs. zidovudine, lamivudine, and efavirenz for HIV. *N Engl J Med* 354:251–60, 2006.

Go JC, Cunha BA. Efavirenz. *Antibiotics for Clinicians* 5:1–8, 2001.

Haas DW, Fessel WJ, Delapenha RA, et al. Therapy with efavirenz plus indinavir in patients with extensive prior nucleoside reverse-transcriptase inhibitor experience: A randomized, double-blind, placebo-controlled trial. *J Infect Dis* 183:392–400, 2001.

la Porte CJ, de Graaff-Teulen MJ, Colbers EP, et al. Effect of efavirenz treatment on the pharmacokinetics of nelfinavir boosted by ritonavir in healthy volunteers. *Br J Clin Pharmacol* 58:632–40, 2004.

Marzolini C, Telenti A, Decosterd LA, et al. Efavirenz plasma levels can predict treatment failure and central nervous system side effects in HIV-1-infected patients. *AIDS* 15:71–5, 2001.

Negredo E, Cruz L, Paredes R, et al. Virological, immunological, and clinical impact of switching from protease inhibitors to nevirapine or to efavirenz in patients with human immunodeficiency virus infection and long-lasting viral suppression. *Clin Infect Dis* 34:504–510, 2002.

Panel on Antiretroviral Guidelines for Adults and Adolescents. Guidelines for the use of antiretroviral agents in HIV-1-infected adults and adolescents. Department of Health and Human Services. December 1, 2009; 1–161. Available at http://www.aidsinfo.nih.gov/ContentFiles/AdultandAdolescentGL.pdf.

Efavirenz + Emtricitabine + Tenofovir disoproxil fumarate (ATRIPLA)

Drug Class: Antiretroviral agent
Usual Dose: 1 tablet (efavirenz 600 mg/emtricitabine 200 mg/tenofovir 300 mg) (PO) QD on an empty stomach
How Supplied: Oral Tablet: Contains 600 mg Efavirenz + 200 mg Emtricitabine + 300 mg Tenofovir Disoproxil Fumarate
Pharmacokinetic Parameters:
Peak serum level: 4.0/1.8 mcg/mL/ 296 ng/mL
Bioavailability: NR/93%/25%
Excreted unchanged: < 1% unchanged and 14–30% as metabolites/86%/32%
Serum half-life (normal/ESRD): (40–55 hrs/ ~ 10 hrs on hemodialysis)/(10 hrs/extended)/ (17 hrs/no data)
Plasma protein binding: 99/< 4/< 0.7%
Volume of distribution (V_d): NR/NR/1.2 L/kg
Primary Mode of Elimination: hepatic/renal/renal
Dosage Adjustments*

CrCl 50–80 mL/min	No change
CrCl 10–50 mL/min	Avoid
CrCl < 10 mL/min	Avoid
Post-HD dose	Avoid
Post-PD dose	Avoid
CVVH dose	Avoid
Mild hepatic insufficiency	No information
Moderate or severe hepatic insufficiency	No information

"Usual dose" assumes normal renal/hepatic function. * For renal insufficiency, give usual dose × 1 followed by maintenance dose per CrCl. For dialysis patients, dose the same as for CrCl < 10 mL/min and give supplemental (post-HD/PD dose) immediately after dialysis. CrCl = creatinine clearance; CVVH = continuous veno-venous hemo-filtration; HD/PD = hemodialysis/peritoneal dialysis. See pp. 190–193 for explanations, p. x for abbreviations

Antiretroviral Dosage Adjustments

Fosamprenavir/ ritonavir	An additional 100 mg/day (300 mg total) of ritonavir is recommended when Atripla is administered with fosamprenavir/ritonavir QD. No change in ritonavir dose when Atripla is administered with fosamprenavir/ritonavir BID
Atazanavir	Avoid
Indinavir	Indinavir 1000 mg TID
Lopinavir/ ritonavir	Increase lopinavir/ritonavir to 600/150 mg (3 tablets) BID
Ritonavir	No information
Saquinavir	Avoid
Didanosine	Avoid
Rifabutin	Rifabutin 450–600 mg QD or 600 mg 2–3x/week if not on protease inhibitor
Rifampin	No change

Drug Interactions: Antiretrovirals, rifabutin (see dose adjustment grid above); astemizole, cisapride, ergotamine, methylergonovine, midazolam, triazolam, St John's wort (↓ efavirenz levels); voriconazole (↓ voriconazole levels; avoid); caspofungin (↓ caspofungin levels); carbamazepine, phenytoin, phenobarbital (monitor anticonvulsant levels; use with caution; potential for ↓ efavirenz levels); statins (may ↓ statin levels); methadone, (↓ methadone levels); clarithromycin (may ↓ clarithromycin effectiveness, consider using azithromycin).

Adverse Effects: Headache, diarrhea, nausea, vomiting, GI upset, lactic acidosis, osteopenia, rash, dizziness, fatigue, lactic acidosis with hepatic steatosis (rare but potentially life-threatening with NRTIs), relapsing type B viral hepatitis, depression, vivid dreams, renal impairment.
Allergic Potential: High
Safety in Pregnancy: D
Comments: Rash/CNS effects usually resolve in a few weeks. Take at bedtime on empty stomach. High fat meals can ↑ efavirenz by 50%. Use with caution in patients with history of seizures (↑ risk of convulsions). Potential for cross-resistance to lamivudine, zalcitabine, abacavir, and didanosine. Low affinity for DNA polymerase-gamma.
Cerebrospinal Fluid Penetration: 1%/no data/no data

REFERENCES:
Gallant JE, DeJesus E, Arribas JR, et al: Tenofovir DF, emtricitabine, and efavirenz vs. zidovudine, lamivudine, and efavirenz for HIV. N Engl J Med 354:251–260, 2006.
Izzedine H, Aymard G, Launay-Vacher V, et al. Pharmacokinetics of efavirenz in a patient on maintenance haemodialysis. AIDS 14:618–619.
Panel on Antiretroviral Guidelines for Adults and Adolescents. Guidelines for the use of antiretroviral agents in HIV-1-infected adults and adolescents. Department of Health and Human Services. December 1, 2009; 1–161. Available at http://www.aidsinfo.nih.gov/ContentFiles/AdultandAdolescentGL.pdf.

Emtricitabine (Emtriva) FTC

Drug Class: Antiretroviral NRTI (nucleoside reverse transcriptase inhibitor)
Usual Dose: 200 mg (PO) QD
How Supplied: Oral Capsule: 200 mg, Oral Solution: 10 mg/mL
Pharmacokinetic Parameters:
Peak serum level: 1.8 mcg/mL
Bioavailability: 93%

"Usual dose" assumes normal renal/hepatic function. * For renal insufficiency, give usual dose × 1 followed by maintenance dose per CrCl. For dialysis patients, dose the same as for CrCl < 10 mL/min and give supplemental (post-HD/PD dose) immediately after dialysis. CrCl = creatinine clearance; CVVH = continuous veno-venous hemo-filtration; HD/PD = hemodialysis/peritoneal dialysis. See pp. 190–193 for explanations, p. x for abbreviations

Excreted unchanged (urine): 86%
Serum half-life (normal/ESRD): 10 hrs/extended
Plasma protein binding: 4%
Primary Mode of Elimination: Renal
Dosage Adjustments*

CrCl ≥ 50 mL/min	200 mg (PO) QD
CrCl 30–49 mL/min	200 mg (PO) q2d
CrCl 15–29 mL/min	200 mg (PO) q3d
CrCl < 15 mL/min	200 mg (PO) q4d
Post-HD dose	200 mg (PO) q4d
Post-PD dose	No information
CVVH dose	No information
Moderate or severe hepatic insufficiency	No change

Drug Interactions: No significant interactions with indinavir, stavudine, zidovudine, famciclovir, tenofovir.
Adverse Effects: Headache, diarrhea, nausea, rash, lactic acidosis with hepatic steatosis (rare, but potentially life-threatening with NRTIs).
Allergic Potential: Low
Safety in Pregnancy: B
Comments: May be taken with or without food. Does not inhibit CYP450 enzymes. Mean intracellular half-life of 39 hours. Potential cross-resistance to lamivudine and zalcitabine. Low affinity for DNA polymerase-gamma.
Cerebrospinal Fluid Penetration: No data

REFERENCES:
Anderson PL. Pharmacologic perspectives for once-daily antiretroviral therapy. *Ann Pharmacother* 38:1924–34, 2004.
Benson CA, van der Horst C, Lamarca A, et al. A randomized study of emtricitabine and lamivudine in stable suppressed patients with HIV. *AIDS* 18:2269–2276, 2004.
Dando TM, Wagstaff AJ. Emtricitabine/tenofovir disoproxil fumarate. *Drugs* 64:2075–82, 2004.
Gallant JE, DeJesus D, Arribas JR, et al. Tenofovir DF, emtricitabine, and efavirenz vs. zidovudine, lamivudine, and efavirenz for HIV. *N Engl J Med* 354:251–60, 2006.
Lim SG, Ng TN, Kung N, et al. A double-blind placebo-controlled study of emtricitabine in chronic hepatitis B. *Arch Intern Med* 166:49–56, 2006.
Panel on Antiretroviral Guidelines for Adults and Adolescents. Guidelines for the use of antiretroviral agents in HIV-1-infected adults and adolescents. Department of Health and Human Services. December 1, 2009; 1–161. Available at http://www.aidsinfo.nih.gov/ContentFiles/AdultandAdolescentGL.pdf.
Saag MS. Emtricitabine, a new antiretroviral agent with activity against HIV and hepatitis B virus. *Clin Infect Dis* 42;128–31, 2006.

Emtricitabine + Tenofovir disoproxil fumarate (Truvada)

Drug Class: Antiretroviral NRTI (nucleoside reverse transcriptase inhibitor) + nucleotide analogue
Usual Dose: One tablet (PO) QD (each tablet contains 200 mg of emtricitabine + 300 mg of tenofovir)
How Supplied: Oral Tablet: Contains 200 mg Emtricitabine + 300 mg Tenofovir Disoproxil Fumarate
Pharmacokinetic Parameters:
Peak serum level: 1.8/0.3 mcg/L
Bioavailability: 93%/27% if fasting (39% with high fat meal)
Excreted unchanged (urine): 86/32%
Serum half-life (normal/ESRD):
(10 hrs/extended)/(17 hrs/no data)
Plasma protein binding: 4/0.7–7.2%
Volume of distribution (V_d): no data/1.3 L/kg

"Usual dose" assumes normal renal/hepatic function. * For renal insufficiency, give usual dose × 1 followed by maintenance dose per CrCl. For dialysis patients, dose the same as for CrCl < 10 mL/min and give supplemental (post-HD/PD dose) immediately after dialysis. CrCl = creatinine clearance; CVVH = continuous veno-venous hemo-filtration; HD/PD = hemodialysis/peritoneal dialysis. See pp. 190–193 for explanations, p. x for abbreviations

Primary Mode of Elimination: Renal/Renal
Dosage Adjustments*

CrCl ≥ 50 mL/min	No change
CrCl 30–49 mL/min	One capsule (PO) q2d
CrCl 15–29 mL/min	Avoid
CrCl < 15 mL/min	Avoid
Post-HD dose	Avoid
Post-PD dose	Avoid
CVVH dose	Avoid
Moderate or severe hepatic insufficiency	No change

Drug Interactions: No significant interactions with indinavir, stavudine, zidovudine, famciclovir, lamivudine, lopinavir/ritonavir, efavirenz, methadone, oral contraceptives. Tenofovir ↑ didanosine levels. Tenofovir reduces systemic exposure to atazanavir; whenever the two are coadministered, the recommended dose of atazanavir is 300 mg once daily with ritonavir 100 mg once daily.
Adverse Effects: Headache, diarrhea, nausea, vomiting, GI upset, rash, lactic acidosis with hepatic steatosis (rare but potentially life-threatening with NRTIs).
Allergic Potential: Low
Safety in Pregnancy: B
Comments: May be taken with or without food. Does not inhibit CYP450 enzymes. Mean intracellular half-life with emtricitabine is 39 hours. Potential cross-resistance to lamivudine, zalcitabine, abacavir, didanosine. Low affinity for DNA polymerase-gamma. Avoid coadministration with didanosine.
Cerebrospinal Fluid Penetration: No data

REFERENCES:
Dando TM, Wagstaff AJ. Emtricitabine/tenofovir disoproxil fumarate. *Drugs* 64:2075–82, 2004.
Gallant JE, DeJesus D, Arribas JR, et al. Tenofovir DF, emtricitabine, and efavirenz vs. zidovudine, lamivudine, and efavirenz for HIV. *N Engl J Med* 354:251–60, 2006.
Panel on Antiretroviral Guidelines for Adults and Adolescents. Guidelines for the use of antiretroviral agents in HIV-1-infected adults and adolescents. Department of Health and Human Services. December 1, 2009; 1–161. Available at http://www.aidsinfo.nih.gov/ContentFiles/AdultandAdolescentGL.pdf.
Website: www.truvada.com

Enfuvirtide (Fuzeon) ENF (T-20)

Drug Class: Antiretroviral fusion inhibitor
Usual Dose: 90 mg (SC) BID
How Supplied: Subcutaneous Powder for Solution: 90 mg
Pharmacokinetic Parameters:
Peak serum level: 4.9 mcg/mL
Bioavailability: 84.3%
Serum half-life (normal/ESRD): 3.8 hrs/no data
Plasma protein binding: 92%
Volume of distribution (V_d): 5.5 L
Primary Mode of Elimination: Metabolized
Dosage Adjustments*

CrCl > 35 mL/min	No change
CrCl < 35 mL/min	No data
Post-HD dose	No data
Post-PD dose	No data
CVVH dose	No data
Moderate or severe hepatic insufficiency	No data

"Usual dose" assumes normal renal/hepatic function. * For renal insufficiency, give usual dose × 1 followed by maintenance dose per CrCl. For dialysis patients, dose the same as for CrCl < 10 mL/min and give supplemental (post-HD/PD dose) immediately after dialysis. CrCl = creatinine clearance; CVVH = continuous veno-venous hemo-filtration; HD/PD = hemodialysis/peritoneal dialysis. See pp. 190–193 for explanations, p. x for abbreviations

Drug Interactions: No clinically significant interactions with other antiretrovirals. Does not inhibit CYP450 enzymes.

Adverse Effects: Local injection site reactions are common. Diarrhea, nausea, fatigue may occur. Laboratory abnormalities include mild/transient eosinophilia. Pneumonia may occur, but cause is unclear and may not be due to drug therapy. Pancreatitis, myalgia, conjunctivitis (rare).

Allergic Potential: Hypersensitivity reactions may occur, including fever, chills, hypotension, rash, ↑ serum transaminases. Do not rechallenge following a hypersensitivity reaction

Safety in Pregnancy: B

Comments: Enfuvirtide interferes with entry of HIV-1 into cells by blocking fusion of HIV-1 and CD4 cellular membranes by binding to HR1 in the gp41 subunit of the HIV-1 envelope glycoprotein. Additive/synergistic with NRTIs, NNRTIs, and PIs, and no cross resistance to other antiretrovirals in cell culture. Compared to background regimen, enfuvirtide ↑ CD4 (71 vs. 35 cells/mm^3) and ↓ HIV-1 RNA (–1.52 log$_{10}$ vs. –0.73 log$_{10}$ copies/mL) at 24 weeks. Reconstitute in 1.1 mL of sterile water. SC injection should be given into upper arm, anterior thigh, or abdomen. Rotate injection sites; do not inject into moles, scars, bruises. After reconstitution, use immediately or refrigerate and use within 24 hours (no preservatives added).

REFERENCES:

Coleman CI, Musial, BL, Ross, J. Enfuvirtide: the first fusion inhibitor for the treatment of patients with HIV-1 infection. *Formulary* 38:204–222, 2003.

Kilby JM, Lalezari JP, Eron JJ, et al. The safety, plasma pharmacokinetics, and antiviral activity of subcutaneous enfuvirtide (T-20), a peptide inhibitor of gp41-mediated virus fusion, in HIV-infected adults. *AIDS Res Hum Retroviruses* 18:685–93, 2002.

Lalezari JP, Eron JJ, Carlson M, et al. A phase II clinical study of the long-term safety and antiviral activity of enfuvirtide-based antiretroviral therapy. *AIDS* 17:691–8, 2003.

Lalezari JP, Henry K, O'Hearn M, et al. TORO 1 Study Group. Enfuvirtide, an HIV-1 fusion inhibitor, for drug-resistant HIV infection in North and South America. *N Engl J Med* 348:2175–85, 2003.

Lazzarin A, Clotet B, Cooper D, et al. TORO 2 Study Group. Efficacy of enfuvirtide in patients infected with drug-resistant HIV-1 in Europe and Australia. *N Engl J Med* 348:2186–95, 2003.

Leao I, Frezzini C, Porter S. Enfuvirtide: a new class of antiretroviral therapy for HIV infection. *Oral Dis* 10:327–9, 2004.

Leen C, Wat C, Nieforth K. Pharmacokinetics of enfuvirtide in a patient with impaired renal function. *Clin Infect Dis* 4:339–55, 2004.

Panel on Antiretroviral Guidelines for Adults and Adolescents. Guidelines for the use of antiretroviral agents in HIV-1-infected adults and adolescents. Department of Health and Human Services. December 1, 2009; 1–161. Available at http://www.aidsinfo.nih.gov/ContentFiles/AdultandAdolescentGL.pdf.

Entecavir (Baraclude) ETV

Drug Class: Anti-hepatitis B agent—Guanosine Nucleoside Analog

Usual Dose: nucleoside-treatment-naïve patients—0.5 mg PO once daily without food; history of hepatitis B viremia while receiving lamivudine or known lamivudine resistant mutations—1 mg PO once daily, without food

How Supplied: Oral Solution: 0.05 mg/mL; Oral Tablet: 0.5 mg, 1 mg

Pharmacokinetic Parameters:

Peak serum level: 4.2 ng/mL (0.5 mg), 8.2 ng/ml (1 mg)

Bioavailability: ~ 100%

Excreted unchanged (urine): 62–73% (urine)

"Usual dose" assumes normal renal/hepatic function. * For renal insufficiency, give usual dose × 1 followed by maintenance dose per CrCl. For dialysis patients, dose the same as for CrCl < 10 mL/min and give supplemental (post-HD/PD dose) immediately after dialysis. CrCl = creatinine clearance; CVVH = continuous veno-venous hemo-filtration; HD/PD = hemodialysis/peritoneal dialysis. See pp. 190–193 for explanations, p. x for abbreviations

Serum half-life (normal/ESRD): 128–149 hrs/ no data

Plasma protein binding: 13%

Volume of distribution (V_d): extensively distributed into tissues

Primary Mode of Elimination: renal

Dosage Adjustments*

	Treatment-naïve (0.5 mg)	Lamivudine-refractory (1 mg)
CrCl > 50 mL/min	0.5 mg QD	1 mg QD
CrCl 30–50 mL/min	0.25 mg QD or 0.5 mg q2d	0.5 mg QD or 1 mg q2d
CrCl 10–30 mL/min	0.15 mg QD or 0.5 mg q3d	0.3 mg QD or 1 mg q3d
CrCl < 10 mL/min	0.05 mg QD or 0.5 mg q7d	0.1 mg QD or 1 mg q7d
Post-HD dose†	0.05 mg QD or 0.5 mg q7d	0.1 mg QD or 1 mg q7d
Post-PD dose†	0.05 mg QD or 0.5 mg q7d	0.1 mg QD or 1 mg q7d
CVVH dose	No data	No data
Mild to moderate hepatic insufficiency	No change	No change
Severe hepatic insufficiency	Mop change	No change

† On dialysis days, give dose after dialysis.

Antiretroviral Dosage Adjustments: None

Drug Interactions: Since entecavir is primarily eliminated by the kidneys, coadministration of entecavir with drugs that reduce renal function or compete for active tubular secretion may increase serum concentrations of either entecavir or the coadministered drug. Coadministration of entecavir with lamivudine, adefovir dipivoxil, or tenofovir disoproxil fumarate did not result in significant drug interactions.

Adverse Effects: Rash has been reported with entecavir therapy during postmarketing surveillance. Lactic acidosis and severe hepatomegaly with steatosis have been reported, predominantly in women, with the use of nucleoside analogs alone or in combination with antiretrovirals, including entecavir. Obesity and prolonged exposure may be risk factors. GI effects: Nausea/vomiting/diarrhea/indigestion have been reported in < 1% of patients. Neurologic effects: dizziness 3%, headache 3%, insomnia < 1%, somnolence < 1%. Renal effects: hematuria 9%. Fatigue 3%.

Allergic Potential: Low—Anaphylactoid reaction has been reported with entecavir therapy during postmarketing surveillance

Safety in Pregnancy: C

Comments: Entecavir should be taken on an empty stomach (at least 2 hours after a meal and 2 hours before the next meal). Oral solution—do not dilute or mix with water or any other liquid. HIV coinfection; entecavir is not recommended in patients who are not receiving concurrent HIV treatment (i.e., highly active antiretroviral therapy) due to the risk of HIV nucleoside reverse transcriptase inhibitor resistance. Lactic acidosis and severe hepatomegaly with steatosis, including fatalities, have been reported with nucleoside analogs; patients with obesity, female gender, prolonged nucleoside exposure, or known risk factors for liver disease may be at increased risk; suspend treatment if signs or symptoms of lactic acidosis or hepatotoxicity

---

"Usual dose" assumes normal renal/hepatic function. * For renal insufficiency, give usual dose × 1 followed by maintenance dose per CrCl. For dialysis patients, dose the same as for CrCl < 10 mL/min and give supplemental (post-HD/PD dose) immediately after dialysis. CrCl = creatinine clearance; CVVH = continuous veno-venous hemo-filtration; HD/PD = hemodialysis/peritoneal dialysis. See pp. 190–193 for explanations, p. x for abbreviations

occur. Entecavir is potent and well tolerated and has extremely low resistance rates in nucleoside/nucleotide analogue-naïve patients.

Cerebrospinal Fluid Penetration: No data

Comments: Entecavir may select for the M184V mutation in HIV. As a result, it is contraindicated in patients with HIV who are not on suppressive ART.

REFERENCES:

Chang TT, Gish RG, deMan R, et al. A comparison of entecavir and lamivudine for HBeAg-positive chronic hepatitis B. *N Engl J Med* 354(10):1001–10, 2006.

Honkoop P, de Man RA. Entecavir: a potent new antiviral drug for hepatitis B. *Expert Opin Investig Drugs* 12(4):683–8, 2003.

Lai CL, Rosmawati M, Lao J. Entecavir is superior to lamivudine in reducing hepatitis B virus DNA in patients with chronic hepatitis B infection. *Gastroenterology* 123:1831–38, 2002.

Lai CL, Shouval D, Lok AS, et al. Entecavir versus lamivudine for patients with HBeAg-negative chronic hepatitis B. *N Engl J Med* 354(10):1011–20, 2006.

Product Information: BARACLUDE® oral tablets, solution, entecavir oral tablets, solution. Bristol-Myers Squibb, Princeton, NJ, 2008.

Sherman M, Yurdaydin C, Sollano J, et al. Entecavir for treatment of lamivudine-refractory, HBeAg-positive chronic hepatitis B. *Gastroenterology* 130(7):2039–49, 2006.

Tenney DJ, Levine SM, Rose RE, et al. Clinical emergence of entecavir-resistant hepatitis B virus requires additional substitutions in virus already resistant to lamivudine. *Antimicrob Agents Chemother* 48(9):3498–3507, 2004.

Website: www.baraclude.com

Etravirine (Intelence) ETR

Drug Class: Antiretroviral NNRTI (non-nucleoside reverse transcriptase inhibitor)

Usual Dose: 200 mg (PO) BID following a meal

How Supplied: Oral Tablet: 100 mg

Pharmacokinetic Parameters:
Peak serum level: 296 ng/mL
Bioavailability: unknown (food increases systemic exposure)
Excreted unchanged: 81–86% (feces); 0% (urine)
Serum half-life (normal/ESRD): 41 hrs/not studied
Plasma protein binding: 99.9%
Volume of distribution (V_d): Not studied

Primary Mode of Elimination: Fecal 93.7%/renal 1.2%

Dosage Adjustments*

CrCl 50–80 mL/min	Not studied
CrCl 10–50 mL/min	Not studied
CrCl < 10 mL/min	Not studied
Post-HD dose	No change
Post-PD dose	No change
CVVH dose	Not studied
Moderate or severe hepatic insufficiency	No change
Co-infection with Hepatitis B or C virus	No change

Antiretroviral Dosage Adjustments

Atazanavir/ritonavir	Avoid
Delavirdine	Avoid (↑ etravirine)
Efavirenz/nevirapine	Avoid (↓ etravirine)
Fosamprenavir/ritonavir	Use with caution (↑ amprenavir)
Lopinavir/ritonavir	Use with caution (↑ etravirine)
Ritonavir (600 mg BID)	Avoid (↓ etravirine)
Darunavir/ritonavir	No change
Rifabutin, Rifampin	Avoid (↓ etravirine)

"Usual dose" assumes normal renal/hepatic function. * For renal insufficiency, give usual dose × 1 followed by maintenance dose per CrCl. For dialysis patients, dose the same as for CrCl < 10 mL/min and give supplemental (post-HD/PD dose) immediately after dialysis. CrCl = creatinine clearance; CVVH = continuous veno-venous hemo-filtration; HD/PD = hemodialysis/peritoneal dialysis. See pp. 190–193 for explanations, p. x for abbreviations

Tipranavir/ritonavir	Avoid (↓ etravirine)
Saquinavir/ritonavir	No change
Maraviroc	600 mg BID
Raltegravir	No change

Drug Interactions: Etravirine is a substrate for the liver enzymes CYP3A4, CYP2C9, and CYP2C19. Coadministration with drugs that inhibit or induce these enzymes may alter the therapeutic effect or adverse reaction profile of etravirine or concomitant drug. Amiodarone, bepridil, disopyramide, flecainide, lidocaine (systemic), mexiletine, propafenone, quinidine (↓ antiarrhythmic levels); warfarin (↑ warfarin levels); carbamazepine, phenobarbital, phenytoin (↓ etravirine levels); antifungals (↑ etravirine levels)—also etravirine decreases itraconazole and ketoconazole levels and increases voriconazole levels but has no effect on fluconazole or posaconazole levels; clarithromycin (↑ etravirine levels, ↓ clarithromycin levels), atorvastatin (↓ atorvastatin levels), sildenafil (↓ sildenafil levels), tadalafil (↓ tadalafil levels), vardenafil (↓ vardenafil levels); etravirine has no effect on methadone levels.

Adverse Effects: Hypertension, rash, abdominal pain, nausea, diarrhea, ↑ liver enzymes AST(SGOT)/ALT(SGPT), myocardial infarction, hypersensitivity reaction.

Allergic Potential: Low (< 2%)

Safety in Pregnancy: B

Comments: Severe and potentially life-threatening skin reactions have been reported, including Stevens-Johnson syndrome, hypersensitivity reaction, and erythema multiforme. Discontinue treatment if severe rash develops. Efficacy in treatment-naïve patients

has not been established. Take with meals; food increases systemic exposure by 50%.

Cerebrospinal Fluid Penetration: No data

REFERENCES:

Lazzarin A, Campbell T, Clotet B, et al. Efficacy and safety of TMC125 (etravirine) in treatment-experienced HIV-1-infected patients in DUET-2: 24-week results from a randomised, double-blind, placebo-controlled trial. *Lancet* 370:39–48, 2007.

Madruga JV, Cahn P, Grinsztejn B, et al. Efficacy and safety of TMC125 (etravirine) in treatment-experienced HIV-1-infected patients in DUET-1: 24-week results from a randomised, double-blind, placebo-controlled trial. *Lancet* 370:29–38, 2007.

Panel on Antiretroviral Guidelines for Adults and Adolescents. Guidelines for the use of antiretroviral agents in HIV-1-infected adults and adolescents. Department of Health and Human Services. December 1, 2009; 1–161. Available at http://www.aidsinfo.nih.gov/ContentFiles/AdultandAdolescentGL.pdf.

Product Information: INTELENCE™ oral tablets, etravirine oral tablets. Tibotec Therapeutics, Inc., Raritan, NJ, 2008.

Fosamprenavir (Lexiva) FPV

Drug Class: Antiretroviral protease inhibitor

Usual Dose: Treatment-naïve patients: 1400 mg BID or 1400 mg + ritonavir 100–200 mg QD or 700 mg + ritonavir 100 mg BID

Treatment-experienced patients: (once daily dosing not recommended) 700 mg + ritonavir 100 mg BID

Pharmacokinetic Parameters:

Peak serum level: 4.8 mcg/mL
Bioavailability: No data
Excreted unchanged (urine): 1%
Serum half-life (normal/ESRD): 7 hrs/no data
Plasma protein binding: 90%
Volume of distribution (V_d): 6.1 L/kg

"Usual dose" assumes normal renal/hepatic function. * For renal insufficiency, give usual dose × 1 followed by maintenance dose per CrCl. For dialysis patients, dose the same as for CrCl < 10 mL/min and give supplemental (post-HD/PD dose) immediately after dialysis. CrCl = creatinine clearance; CVVH = continuous veno-venous hemo-filtration; HD/PD = hemodialysis/peritoneal dialysis. See pp. 190–193 for explanations, p. x for abbreviations

Primary Mode of Elimination: Hepatic
Dosage Adjustments*

CrCl 50–80 mL/min	No change
CrCl 10–50 mL/min	No change
CrCl < 10 mL/min	No change
Post-HD or PD dose	No change
CVVH dose	No change
Mild-moderate hepatic insufficiency (Child-Pugh score 5–8)	700 mg (PO) BID if given without ritonavir; no data with ritonavir
Severe hepatic insufficiency (Child-Pugh score 9–12)	Avoid

Antiretroviral Dosage Adjustments:

Didanosine	Administer didanosine 1 hour apart
Delavirdine	Avoid combination
Efavirenz	Fosamprenavir 700 mg BID + ritonavir 100 mg BID + efavirenz; fosamprenavir 1400 mg QD + ritonavir 200 mg QD + efavirenz; no data for fosamprenavir 1400 mg BID + efavirenz
Indinavir	No information
Lopinavir/ ritonavir	Avoid
Nelfinavir	No information
Nevirapine	(FPV 700 mg + RTV 100 mg) BID NVP standard
Saquinavir	No information

Rifampin	Avoid combination
Rifabutin	Reduce usual rifabutin dose by 50% (or 75% if given with fosamprenavir plus ritonavir; max. 150 mg q2d)
Etravirine	Avoid combination
Maraviroc	150 mg BID
Raltegravir	No data

Drug Interactions: Antiretrovirals (see dose adjustment grid, above). Contraindicated with: ergot derivatives, cisapride, midazolam, triazolam, pimozide, flecainide and propafenone (if administered with ritonavir). Do not coadminister with: rifampin, lovastatin, simvastatin, St. John's wort, delavirdine. Dose reduction (of other drug): atorvastatin, rifabutin, sildenafil, vardenafil, ketoconazole, itraconazole. Concentration monitoring (of other drug): amiodarone, systemic lidocaine, quinidine, warfarin (INR), tricyclic antidepressants, cyclosporin, tacrolimus, sirolimus. H_2 blockers and proton pump inhibitors interfere with absorption. Sildenafil (do not give > 25 mg/48 hrs); tadalafil (max. 10 mg/72 hrs); vardenafil (max. 2.5 mg/72 hrs).
Adverse Effects: Rash, Stevens-Johnson syndrome (rare), GI upset, headache, depression, diarrhea, hyperglycemia (including worsening diabetes, new-onset diabetes, DKA), ↑ cholesterol/triglycerides (evaluate risk for coronary disease/pancreatitis), fat redistribution, ↑ SGOT/SGPT, possible increased bleeding in hemophilia; potential increased risk of myocardial infarction has been reported.
Allergic Potential: High. Fosamprenavir is a sulfonamide; use with caution in patients with sulfonamide allergies
Safety in Pregnancy: C

"Usual dose" assumes normal renal/hepatic function. * For renal insufficiency, give usual dose × 1 followed by maintenance dose per CrCl. For dialysis patients, dose the same as for CrCl < 10 mL/min and give supplemental (post-HD/PD dose) immediately after dialysis. CrCl = creatinine clearance; CVVH = continuous veno-venous hemo-filtration; HD/PD = hemodialysis/peritoneal dialysis. See pp. 190–193 for explanations, p. x for abbreviations

Comments: Usually given in conjunction with ritonavir. May be taken with or without food. Fosamprenavir is a prodrug that is rapidly hydrolyzed to amprenavir by gut epithelium during absorption. Amprenavir inhibits CYP3A4. Fosamprenavir contains a sulfonamide moiety (as do darunavir and tipranavir).

REFERENCES:

Becker S, Thornton L. Fosamprenavir: advancing HIV protease inhibitor treatment options. *Expert Opin Pharmacother* 5:1995–2005, 2004.

Chapman TM, Plosker GL, Perry CM. Fosamprenavir: a review of its use in the management of antiretroviral therapy-naïve patients with HIV infection. *Drugs* 64:2101–24, 2004.

Lexiva (fosamprenavir) approved. *AIDS Treat News* 31;2, 2003.

Panel on Antiretroviral Guidelines for Adults and Adolescents. Guidelines for the use of antiretroviral agents in HIV-1-infected adults and adolescents. Department of Health and Human Services. December 1, 2009; 1–161. Available at http://www.aidsinfo.nih.gov/ContentFiles/AdultandAdolescentGL.pdf.

Rodriguez-French A, Boghossian J, Gray GE, et al. The NEAT study: a 48-week open-label study to compare the antiviral efficacy and safety of GW433908 versus nelfinavir in antiretroviral therapy-naïve HIV-1-infected patients. *J Acquir Immune Defic Syndr* 35:22–32, 2004.

Indinavir (Crixivan) IDV

Drug Class: Antiretroviral protease inhibitor
Usual Dose: 800 mg (PO) TID
How Supplied: Oral Capsule: 100 mg, 200 mg, 400 mg
Pharmacokinetic Parameters:
Peak serum level: 252 mcg/mL
Bioavailability: 65% (77% with food)
Excreted unchanged (urine): < 20%
Serum half-life (normal/ESRD): 2 hrs/no data
Plasma protein binding: 60%

Volume of distribution (V_d): No data
Primary Mode of Elimination: Hepatic
Dosage Adjustments*

CrCl 50–80 mL/min	No change
CrCl 10–50 mL/min	No change
CrCl < 10 mL/min	No change
Post-HD dose	None
Post-PD dose	None
CVVH dose	No change
Moderate hepatic insufficiency	600 mg (PO) TID
Severe hepatic insufficiency	400 mg (PO) TID

Antiretroviral Dosage Adjustments

Didanosine	Administer didanosine 1 hour apart
Delavirdine	Indinavir 600 mg TID
Efavirenz	Indinavir 1000 mg TID or IDV 800 mg + RTV 100–200 mg BID
Lopinavir/ ritonavir	Indinavir 600 mg BID
Nelfinavir	Limited data for indinavir 1200 mg BID + nelfinavir 1250 mg BID
Nevirapine	Indinavir 1000 mg TID or IDV 800 mg + RTV 100–200 mg BID
Ritonavir	Indinavir 800 mg BID + ritonavir 100–200 mg BID, or 400 mg BID of each drug

---

"Usual dose" assumes normal renal/hepatic function. * For renal insufficiency, give usual dose × 1 followed by maintenance dose per CrCl. For dialysis patients, dose the same as for CrCl < 10 mL/min and give supplemental (post-HD/PD dose) immediately after dialysis. CrCl = creatinine clearance; CVVH = continuous veno-venous hemo-filtration; HD/PD = hemodialysis/peritoneal dialysis. See pp. 190–193 for explanations, p. x for abbreviations

Saquinavir	No information
Rifampin	Avoid combination
Rifabutin	Indinavir 1000 mg TID; rifabutin 150 mg QD or 300 mg 2–3x/week
Etravirine	Avoid combination
Maraviroc	150 mg BID
Raltegravir	No information

Drug Interactions: Antiretrovirals, rifabutin, rifampin (see dose adjustment grid, above); astemizole, terfenadine, benzodiazepines, cisapride, ergot alkaloids, statins, St. John's wort (avoid if possible); calcium channel blockers (↑ calcium channel blocker levels); carbamazepine, phenobarbital, phenytoin (↓ indinavir levels, ↑ anticonvulsant levels; monitor); tenofovir (↓ indinavir levels, ↑ tenofovir levels); clarithromycin, erythromycin, telithromycin (↑ indinavir and macrolide levels); didanosine (administer indinavir on empty stomach 1 hour apart); ethinyl estradiol, norethindrone (↑ interacting drug levels; no dosage adjustment); grapefruit juice (↓ indinavir levels); itraconazole, ketoconazole (↑ indinavir levels); sildenafil (↑ or ↓ sildenafil levels; do not exceed 25 mg in 48 hrs); tadalafil (max. 10 mg/72 hrs), vardenafil (max 2.5 mg/72 hrs); theophylline (↓ theophylline levels); fluticasone nasal spray (avoid concomitant use).

Adverse Effects: Nephrolithiasis, nausea, vomiting, diarrhea, anemia, leukopenia, headache, insomnia, hyperglycemia (including worsening diabetes, new-onset diabetes, DKA), ↑ SGOT/SGPT, ↑ indirect bilirubin (2° to drug-induced Gilbert's syndrome; inconsequential), fat redistribution, lipid abnormalities (evaluate risk of coronary disease/pancreatitis), abdominal pain, possible ↑ bleeding in hemophilia, dry skin, chelitis, paronychiae.

Allergic Potential: Low

Safety in Pregnancy: C

Comments: Renal stone formation may be prevented/minimized by adequate hydration (1–3 liters water daily); ↑ risk of nephrolithiasis with alcohol. Take 1 hour before or 2 hours after meals (may take with skim milk or low-fat meal). Separate dosing with ddI by 1 hour.

Cerebrospinal Fluid Penetration: 16%

REFERENCES:

Acosta EP, Henry K, Baken L, et al. Indinavir concentrations and antiviral effect. *Pharmacotherapy* 19:708–712, 1999.

Antinori A, Giancola MI, Griserri S, et al. Factors influencing virological response to antiretroviral drugs in cerebrospinal fluid of advanced HIV-1-infected patients. *AIDS* 16:1867–76, 2002.

Deeks SG, Smith M, Holodniy M, et al. HIV-1 protease inhibitors: A review for clinicians. *JAMA* 277:145–53, 1997.

DiCenzo R, Forrest A, Fischl MA, et al. Pharmacokinetics of indinavir and nelfinavir in treatment-naïve, human immunodeficiency virus-infected subjects. *Antimicrob Agents Chemother* 48:918–23, 2004.

Go J, Cunha BA. Indinavir: A review. *Antibiotics for Clinicians* 3:81–87, 1999.

Justesen US, Andersen AB, Klitgaard NA, et al. Pharmacokinetic interaction between rifampin and the combination of indinavir and low-dose ritonavir in HIV-infected patients. *Clin Infect Dis* 38:426–9, 2004.

Kopp JB, Falloon J, Filie A, et al. Indinavir-associated intestinal nephritis and urothelial inflammation: clinical and cytologic findings. *Clin Infect Dis* 34:1122–8, 2002.

Meraviglia P, Angeli E, Del Sorbo F, et al. Risk factors for indinavir-related renal colic in HIV patients: predicative value of indinavir dose-body mass index. *AIDS* 16:2089–93, 2002.

"Usual dose" assumes normal renal/hepatic function. * For renal insufficiency, give usual dose × 1 followed by maintenance dose per CrCl. For dialysis patients, dose the same as for CrCl < 10 mL/min and give supplemental (post-HD/PD dose) immediately after dialysis. CrCl = creatinine clearance; CVVH = continuous veno-venous hemo-filtration; HD/PD = hemodialysis/peritoneal dialysis. See pp. 190–193 for explanations, p. x for abbreviations

McDonald CK, Kuritzkes DR. Human immunodeficiency virus type 1 protease inhibitors. Arch Intern Med 157:951–9, 1997.

Panel on Antiretroviral Guidelines for Adults and Adolescents. Guidelines for the use of antiretroviral agents in HIV-1-infected adults and adolescents. Department of Health and Human Services. December 1, 2009; 1–161. Available at http://www.aidsinfo.nih.gov/ContentFiles/AdultandAdolescentGL.pdf.

Lamivudine (Epivir) 3TC

Drug Class: Antiretroviral NRTI (nucleoside reverse transcriptase inhibitor); antiviral (Hepatitis B Virus)
Usual Dose: 150 mg (PO) BID or 300 mg (PO) QD (HIV); 100 mg (PO) QD (HBV)
How Supplied:
Epivir A/F—Oral Solution: 10 mg/mL
Epivir HBV—Oral Solution: 5 mg/mL
Epivir—Oral Solution: 10 mg/mL
Oral Tablet: 150, 300 mg
Pharmacokinetic Parameters:
Peak serum level: 1.5 mcg/mL
Bioavailability: 86%
Excreted unchanged (urine): 71%
Serum half-life (normal/ESRD): 5–7/20 hrs
Plasma protein binding: 36%
Volume of distribution (V_d): 1.3 L/kg
Primary Mode of Elimination: Renal
Dosage Adjustments*

CrCl 30–50 mL/min	150 mg (PO) QD
CrCl 15–30 mL/min	100 mg (PO) QD
CrCl 5–15 mL/min	50 mg (PO) QD
CrCl < 5 mL/min	25 mg (PO) QD
Post-HD dose	No information
Post-PD dose	No information

CVVH dose	No information
Moderate hepatic insufficiency	No change
Severe hepatic insufficiency	No information

Drug Interactions: Didanosine, zalcitabine (↑ risk of pancreatitis); TMP-SMX (↑ lamivudine levels); zidovudine (↑ lamivudine levels).
Adverse Effects: Drug fever/rash, abdominal pain/diarrhea, nausea, vomiting, anemia, leukopenia, photophobia, depression, cough, nasal complaints, headache, dizziness, peripheral neuropathy, pancreatitis, myalgias, lactic acidosis with hepatic steatosis (rare, but potentially life-threatening toxicity with NRTIs).
Allergic Potential: Low
Safety in Pregnancy: C
Comments: Potential cross resistance with didanosine. Prevents development of AZT resistance and restores AZT susceptibility. May be taken with or without food. Effective against HBV, but HBV may reactivate after lamivudine therapy is stopped. Also a component of Combivir, Trizivir, and Epzicom.
Cerebrospinal Fluid Penetration: 15%

REFERENCES:
Benson CA, van der Horst C, Lamarca A, et al. A randomized study of emtricitabine and lamivudine in stable suppressed patients with HIV. *AIDS* 18:2269–76, 2004.

Eron JJ, Benoit SL, Jemsek J, et al. Treatment with lamivudine, zidovudine, or both in HIV-positive patients with 200 to 500 CD4 cells per cubic millimeter. *N Engl J Med* 333:1662–9, 1995.

Lai CI, Chien RN. Leung NW, et al. A one-year trial of lamivudine for chronic hepatitis B. *N Engl J Med* 339:61–8, 1998.

"Usual dose" assumes normal renal/hepatic function. * For renal insufficiency, give usual dose × 1 followed by maintenance dose per CrCl. For dialysis patients, dose the same as for CrCl < 10 mL/min and give supplemental (post-HD/PD dose) immediately after dialysis. CrCl = creatinine clearance; CVVH = continuous veno-venous hemo-filtration; HD/PD = hemodialysis/peritoneal dialysis. See pp. 190–193 for explanations, p. x for abbreviations

Lau GK, He ML, Fong DY, et al. Preemptive use of lamivudine reduces hepatitis B exacerbation after allogeneic hematopoietic cell transplantation. *Hepatology* 36:702–9, 2002.

Leung N. Lamivudine for chronic hepatitis B. *Expert Rev Anti Infect Ther* 2:173–80, 2004.

Liaw YF, Sung JY, Chow WC, et al. Lamivudine for patients with chronic hepatitis B and advanced liver disease. *N Engl J Med* 351:1521–31, 2004.

Lu Y, Wang B, Yu L, et al. Lamivudine in prevention and treatment of recurrent HBV after liver transplantation. *Hepatobiliary Pancreat Dis Int* 3:504–7, 2004.

Marrone A, Zampino R, D'Onofrio M, et al. Combined interferon plus lamivudine treatment in young patients with dual HBV (HbeAg positive) and HCV chronic infection. *J Hepatol* 41:1064–5, 2004.

Murphy RL, Brun S, Hicks C, et al. ABT-378/ritonavir plus stavudine and lamivudine for the treatment of antiretroviral-naïve adults with HIV-1 infection: 48-week results. *AIDS* 15:F1–9, 2001.

Panel on Antiretroviral Guidelines for Adults and Adolescents. Guidelines for the use of antiretroviral agents in HIV-1-infected adults and adolescents. Department of Health and Human Services. December 1, 2009; 1–161. Available at http://www.aidsinfo.nih.gov/ContentFiles/AdultandAdolescentGL.pdf.

Perry CM, Faulds D. Lamivudine. A review of its antiviral activity, pharmacokinetic properties and therapeutic efficacy in the management of HIV infection. *Drugs* 53:657–80, 1997.

Rivkina A, Rybalov S. Chronic hepatitis B: current and future treatment options. *Pharmacotherapy* 22:721–37, 2002.

Schmilovitz-Weiss H, Ben-Ari Z, Sikuler E, et al. Lamivudine treatment for acute severe hepatitis B: a pilot study. *Liver Int* 24:547–51, 2004.

Staszewski S, Morales-Ramirez J, Trashima KT, et al. Efavirenz plus zidovudine and lamivudine, efavirenz plus indinavir, and indinavir plus zidovudine and lamivudine in the treatment of HIV-1 infection in adults. *N Engl J Med* 341:1865–1873, 1999.

Lamivudine + Zidovudine (Combivir)

Drug Class: Antiretroviral NRTIs combination
Usual Dose: Combivir tablet = 150 mg lamivudine + 300 mg zidovudine. Usual dose = 1 tablet (PO) BID
How Supplied: Oral Tablet: Contains 150 mg Lamivudine + 300 mg Zidovudine
Pharmacokinetic Parameters:
Peak serum level: 2.6/1.2 mcg/mL
Bioavailability: 82/60%
Excreted unchanged (urine): 86/64%
Serum half-life (normal/ESRD): (6/1.1)/(20/2.2) hrs
Plasma protein binding: < 36/< 38%
Volume of distribution (V_d): 1.3/1.6 L/kg
Primary Mode of Elimination: Renal
Dosage Adjustments*

CrCl 50–80 mL/min	No change
CrCl 10–50 mL/min	Avoid
CrCl < 10 mL/min	Avoid
Post-HD dose	Avoid
Post-PD dose	Avoid
CVVH dose	Avoid
Moderate hepatic insufficiency	Avoid
Severe hepatic insufficiency	Avoid

Drug Interactions: Atovaquone (↑ zidovudine levels); stavudine (antagonist to stavudine; avoid combination); ganciclovir, doxorubicin (neutropenia); tipranavir (↓ zidovudine levels); TMP-SMX (↑ lamivudine and zidovudine levels); vinca alkaloids (neutropenia).
Adverse Effects: Most common (> 5%): nausea, vomiting, diarrhea, anorexia,

"Usual dose" assumes normal renal/hepatic function. * For renal insufficiency, give usual dose × 1 followed by maintenance dose per CrCl. For dialysis patients, dose the same as for CrCl < 10 mL/min and give supplemental (post-HD/PD dose) immediately after dialysis. CrCl = creatinine clearance; CVVH = continuous veno-venous hemo-filtration; HD/PD = hemodialysis/peritoneal dialysis. See pp. 190–193 for explanations, p. x for abbreviations

insomnia, fever/chills, headache, malaise/ fatigue. Others (less common): peripheral neuropathy, myopathy, steatosis, pancreatitis. Lab abnormalities: mild hyperglycemia, anemia, LFT elevations, hypertriglyceridemia, leukopenia.
Allergic Potential: Low
Safety in Pregnancy: C
Cerebrospinal Fluid Penetration:
Lamivudine = 12%; zidovudine = 60%

REFERENCES:

Drugs for AIDS and associated infections. Med Lett Drug Ther 35:79–86, 1993.

Hirsch MS, D'Aquila RT. Therapy for human immunodeficiency virus infection. N Engl J Med 328:1685–95, 1993.

McLeod GX, Hammer SM. Zidovudine: Five years later. Ann Intern Med 117:487–510, 1992.

Panel on Antiretroviral Guidelines for Adults and Adolescents. Guidelines for the use of antiretroviral agents in HIV-1-infected adults and adolescents. Department of Health and Human Services. December 1, 2009; 1–161. Available at http://www.aidsinfo.nih.gov/ ContentFiles/AdultandAdolescentGL.pdf.

Staszewski S, Morales-Ramirez J, Trashima KT, et al. Efavirenz plus zidovudine and lamivudine, efavirenz plus indinavir, and indinavir plus zidovudine and lamivudine in the treatment of HIV-1 infection in adults. N Engl J Med 341:1865–1873, 1999.

Lopinavir + Ritonavir (Kaletra) LPV/r

Drug Class: Antiretroviral protease inhibitor combination
Usual Dose: Therapy-naïve: 400/10 mg (2 tablets or 5 mL solution) BID or 800/200 mg (4 tablets or 10 mL solution) QD. Therapy-experienced: 400/100 mg BID. New tablet formulation (lopinavir 200 mg + ritonavir 50 mg) replaces capsules (lopinavir 133.3 mg + ritonavir 33.3 mg), resulting in reduction in total number of pills from 6 capsules to 4 tablets per day. Also available as an oral solution (lopinavir 400 mg + ritonavir 100 mg per 5 mL)
How Supplied: Oral Solution: Contains 80 mg/ mL Lopinavir + 20 mg/mL Ritonavir; Oral Tablet: Available as 100 mg Lopinavir + 25 mg Ritonavir, or 200 mg Lopinavir + 50 mg Ritonavir
Pharmacokinetic Parameters:
Peak serum level: 9.6/≤ 1 mcg/mL
Bioavailability: No data
Excreted unchanged (urine): 3%
Serum half-life (normal/ESRD): 5-6/5-6 hrs
Plasma protein binding: 99%
Volume of distribution (V_d): No data/0.44 L/kg
Primary Mode of Elimination: Hepatic
Dosage Adjustments*

CrCl 50–80 mL/min	No change
CrCl 10–50 mL/min	No change
CrCl < 10 mL/min	No change
Post-HD dose	None
Post-PD dose	None
CVVH dose	No change
Moderate hepatic insufficiency	No change
Severe hepatic insufficiency	Avoid

Antiretroviral Dosage Adjustments

Fosamprenavir	Avoid
Delavirdine	No information
Efavirenz	LPV/r tablets 500/125 mg‡ BID; LPV/r oral solution 533/133 mg BID

"Usual dose" assumes normal renal/hepatic function. * For renal insufficiency, give usual dose × 1 followed by maintenance dose per CrCl. For dialysis patients, dose the same as for CrCl < 10 mL/min and give supplemental (post-HD/PD dose) immediately after dialysis. CrCl = creatinine clearance; CVVH = continuous veno-venous hemo-filtration; HD/PD = hemodialysis/peritoneal dialysis. See pp. 190–193 for explanations, p. x for abbreviations

Indinavir	Indinavir 600 mg BID
Nelfinavir	Same as for efavirenz
Nevirapine	Same as for efavirenz
Rifabutin	Max. dose of rifabutin 150 mg QOD (every other day) or 3 times per week
Saquinavir	Saquinavir 1000 mg BID
Etravirine	No change
Maraviroc	150 mg BID
Raltegravir	No information

Drug Interactions: Antiretrovirals, rifabutin, (see dose adjustment grid, above); astemizole, terfenadine, benzodiazepines, cisapride, ergotamine, flecainide, pimozide, propafenone, rifampin, statins, St. John's wort (avoid if possible); tenofovir (↓ lopinavir levels, ↑ tenofovir levels). ↓ effectiveness of oral contraceptives. Insufficient data on other drug interactions listed for ritonavir alone.

Adverse Effects: Diarrhea (very common), headache, nausea, vomiting, asthenia, ↑ SGOT/SGPT, hepatotoxicity, abdominal pain, pancreatitis, paresthesias, hyperglycemia (including worsening diabetes, new-onset diabetes, DKA), ↑ cholesterol/triglycerides (evaluate risk for coronary disease, pancreatitis), ↑ CPK, ↑ uric acid, fat redistribution, possible increased bleeding in hemophilia. Oral solution contains 42.4% alcohol. May prolong PR and QT interval; use with caution in patients with underlying structural heart disease, preexisting conduction system abnormalities, ischemic heart disease, or cardiomyopathies.

Allergic Potential: Low

Safety in Pregnancy: C

Comments: Tablet formulation does not require refrigeration and may be taken with or without food. With oral solution, Lopinavir serum concentrations with moderately fatty meals are increased 54%.

REFERENCES:

Benson CA, Deeks SG, Brun SC, et al. Safety and antiviral activity at 48 weeks of lopinavir/ritonavir plus nevirapine and 2 nucleoside reverse-transcriptase inhibitors in human immunodeficiency virus type 1-infected protease inhibitor-experienced patients. J Infect Dis 185:599–607, 2002.

Manfredi R, Calza L, Chiodo F. First-line efavirenz versus lopinavir-ritonavir-based highly active antiretroviral therapy for naïve patients. AIDS 18:2331–2333, 2004.

Panel on Antiretroviral Guidelines for Adults and Adolescents. Guidelines for the use of antiretroviral agents in HIV-1-infected adults and adolescents. Department of Health and Human Services. December 1, 2009; 1–161. Available at http://www.aidsinfo.nih.gov/ContentFiles/AdultandAdolescentGL.pdf.

Riddler S, et al. Initial treatment for HIV infection—an embarrassment of riches. N Engl J Med 358(20): 2095–2106. May 15, 2008.

Walmsley S, Bernstein B, King M, et al. Lopinavir-ritonavir versus nelfinavir for the initial treatment of HIV infection. N Engl J Med 346:2039–46, 2002.

Website: www.kaletra.com

Maraviroc (Selzentry) MVC

Drug Class: HIV-1 chemokine receptor 5 (CCR5) antagonist

Usual Dose: 150 mg, 300 mg, or 600 mg (PO) BID, depending on concomitant medications (see below), in CCR5-tropic HIV-1 isolates. Available in 150 mg and 300 mg tablets

How Supplied: Oral Tablet: 150 mg, 300 mg

Pharmacokinetic Parameters:

Peak serum level: 266–618 mcg/mL
Bioavailability: 23–33%
Excreted unchanged: 20% (urine); 76% (feces)
Serum half-life (normal/ESRD): 14–18 hrs/not studied

"Usual dose" assumes normal renal/hepatic function. * For renal insufficiency, give usual dose × 1 followed by maintenance dose per CrCl. For dialysis patients, dose the same as for CrCl < 10 mL/min and give supplemental (post-HD/PD dose) immediately after dialysis. CrCl = creatinine clearance; CVVH = continuous veno-venous hemo-filtration; HD/PD = hemodialysis/peritoneal dialysis. See pp. 190–193 for explanations, p. x for abbreviations

Plasma protein binding: 76%
Volume of distribution (V_d): 194 L
Primary Mode of Elimination: Fecal/renal
Dosage Adjustments*

CrCl 50–80 mL/min	No change
CrCl 10–25 mL/min	Use caution
CrCl < 10 mL/min	Use caution
Post-HD dose	No information
Post-PD dose	No information
CVVH dose	No information
Mild hepatic insufficiency	No information
Moderate or severe hepatic insufficiency	No information

Antiretroviral Dosage Adjustments

Protease inhibitors (except tipranavir/ritonavir), delavirdine, ketoconazole, itraconazole, clarithromycin, nefazodone, telithromycin	150 mg (PO) BID
Tipranavir/ritonavir, nevirapine, all NRTIs and enfuvirtide	300 mg (PO) BID
Efavirenz, rifampin, carbamazepine, phenobarbital, phenytoin	600 mg (PO) BID

Drug Interactions: Maraviroc is a substrate of CYP3A and P-glycoprotein and is likely to be modulated by inhibitors and inducers of these enzymes/transporters.
Adverse Effects: Hepatotoxicity has been reported. A systemic allergic reaction (e.g., pruritic rash, eosinophilia, or elevated IgE) prior to the development of hepatotoxicity may occur. Other adverse effects: cough, infection, upper respiratory tract infection, rash, pyrexia, dizziness, abdominal pain, musculoskeletal symptoms (joint/muscle pain). Myocardial infarction/ischemia reported in < 2% in clinical trials.
Allergic Potential: Low
Safety in Pregnancy: B
Comments: Indicated for treatment-experienced adult patients infected with only cellular chemokine receptor (CCR) 5-tropic HIV-1 virus detectable who have evidence of viral replication and HIV-1 strains resistant to multiple antiretroviral agents. Used in combination with other antiretroviral agents.Trofile phenotype test (performed at Monogram) is needed to confirm infection with CCR5-tropic HIV-1 (also known as "R5 virus").
Cerebrospinal Fluid Penetration: No data

REFERENCES:
Dorr P, Westby M, Dobbs S, et al. Maraviroc (UK-427, 857), a potent, orally bioavailable, and selective small-molecule inhibitor of chemokine receptor CCR5 with broad-spectrum anti-human immunodeficiency virus type 1 activity. *Antimicrob Agents Chemother* 49:4721–4732, 2005.
Gulick R. Maraviroc for previously treated patients with R5 HIV-1 infection, *N Engl J Med* 359(14):1429–41. Oct 2, 2008.
Fätkenheuer G. Subgroup analyses of maraviroc in previously treated R5 HIV-1 infection. *N Engl J Med* 359(14):1442–55. Oct 2, 2008.
Lederman MM, Penn-Nicholson A, Cho M, et al. Biology of CCR5 and its role in HIV infection and treatment. *JAMA* 296:815–826, 2006.
Panel on Antiretroviral Guidelines for Adults and Adolescents. Guidelines for the use of antiretroviral agents in HIV-1-infected adults and adolescents. Department of Health and Human Services. December 1, 2009; 1–161. Available at http://www.aidsinfo.nih.gov/ContentFiles/AdultandAdolescentGL.pdf.
Product Information: SELZENTRY(R) oral tablets, maraviroc oral tablets. Pfizer Labs, New York, NY, 2007.
Website: www.selzentry.com

"Usual dose" assumes normal renal/hepatic function. * For renal insufficiency, give usual dose × 1 followed by maintenance dose per CrCl. For dialysis patients, dose the same as for CrCl < 10 mL/min and give supplemental (post-HD/PD dose) immediately after dialysis. CrCl = creatinine clearance; CVVH = continuous veno-venous hemo-filtration; HD/PD = hemodialysis/peritoneal dialysis. See pp. 190–193 for explanations, p. x for abbreviations

Nelfinavir (Viracept) NFV

Drug Class: Antiretroviral protease inhibitor
Usual Dose: 1250 mg (PO) BID (two 625-mg tablets per dose) with meals, or five 250-mg tabs or 750 mg (three 250-mg tabs) (PO) TID
How Supplied: Oral Powder for Suspension: 50 mg/gm, Oral Tablet: 250 mg, 625 mg
Pharmacokinetic Parameters:
Peak serum level: 35 mcg/mL
Bioavailability: 20–80%
Excreted unchanged (urine): 1–2%
Serum half-life (normal/ESRD): 4 hrs/no data
Plasma protein binding: 98%
Volume of distribution (V_d): 5 L/kg
Primary Mode of Elimination: Hepatic
Dosage Adjustments*

CrCl 50–80 mL/min	No change
CrCl 10–50 mL/min	No change
CrCl < 10 mL/min	No change
Post-HD dose	None
Post-PD dose	None
CVVH dose	No change
Moderate hepatic insufficiency	No information
Severe hepatic insufficiency	No information—use caution

Antiretroviral Dosage Adjustments

Delavirdine	No information (monitor for neutropenia)
Efavirenz	No changes
Indinavir	Limited data for nelfinavir 1250 mg BID + indinavir 1200 mg BID

Lopinavir/ ritonavir	Nelfinavir 1000 mg BID or lopinavir/r 600/150 mg BID
Nevirapine	No changes
Ritonavir	No information
Saquinavir	Saquinavir 1200 mg BID
Rifampin	Avoid combination
Rifabutin	Nelfinavir 1250 mg BID; rifabutin 150 mg QD or 300 mg 2–3x/week
Etravirine	No data
Maraviroc	150 mg BID
Raltegravir	No data

Drug Interactions: Antiretrovirals, rifabutin, rifampin (see dose adjustment grid, above); amiodarone, quinidine, astemizole, terfenadine, benzodiazepines, cisapride, ergot alkaloids, statins, St. John's wort (avoid if possible); carbamazepine, phenytoin, phenobarbital (↓ nelfinavir levels, ↑ anticonvulsant levels; monitor); caspofungin (↓ caspofungin levels, may ↓ caspofungin effect); clarithromycin, erythromycin, telithromycin (↑ nelfinavir and macrolide levels); didanosine (dosing conflict with food; give nelfinavir with food 2 hours before or 1 hour after didanosine); itraconazole, voriconazole, ketoconazole (↑ nelfinavir levels); lamivudine (↑ lamivudine levels); methadone (may require ↑ methadone dose); oral contraceptives, zidovudine (↓ zidovudine levels); sildenafil (↑ or ↓ sildenafil levels; do not exceed 25 mg in 48 hrs, tadalafil (max. 10 mg/72 hrs, vardenafil (max. 2.5 mg/72 hrs).
Adverse Effects: Impaired concentration, nausea, abdominal pain, secretory diarrhea, ↑ SGOT/SGPT, rash, ↑ cholesterol/triglycerides

---

"Usual dose" assumes normal renal/hepatic function. * For renal insufficiency, give usual dose × 1 followed by maintenance dose per CrCl. For dialysis patients, dose the same as for CrCl < 10 mL/min and give supplemental (post-HD/PD dose) immediately after dialysis. CrCl = creatinine clearance; CVVH = continuous veno-venous hemo-filtration; HD/PD = hemodialysis/peritoneal dialysis. See pp. 190–193 for explanations, p. x for abbreviations

(evaluate risk for coronary disease/pancreatitis), fat redistribution, hyperglycemia (including worsening diabetes, new-onset diabetes, DKA), possible increased bleeding in hemophilia.

Allergic Potential: Low

Safety in Pregnancy: B

Comments: Take with food (absorption increased 300%). New 625-mg tablet available.

Cerebrospinal Fluid Penetration: Undetectable

REFERENCES:

Albrecht MA, Bosch RJ, Hammer SM, et al. Nelfinavir, efavirenz, or both after the failure of nucleoside treatment of HIV infection. *N Engl J Med* 345: 398–407, 2001.

Clotet B, Ruiz L, Martinez-Picado J, et al. Prevalence of HIV protease mutations on failure of nelfinavir-containing HAART: a retrospective analysis of four clinical studies and two observational cohorts. *HIV Clin Trials* 3:316–23, 2002.

Deeks SG, Smith M, Holodniy M, et al. HIV-1 protease inhibitors: A review for clinicians. *JAMA* 277: 145–53, 1997.

DiCenzo R, Forrest A, Fischl MA, et al. Pharmacokinetics of indinavir and nelfinavir in treatment-naïve, human immunodeficiency virus-infected subjects. *Antimicrob Agents Chemother* 48:918–23, 2004.

Go J, Cunha BA. Nelfinavir: a review. *Antibiotics for Clinicians* 4:17–23, 2000.

Kaul DR, Cinti SK, Carver PL, et al. HIV protease inhibitors: Advances in therapy and adverse reactions, including metabolic complications. *Pharmacotherapy* 19:281–98, 1999.

Panel on Antiretroviral Guidelines for Adults and Adolescents. Guidelines for the use of antiretroviral agents in HIV-1-infected adults and adolescents. Department of Health and Human Services. December 1, 2009; 1–161. Available at http://www.aidsinfo.nih.gov/ContentFiles/AdultandAdolescentGL.pdf.

Perry CM, Benfield P. Nelfinavir. *Drugs* 54:81–7, 1997.

Simpson KN, Luo MP, Chumney E, et al. Cost-effective of lopinavir/ritonavir versus nelfinavir as the first-line highly active antiretroviral therapy regimen for HIV infection. HIV Clin Trials 5: 294–304, 2004.

Walmsley S, Bernstein B, King M, et al. Lopinavir-ritonavir versus nelfinavir for the initial treatment of HIV infection. *N Engl J Med* 346:2039–46, 2002.

Website: www.viracept.com

Nevirapine (Viramune) NVP

Drug Class: Antiretroviral NNRTI (non-nucleoside reverse transcriptase inhibitor)

Usual Dose: 200 mg (PO) QD × 2 weeks, then 200 mg (PO) BID

How Supplied:

Viramune O/S—Oral Suspension: 50 mg/5 mL

Viramune—Oral Suspension: 50 mg/5 mL, Oral Tablet: 200 mg

Pharmacokinetic Parameters:

Peak serum level: 0.9–3.6 mcg/mL

Bioavailability: 90%

Excreted unchanged (urine): 5%

Serum half-life (normal/ESRD): 40 hrs/no data

Plasma protein binding: 60%

Volume of distribution (V_d): 1.4 L/kg

Primary Mode of Elimination: Hepatic

Dosage Adjustments*

CrCl > 20 mL/min	No change
CrCl < 20 mL/min	No change; use caution
Post-HD dose	200 mg (PO)
Post-PD dose	None
CVVH dose	No change
Moderate hepatic insufficiency	Use caution
Severe hepatic insufficiency	Avoid

"Usual dose" assumes normal renal/hepatic function. * For renal insufficiency, give usual dose × 1 followed by maintenance dose per CrCl. For dialysis patients, dose the same as for CrCl < 10 mL/min and give supplemental (post-HD/PD dose) immediately after dialysis. CrCl = creatinine clearance; CVVH = continuous veno-venous hemo-filtration; HD/PD = hemodialysis/peritoneal dialysis. See pp. 190–193 for explanations, p. x for abbreviations

Antiretroviral Dosage Adjustments

Delavirdine	No information
Efavirenz	Avoid combination
Indinavir	Indinavir 1000 mg TID
Lopinavir/ ritonavir (l/r)	Consider l/r 600/150 mg BID in PI-experienced patients
Nelfinavir	No information
Ritonavir	No changes
Saquinavir	No information
Rifampin	Not recommended
Rifabutin	Use caution
Etravirine	Avoid combination
Maraviroc	Without PI MVC 300 mg BID with PI (except TPV/r) MVC 150 mg BID
Raltegravir	No data

Drug Interactions: Antiretrovirals, rifabutin, rifampin (see dose adjustment grid, above); carbamazepine, phenobarbital, phenytoin (monitor anticonvulsant levels); caspofungin (↓ caspofungin levels, may ↓ caspofungin effect); ethinyl estradiol (↓ ethinyl estradiol levels; use additional/alternative method); ketoconazole (avoid); voriconazole (↑ nevirapine levels); methadone (↓ methadone levels; titrate methadone dose to effect); tacrolimus (↓ tacrolimus levels).

Adverse Effects: Drug fever/rash (may be severe; usually occurs within 6 weeks), Stevens-Johnson syndrome, ↑ SGOT/SGPT, *fatal hepatitis*, headache, diarrhea, leukopenia, stomatitis, peripheral neuropathy, paresthesias. Greater risk of fatal hepatitis and Stevens-Johnson

syndrome when CD4 > 400/mm^3 (males) or > 250/mm^3 (females) (monitor patients intensely for first 18 weeks of therapy).
Allergic Potential: High
Safety in Pregnancy: B
Comments: Absorption not affected by food. Not to be used for post-exposure prophylaxis because of potential for fatal hepatitis.
Cerebrospinal Fluid Penetration: 45%

REFERENCES:

D'Aquila RT, Hughes MD, Johnson VA, et al. Nevirapine, zidovudine, and didanosine compared with zidovudine and didanosine in patients with HIV-1 infection. *Ann Intern Med* 124:1019–30, 1996.

Hammer SM, Kessler HA, Saag MS. Issues in combination antiretroviral therapy: a review. *J Acquired Immune Defic Syndr* 7:24–37, 1994.

Havlir DV, Lange JM. New antiretrovirals and new combinations. *AIDS* 12:165–74, 1998.

Herzmann C, Karcher H. Nevirapine plus zidovudine to prevent mother-to-child transmission of HIV. *N Engl J Med* 351:2013–5, 2004.

Johnson S, Chan J, Bennett CL. Hepatotoxicity after prophylaxis with a nevirapine-containing antiretroviral regimen. *Ann Intern Med* 137:146–7, 2002.

Milinkovic A, Martinez E. Nevirapine in the treatment of HIV. *Expert Rev Anti Infect Ther* 2:367–73, 2004.

Montaner JS, Reiss P, Cooper D, et al. A randomized, double-blind trial comparing combinations of nevirapine, didanosine, and zidovudine for HIV-infected patients: the INCAS trial. Italy, the Netherlands, Canada and Australia Study. *J Am Med Assoc* 279:930–937, 1998.

Negredo E, Ribalta J, Paredes R, et al. Reversal of atherogenic lipoprotein profile in HIV-1 infected patients with lipodystrophy after replacing protease inhibitors by nevirapine. *AIDS* 16:1383–9, 2002.

Panel on Antiretroviral Guidelines for Adults and Adolescents. Guidelines for the use of antiretroviral agents in HIV-1-infected adults and adolescents. Department of Health and Human Services. December 1, 2009; 1–161. Available at http://www.aidsinfo.nih.gov/ContentFiles/AdultandAdolescentGL.pdf.

"Usual dose" assumes normal renal/hepatic function. * For renal insufficiency, give usual dose × 1 followed by maintenance dose per CrCl. For dialysis patients, dose the same as for CrCl < 10 mL/min and give supplemental (post-HD/PD dose) immediately after dialysis. CrCl = creatinine clearance; CVVH = continuous veno-venous hemo-filtration; HD/PD = hemodialysis/peritoneal dialysis. See pp. 190–193 for explanations, p. x for abbreviations

Weverling GJ, Lange JM, Jurriaans S, et al. Alternative
    multidrug regimen provides improved suppression
    of HIV-1 replication over triple therapy. *AIDS*
    12:117–22, 1998.
Website: www.viramune.com

Raltegravir (Isentress) RAL

Drug Class: HIV-1 integrase inhibitor
Usual Dose: 400 mg (PO) BID
How Supplied: Oral Tablet: 400 mg
Pharmacokinetic Parameters:
Peak serum level: 6.5 μM
Bioavailability: ~ 32% (20–43%)
Excreted unchanged: 51% (feces); 9% (urine)
Serum half-life (normal/ESRD): 9–12 hrs/no data
Plasma protein binding: 83%
Volume of distribution (V_d): not studied
Primary Mode of Elimination: Fecal/renal
Dosage Adjustments*

CrCl 50–80 mL/min	No change
CrCl 10–50 mL/min	No change
CrCl < 10 mL/min	No information
Post-HD dose	No information
Post-PD dose	No information
CVVH dose	No information
Mild/moderate hepatic insufficiency	No change
Severe hepatic insufficiency	No information

Antiretroviral Dosage Adjustments

Atazanavir	No change
Atazanavir/ritonavir	No change
Efavirenz	No change
Rifampin	Raltegravir 800 mg BID
Ritonavir	No change
Tenofovir	No change
Tipranavir/ritonavir	No change
Etravirine	No changes
Nevirapine	No data
Maraciroc	No changes

Drug Interactions: Rifampin (↓ raltegravir levels, use with caution). Omeprazole (↑ raltegravir levels, no adjustment needed). In vitro, raltegravir does not inhibit CYP1A2, CYP2B6, CYP2C8, CYP2C9, CYP2C19, CYP2D6 or CYP3A and does not induce CYP3A4. In addition, raltegravir does not inhibit P-glycoprotein-mediated transport. Raltegravir is therefore not expected to affect the pharmacokinetics of drugs that are substrates of these enzymes or P-glycoprotein (e.g., protease inhibitors, NNRTIs, methadone, opioid analgesics, statins, azole antifungals, proton pump inhibitors, oral contraceptives, anti-erectile dysfunction agents).
Adverse Effects: Nausea, headache, diarrhea, pyrexia.
Allergic Potential: Low
Safety in Pregnancy: C
Comments: May be taken with or without food. CPK elevations, myopathy, and rhabdomyolysis have been reported—use with caution in patients at increased risk for myopathy or rhabdomyolysis, such as those receiving concomitant medications known to cause these conditions (e.g., statins). Raltegravir is indicated for treatment-naïve and treatment-experienced adult patients who have evidence of viral replication and HIV-1 strains resistant to multiple antiretroviral agents. Treatment experienced patients who

----
"Usual dose" assumes normal renal/hepatic function. * For renal insufficiency, give usual dose × 1 followed by maintenance dose per CrCl. For dialysis patients, dose the same as for CrCl < 10 mL/min and give supplemental (post-HD/PD dose) immediately after dialysis. CrCl = creatinine clearance; CVVH = continuous veno-venous hemo-filtration; HD/PD = hemodialysis/peritoneal dialysis. See pp. 190–193 for explanations, p. x for abbreviations

switch to raltegravir must have a least two other fully active agents in their regimen.

Cerebrospinal Fluid Penetration: No data

REFERENCES:

Cooper, OA. Subgroup and resistance analyses of raltegravir for resistant HIV-1 infection. *N Engl J Med* 359(4):355–65. Jul 24, 2008.

Eron JJ, Young B, Cooper DA, et al. Switch to a raltegravir-based regimen versus continuation of a lopinavir-ritonavir-based regimen in stable HIV-infected patients with suppressed viraemia (SWITCHMRK 1 and 2): two multicentre, double-blind, randomised controlled trials. *Lancet.* Jan 30;375(9712):396–407.

Grinsztejn B, Nguyen BY, Katlama C, et al. Safety and efficacy of the HIV-1 integrase inhibitor raltegravir (MK-0518) in treatment-experienced patients with multidrug-resistant virus: a phase II randomised controlled trial. *Lancet* 369:1261–69, 2007.

Iwamoto M, Wenning LA, Nguyen BY, et al. Effects of omeprazole on plasma levels of raltegravir. *Clin Infect Dis.* Feb 15 2009;48(4):489–492.

Iwamoto M, Wenning LA, Petry AS, et al. Safety, tolerability, and pharmacokinetics of raltegravir after single and multiple doses in healthy subjects. *Clin Pharmacol Ther* 83:293–9, 2007.

Kassahun K, McIntosh I, Cui D, et al. Metabolism and Disposition in Humans of Raltegravir (MK-0518), an Anti-AIDS Drug Targeting the HIV-1 Integrase Enzyme. *Drug Metab Dispos Epub*: 1–28, 2007.

Lennox JL, DeJesus E, Lazzarin A, et al. Safety and efficacy of raltegravir-based versus efavirenz-based combination therapy in treatment-naïve patients with HIV-1 infection: a multicentre, double-blind randomised controlled trial. *Lancet.* Sep 5 2009;374(9692):796–806.

Markowitz M, Morales-Ramirez JO, Nguyen BY, et al. Antiretroviral activity, pharmacokinetics, and tolerability of MK-0518, a novel inhibitor of HIV-1 integrase, dosed as monotherapy for 10 days in treatment-naïve HIV-1-infected individuals. *J Acquir Immune Defic Syndr* 43:509–15, 2006.

Palmisano L, Role of integrase inhibitors in the treatment of HIV disease. *Expert Rev Anti Infect Ther* 5:67–75, 2007.

Panel on Antiretroviral Guidelines for Adults and Adolescents. Guidelines for the use of antiretroviral agents in HIV-1-infected adults and adolescents. Department of Health and Human Services. December 1, 2009; 1–161. Available at http://www.aidsinfo.nih.gov/ContentFiles/AdultandAdolescentGL.pdf.

Product Information. ISENTRESS oral tablets, raltegravir oral tablets. Merck & Co, Inc, Whitehouse Station, NJ, 2007.

Steigbigel RT. Raltegravir with optimized background therapy for resistant HIV-1 infection. *N Engl J Med* 359(4):339–54. Jul 24, 2008.

Wenning LA, Hanley WD, Brainard DM, et al. Effect of rifampin, a potent inducer of drug-metabolizing enzymes, on the pharmacokinetics of raltegravir. *Antimicrob Agents Chemother.* Jul 2009;53(7): 2852–2856.

Ritonavir (Norvir) RTV

Drug Class: Antiretroviral protease inhibitor
Usual Dose: 600 mg (PO) BID (see comments)
How Supplied: Oral Capsule, Liquid Filled: 100 mg; Oral Solution: 80 mg/mL; Oral Tablet (heat stable) 100 mg
Pharmacokinetic Parameters:
Peak serum level: 11 mcg/mL
Bioavailability: No data
Excreted unchanged (urine): 3.5%
Serum half-life (normal/ESRD): 4 hrs/no data
Plasma protein binding: 99%
Volume of distribution (V_d): 0.41 L/kg
Primary Mode of Elimination: Hepatic
Dosage Adjustments*

CrCl 50–80 mL/min	No change
CrCl 10–50 mL/min	No change
CrCl < 10 mL/min	No change
Post-HD dose	None
Post-PD dose	None

"Usual dose" assumes normal renal/hepatic function. * For renal insufficiency, give usual dose × 1 followed by maintenance dose per CrCl. For dialysis patients, dose the same as for CrCl < 10 mL/min and give supplemental (post-HD/PD dose) immediately after dialysis. CrCl = creatinine clearance; CVVH = continuous veno-venous hemo-filtration; HD/PD = hemodialysis/peritoneal dialysis. See pp. 190–193 for explanations, p. x for abbreviations

CVVH dose	None
Moderate hepatic insufficiency	No change
Severe hepatic insufficiency	No change; use caution

Antiretroviral Dosage Adjustments

Atazanavir	Ritonavir 100 mg QD + atazanavir 300 mg QD with food
Delavirdine	Delavirdine: no change; ritonavir: no information
Efavirenz	Ritonavir 600 mg BID (500 mg BID for intolerance)
Indinavir	Ritonavir 100–200 mg BID + indinavir 800 mg BID, or 400 mg BID of each drug
Nelfinavir	Ritonavir 400 mg BID + nelfinavir 500–750 mg BID
Nevirapine	No changes
Saquinavir	Ritonavir 400 mg BID + saquinavir 400 mg BID
Ketoconazole	Caution; do not exceed ketoconazole 200 mg QD
Rifampin	Avoid
Rifabutin	150 mg q2d or 3x/week

Drug Interactions: Antiretrovirals, rifabutin, rifampin (see dose adjustment grid, above); alprazolam, diazepam, estazolam, flurazepam, midazolam, triazolam, zolpidem, meperidine, propoxyphene, piroxicam, quinidine, amiodarone, encainide, flecainide, propafenone, astemizole, bepridil, bupropion, cisapride, clorazepate, clozapine, pimozide, St. John's wort, terfenadine (avoid); alfentanil, fentanyl, hydrocodone, tramadol, disopyramide, lidocaine, mexiletine, erythromycin, clarithromycin, warfarin, dronabinol, ondansetron, metoprolol, pindolol, propranolol, timolol, amlodipine, diltiazem, felodipine, isradipine, nicardipine, nifedipine, nimodipine, nisolidipine, nitrendipine, verapamil, etoposide, paclitaxel, tamoxifen, vinblastine, vincristine, loratadine, tricyclic antidepressants, paroxetine, nefazodone, sertraline, trazodone, fluoxetine, venlafaxine, fluvoxamine, cyclosporine, tacrolimus, chlorpromazine, haloperidol, perphenazine, risperidone, thioridazine, clozapine, pimozide, methamphetamine ($\uparrow$ interacting drug levels); voriconazole ($\downarrow$ voriconazole levels); telithromycin ($\uparrow$ ritonavir levels); codeine, hydromorphone, methadone, morphine, ketoprofen, ketorolac, naproxen, diphenoxylate, oral contraceptives, theophylline ($\downarrow$ interacting drug levels); carbamazepine, phenytoin, phenobarbital, clonazepam, dexamethasone, prednisone ($\downarrow$ ritonavir levels, $\uparrow$ interacting drug levels; monitor anticonvulsant levels); metronidazole (disulfiram-like reaction); tenofovir, tobacco ($\downarrow$ ritonavir levels); sildenafil (do not exceed 25 mg in 48 hrs); tadalafil (max. 10 mg/ 72 hrs); vardenafil (max. 2.5 mg/72 hrs).

Adverse Effects: Anorexia, anemia, leukopenia, hyperglycemia (including worsening diabetes, new-onset diabetes, DKA), $\uparrow$ cholesterol/ triglycerides (evaluate risk for coronary disease/ pancreatitis), fat redistribution, $\uparrow$ CPK, nausea, vomiting, diarrhea, abdominal pain, circumoral/ extremity paresthesias, $\uparrow$ SGOT/SGPT, pancreatitis, taste perversion, possible increased bleeding in hemophilia.

Allergic Potential: Low

Safety in Pregnancy: B

"Usual dose" assumes normal renal/hepatic function. * For renal insufficiency, give usual dose × 1 followed by maintenance dose per CrCl. For dialysis patients, dose the same as for CrCl < 10 mL/min and give supplemental (post-HD/PD dose) immediately after dialysis. CrCl = creatinine clearance; CVVH = continuous veno-venous hemo-filtration; HD/PD = hemodialysis/peritoneal dialysis. See pp. 190–193 for explanations, p. x for abbreviations

Comments: Usually used at low dose (100–200 mg/day) as pharmacokinetic "booster" of other PIs. GI intolerance decreases over time. Take with food if possible (serum levels increase 15%, fewer GI side effects). Dose escalation regimen: day 1–2 (300 mg BID), day 3–5 (400 mg BID), day 6–13 (500 mg BID), day 14 (600 mg BID). Separate dosing from ddI by 2 hours. Refrigerate capsules (not oral solution) if temperature to exceed 78°F. Do not refrigerate oral tablets, they are heat stable. Tablets are not bioequivalent to capsules and patients may experience more GI side effects when switched to tablet formulation.

Cerebrospinal Fluid Penetration: < 10%

REFERENCES:

Cameron DW, Japour AJ, Xu Y, et al. Ritonavir and saquinavir combination therapy for the treatment of HIV infection. *AIDS* 13:213–24, 1999.

Deeks SG, Smith M, Holodniy M, et al. HIV-1 protease inhibitors: a review for clinicians. *JAMA* 277: 145–53, 1997.

Kaul DR, Cinti SK, Carver PL, et al. HIV protease inhibitors: advances in therapy and adverse reactions, including metabolic complications. *Pharmacotherapy* 19:281–98, 1999.

Lea AP, Faulds D. Ritonavir. *Drugs* 52:541–6, 1996.

McDonald CK, Kuritzkes DR. Human immunodeficiency virus type 1 protease inhibitors. *Arch Intern Med* 157:951–9, 1997.

Panel on Antiretroviral Guidelines for Adults and Adolescents. Guidelines for the use of antiretroviral agents in HIV-1-infected adults and adolescents. Department of Health and Human Services. December 1, 2009; 1–161. Available at http://www.aidsinfo.nih.gov/ContentFiles/AdultandAdolescentGL.pdf.

Piliero PJ. Interaction between ritonavir and statins. *Am J Med* 112:510–1, 2002.

Rathbun RC, Rossi DR. Low-dose ritonavir for protease inhibitor pharmacokinetic enhancement. *Ann Pharmacother* 36:702–6, 2002.

Shepp DH, Stevens RC. Ritonavir boosting of HIV protease inhibitors. *Antibiotics for Clinicians* 9:301–11, 2005.

Website: www.TreatHIV.com

Saquinavir (Invirase) SQV

Drug Class: Antiretroviral protease inhibitor

Usual Dose: 1000 mg (PO) BID (see comments) with ritonavir 100 mg (PO) BID, or 400 mg (PO) BID with ritonavir 400 mg (PO) BID

How Supplied: Oral Capsule: 200 mg; Oral Tablet: 500 mg

Pharmacokinetic Parameters:

Peak serum level: 0.07 mcg/mL
Bioavailability: hard-gel (4%)
Excreted unchanged (urine): 13%
Serum half-life (normal/ESRD): 13 hrs/no data
Plasma protein binding: 98%
Volume of distribution (V_d): 10 L/kg

Primary Mode of Elimination: Hepatic

Dosage Adjustments*

CrCl 50–80 mL/min	No change
CrCl 10–50 mL/min	No change
CrCl < 10 mL/min	No change
Post-HD dose	None
Post-PD dose	None
CVVH dose	No change
Moderate hepatic insufficiency	No change
Severe hepatic insufficiency	Use caution

Antiretroviral Dosage Adjustments

Darunavir	Avoid
Delavirdine	No Information

"Usual dose" assumes normal renal/hepatic function. * For renal insufficiency, give usual dose × 1 followed by maintenance dose per CrCl. For dialysis patients, dose the same as for CrCl < 10 mL/min and give supplemental (post-HD/PD dose) immediately after dialysis. CrCl = creatinine clearance; CVVH = continuous veno-venous hemo-filtration; HD/PD = hemodialysis/peritoneal dialysis. See pp. 190–193 for explanations, p. x for abbreviations

Efavirenz	(SQV 1,000 mg + RTV 100 mg) BID
Indinavir	No information
Lopinavir/ritonavir 3 capsules BID	Saquinavir 500 mg BID
Nelfinavir	Saquinavir 1 gm BID or 1200 mg BID
Nevirapine	(SQV 1,000 mg + RTV 100 mg) BID
Ritonavir	Ritonavir 100 mg BID + saquinavir 1 gm BID
Rifampin	Contraindicated
Rifabutin	Avoid
Etravirine	(SQV 1,000 mg + RTV 100 mg) BID
Maraviroc	300 mg BID
Raltegravir	No data

Drug Interactions: Antiretrovirals, rifabutin, rifampin (see dose adjustment grid, above); astemizole, terfenadine, benzodiazepines, cisapride, ergotamine, statins, St. John's wort (avoid if possible); carbamazepine, phenytoin, phenobarbital, dexamethasone, prednisone (↓ saquinavir levels, ↑ interacting drug levels; monitor anticonvulsant levels); clarithromycin, erythromycin, telithromycin (↑ saquinavir and macrolide levels); grapefruit juice, itraconazole, voriconazole, ketoconazole (↑ saquinavir levels); sildenafil (do not give > 25 mg/48 hrs); tadalafil (max. 10 mg/72 hrs), vardenafil (max. 2.5 mg/ 72 hrs).

Adverse Effects: Anorexia, headache, anemia, leukopenia, hyperglycemia (including worsening diabetes, new-onset diabetes, DKA),

↑ cholesterol/triglycerides (evaluate risk for coronary disease/pancreatitis), ↑ SGOT/SGPT, hyperuricemia, fat redistribution, possible increased bleeding in hemophilia. May cause QT interval prolongation when combined with ritonavir.

Allergic Potential: Low

Safety in Pregnancy: B

Comments: Take with food. Avoid garlic supplements, which ↓ saquinavir levels ~ 50%. Boosted dose: 1 gm saquinavir/100 mg ritonavir (PO) BID. Preferred formulation is 500 mg hard-gel capsule (Invirase 500). Soft-gel capsules (Fortovase) no longer available.

Cerebrospinal Fluid Penetration: < 1%

REFERENCES:

Borck C. Garlic supplements and saquinavir. *Clin Infect Dis* 35:343, 2002.

Cameron DW, Japour AJ, Xu Y, et al. Ritonavir and saquinavir combination therapy for the treatment of HIV infection. *AIDS* 13:213–24, 1999.

Cardiello PF, van Heeswijk RP, Hassink EA, et al. Simplifying protease inhibitor therapy with once-daily dosing of saquinavir soft-gelatin capsules/ritonavir (1600/100 mg): HIVNAT 001.3 study. *J Acquir Immune Defic Syndr* 29:464–70, 2002.

Hsu A, Granneman GR, Cao G, et al. Pharmacokinetic interactions between two human immunodeficiency virus protease inhibitors, ritonavir and saquinavir. *Clin Pharmacol Ther* 63:453–64, 1998.

Murphy RL, Brun S, Hicks C, et al. ABT-378/ritonavir plus stavudine and lamivudine for the treatment of antiretroviral-naïve adults with HIV-1 infection: 48-week results. *AIDS* 15:F1–9, 2001.

Noble S, Faulds D. Saquinavir: a review of its pharmacology and clinical potential in the management of HIV infection. *Drugs* 52:93–112, 1996.

Panel on Antiretroviral Guidelines for Adults and Adolescents. Guidelines for the use of antiretroviral agents in HIV-1-infected adults and adolescents. Department of Health and Human Services. December 1, 2009; 1–161. Available at

---

"Usual dose" assumes normal renal/hepatic function. * For renal insufficiency, give usual dose × 1 followed by maintenance dose per CrCl. For dialysis patients, dose the same as for CrCl < 10 mL/min and give supplemental (post-HD/PD dose) immediately after dialysis. CrCl = creatinine clearance; CVVH = continuous veno-venous hemo-filtration; HD/PD = hemodialysis/peritoneal dialysis. See pp. 190–193 for explanations, p. x for abbreviations

http://www.aidsinfo.nih.gov/ContentFiles/
AdultandAdolescentGL.pdf.

Perry CM, Noble S. Saquinavir soft-gel capsule
formation: a review of its use in patients with HIV
infection. *Drugs* 55:461–86, 1998.

Vella S, Floridia M. Saquinavir: Clinical pharmacology and
efficacy. *Clin Pharmacokinet* 34:189–201, 1998. http://
www.fda.gov/Safety/MedWatch/SafetyInformation/
SafetyAlertsforHumanMedicalProducts/ucm201563.htm

Website: www.fortovase.com

Stavudine (Zerit) d4t

Drug Class: Antiretroviral NRTI (nucleoside
reverse transcriptase inhibitor)
Usual Dose: ≥ 60 kg: 40 mg (PO) BID;
< 60 kg: 30 mg (PO) BID
How Supplied:
Generic—Oral Capsule: 15 mg, 20 mg,
30 mg, 40 mg
Zerit—Oral Capsule: 15 mg, 20 mg, 30 mg,
40 mg, Oral Powder for Suspension: 1 mg/mL
Pharmacokinetic Parameters:
Peak serum level: 4.2 mcg/mL
Bioavailability: 86%
Excreted unchanged (urine): 40%
Serum half-life (normal/ESRD): 1.0/5.1 hrs
Plasma protein binding: 0%
Volume of distribution (V_d): 0.5 L/kg
Primary Mode of Elimination: Renal
Dosage Adjustments* ≥ 60 kg/(≤ 60 kg)

CrCl 50–80 mL/min	40 mg (PO) BID (30 mg [PO] BID)
CrCl 25–50 mL/min	20 mg (PO) BID (15 mg [PO] BID)
CrCl ~ 10–25 mL/min	20 mg (PO) QD (15 mg [PO] QD)
Post-HD dose	20 mg (PO) (15 mg [PO])

Post-PD dose	No information
CVVH dose	20 mg (PO) QD (15 mg [PO] QD)
Moderate hepatic insufficiency	No change
Severe hepatic insufficiency	No change

Drug Interactions: Ribavirin (↓ stavudine
efficacy, ↑ risk of lactic acidosis); zidovudine
(↓ stavudine levels); dapsone, INH, other
neurotoxic agents (↑ risk of neuropathy),
didanosine (↑ risk of neuropathy, lactic
acidosis).
Adverse Effects: Drug fever/rash, nausea,
vomiting, GI upset, diarrhea, headache, insomnia,
dose dependent peripheral neuropathy,
myalgias, pancreatitis, ↑ SGOT/SGPT, ↑
cholesterol, facial fat pad wasting, lipodystrophy,
thrombocytopenia, leukopenia, lactic acidosis
with hepatic steatosis (rare, but potentially life-
threatening toxicity with use of NRTIs).
Allergic Potential: Low
Safety in Pregnancy: C
Comments: Pancreatitis may be severe/
fatal. Avoid coadministration with AZT or ddC.
Decrease dose in patients with peripheral
neuropathy to 20 mg (PO) BID. Pregnant
women may be at increased risk for lactic
acidosis/liver damage when stavudine is used
with didanosine (ddI).
Cerebrospinal Fluid Penetration: 30%

REFERENCES:
Berasconi E, Boubaker K, Junghans C, et al
Abnormalities of body fat distribution in HIV-infected
persons treated with antiretroviral drugs: the Swiss
HIV Cohort Study. *J Acquir Immune Defic Syndr*
31:50–5, 2002.

"Usual dose" assumes normal renal/hepatic function. * For renal insufficiency, give usual dose × 1 followed by maintenance dose per CrCl. For dialysis patients, dose the same as for CrCl < 10 mL/min and give supplemental (post-HD/PD dose) immediately after dialysis. CrCl = creatinine clearance; CVVH = continuous veno-venous hemo-filtration; HD/PD = hemodialysis/peritoneal dialysis. See pp. 190–193 for explanations, p. x for abbreviations

Dudley MN, Graham KK, Kaul S, et al. Pharmacokinetics of stavudine in patients with AIDS and AIDS-related complex. *J Infect Dis* 166:480–5, 1992.

FDA notifications. FDA changes information for stavudine label. *Aids Alert* 17:67, 2002.

Joly V, Flandre P, Meiffredy V, et al. Efficacy of zidovudine compared to stavudine, both in combination with lamivudine and indinavir, in human immunodeficiency virus-infected nucleoside-experienced patients with no prior exposure to lamivudine, stavudine, or protease inhibitors (Novavir trial). *Antimicrob Agents Chemother* 46:1906–13, 2002.

Lea AP, Faulds D. Stavudine: A review of its pharmacodynamic and pharmacokinetic properties and clinical potential in HIV infection. *Drugs* 51: 846–64, 1996.

Miller KD, Cameron M, Wood LV, et al. Lactic acidosis and hepatic steatosis associated with use of stavudine: report of four cases. Ann Intern Med 133:192–96, 2000.

Murphy RL, Brun S, Hicks C, et al. ABT-378/ritonavir plus stavudine and lamivudine for the treatment of antiretroviral-naïve adults with HIV-1 infection: 48-week results. *AIDS* 15:F1–9, 2001.

Panel on Antiretroviral Guidelines for Adults and Adolescents. Guidelines for the use of antiretroviral agents in HIV-1-infected adults and adolescents. Department of Health and Human Services. December 1, 2009; 1–161. Available at http://www.aidsinfo.nih.gov/ContentFiles/ AdultandAdolescentGL.pdf.

Website: www.zerit.com

Telbivudine (Tyzeka) LDT

Drug Class: Anti-Hepatitis B agent (nucleoside reverse transcriptase inhibitor)

Usual Dose: 600 mg (PO) QD

How Supplied: Oral Tablet: 600 mg

Pharmacokinetic Parameters:

Peak serum level: 3.69 mcg/mL

Bioavailability: The absolute bioavailability is unknown

Excreted unchanged: 0% (feces), 42% (urine)

Serum half-life (normal/ESRD): 40–49 hrs/ no data

Plasma protein binding: 3.3%

Volume of distribution (V_d): not studied

Primary Mode of Elimination: Renal

Dosage Adjustments*

CrCl 50–80 mL/min	No change
CrCl 30–49 mL/min	600 mg q2d
CrCl < 30 mL/min	600 mg q3d
ESRD	600 mg q4d
Post-HD dose	Give dose after HD
Post-PD dose	Not studied
CVVH dose	Not studied
Mild to moderate hepatic insufficiency	No change
Severe hepatic insufficiency	No change

Antiretroviral Dosage Adjustments: None

Drug Interactions: Telbivudine Use with Peginterferon Alfa-2a: Increased Risk of Peripheral Neuropathy. Telbivudine is not metabolized by the liver and it is not a substrate or inhibitor of the cytochrome P450 enzyme system, and no drug other drug interactions have been established.

Adverse Effects: Boxed Warnings; Lactic acidosis/hepatomegaly, including fatal cases, have been reported with the use of nucleoside analogues alone or in combination with other antiretrovirals. Signs/symptoms of lactic acidosis include; nausea, vomiting, abdominal pain, tachypnea, decreased renal function, or decreased liver function. Severe acute exacerbations of hepatitis B have been reported in patients who have discontinued anti-hepatitis B therapy. Myopathy has also been associated with telbivudine use. Other less serious adverse

---

"Usual dose" assumes normal renal/hepatic function. * For renal insufficiency, give usual dose × 1 followed by maintenance dose per CrCl. For dialysis patients, dose the same as for CrCl < 10 mL/min and give supplemental (post-HD/PD dose) immediately after dialysis. CrCl = creatinine clearance; CVVH = continuous veno-venous hemo-filtration; HD/PD = hemodialysis/peritoneal dialysis. See pp. 190–193 for explanations, p. x for abbreviations

effects include: abdominal pain, dizziness, headache, nasopharyngitis, malaise, and fatigue.
Allergic Potential: Low
Safety in Pregnancy: B
Comments: May be administered without regard to food. Telbivudine does not exhibit any clinically relevant activity against HIV type 1. The efficacy and safety in patients co-infected with HIV, hepatitis C virus, hepatitis D virus, a history or signs of hepatic decompensation, or a history of alcohol or illicit substance abuse within the preceding 2 years are unknown. Severe, acute exacerbation of hepatitis B may occur upon discontinuation. Monitor liver function several months after stopping treatment; re-initiation of anti-hepatitis B therapy may be required.
Cerebrospinal Fluid Penetration: no data

REFERENCES:
Chan HL, Heathcote EJ, Marcellin P. Treatment of hepatitis B e antigen positive chronic hepatitis with telbivudine or adefovir: a randomized trial. *Ann Intern Med* 147(11):745–54, 2007.
Gane E, Lai CL, Liaw YF, et al. Phase III comparison of telbivudine vs lamivudine in HBeAg-positive patients with chronic hepatitis B: efficacy, safety, and predictors of response at 1 year. *J Hepatol* 44 (suppl 2):S183–S184, 2006.
Lai CL, Gane E, Liaw YF, et al. Maximal early HBV suppression is predictive of optimal virologic and clinical efficacy in nucleoside-treated hepatitis B patients: scientific observations from a large multinational trial (the GLOBE study). *Hepatology* 42(S1):232A–3A, 2005.
Lai CL, Gane E, Liaw YF, et al. Telbivudine (LdT) vs. lamivudine for chronic hepatitis B: first-year results from the international phase III GLOBE trial. *Hepatology* 42(Supp 1):748A, 2005.
Lai CL, Gane E, Liaw YF, et al. Telbivudine versus lamivudine in patients with chronic hepatitis B. *N Engl J Med* 357(25):2576–88, 2007.
Lai CL, Leung N, Teo EK, et al. A 1-year trial of telbivudine, lamivudine, and the combination in patients with hepatitis B e antigen-positive chronic hepatitis B. *Gastroenterology* 129(2):528–36, 2005.
Product Information: TYZEKA(TM) oral tablets, telbivudine oral tablets. Novartis Pharmaceuticals Corporation, East Hanover, NJ, 2006.
Zhou X, Marbury TC, Alcorn HW, et al. Pharmacokinetics of telbivudine in subjects with various degrees of hepatic impairment. *Antimicrob Agents Chemother* 50(5):1721–26, 2006.
Zhou XJ, Lloyd DM, Chao GC, et al. Absence of food effect on the pharmacokinetics of telbivudine following oral administration in healthy subjects. *J Clin Pharmacol* 46(3):275–81, 2006.
Zhou XJ, Myers M, Chao G, et al. Clinical pharmacokinetics of telbivudine, a potent antiviral for hepatitis B, in subjects with impaired hepatic or renal function. *J Hepatol* 40(Suppl 1):452, 2004.
Website: www.tyzeka.com

Tenofovir disoproxil fumarate (Viread) TDF

Drug Class: Antiretroviral (nucleotide analogue) (HIV) (HBV)
Usual Dose: 300 mg (PO) QD (HIV); 300 mg (PO) QD (HBV)
How Supplied: Oral Tablet: 300 mg
Pharmacokinetic Parameters:
Peak serum level: 0.29 mcg/mL
Bioavailability: 25%/39% (fasting/high-fat meal)
Excreted unchanged (urine): 32%
Serum half-life (normal/ESRD): 17 hrs/no data
Plasma protein binding: 0.7–7.2%
Volume of distribution (V_d): 1.3 L/kg
Primary Mode of Elimination: Renal
Dosage Adjustments*

CrCl ≥ 50 mL/min	No change
CrCl 30–49 mL/min	300 mg (PO) q2d
CrCl 10–29 mL/min	300 mg (PO) 2x/week

"Usual dose" assumes normal renal/hepatic function. * For renal insufficiency, give usual dose × 1 followed by maintenance dose per CrCl. For dialysis patients, dose the same as for CrCl < 10 mL/min and give supplemental (post-HD/PD dose) immediately after dialysis. CrCl = creatinine clearance; CVVH = continuous veno-venous hemo-filtration; HD/PD = hemodialysis/peritoneal dialysis. See pp. 190–193 for explanations, p. x for abbreviations

CrCl < 10 mL/min	No information
Post-HD dose	300 mg q7d or after 12 hours on HD
Post-PD dose	No information
CVVH dose	No information
Moderate hepatic insufficiency	No change
Severe hepatic insufficiency	No change

Drug Interactions: Didanosine (if possible, avoid concomitant didanosine due to impaired CD4 response and increased risk of virologic failure); valganciclovir (↑ tenofovir levels); atazanavir, lopinavir/ritonavir (↑ tenofovir levels) (↓ atazanavir levels; use atazanavir 300 mg/ ritonavir 100 mg with tenofovir); no clinically significant interactions with lamivudine, efavirenz, methadone, oral contraceptives. Not a substrate/ inhibitor of cytochrome P-450 enzymes.

Adverse Effects: Mild nausea, vomiting, GI upset, asthenia, headache, diarrhea, lactic acidosis with hepatic steatosis (rare, but potentially life-threatening with NRTIs), renal tubular acidosis, acute renal failure, and Fanconi syndrome have been reported, ↓ bone density (clinical significance unknown).

Allergic Potential: Low

Safety in Pregnancy: B

Comments: Eliminated by glomerular filtration/tubular secretion. May be taken with or without food. If possible, avoid concomitant didanosine (see drug interactions).

Cerebrospinal Fluid Penetration: No data

REFERENCES:

Gallant JE, DeJesus D, Arribas JR, et al. Tenofovir DF, emtricitabine, and efavirenz vs. zidovudine, lamivudine, and efavirenz for HIV. N Engl J Med 354:251–60, 2006.

Gallant JE. Efficacy and safety of tenofovir DF vs. stavudine in combination therapy in antiretroviral-naïve patients: a 3-year randomized trial. JAMA 292: 191–201, 2004.

Gallant JE, Deresinski S. Tenofovir disoproxil fumarate. Clin Infect Dis 37:944–50, 2003.

Jullien V, Treluye JM, Rey E, et al. Population pharmacokinetics of tenofovir in human immunodeficiency virus-infected patients taking highly active antiretroviral therapy. Antimicrobial Agents and Chemotherapy 49:3361–66, 2005.

Marcellin P, Heathcote EJ, Buti M, et al: Tenofovir disoproxil fumarate versus adefovir dipivoxil for chronic hepatitis B. N Engl J Med 2008; 359(23):2442–2455.

Nelson M, Portsmouth S, Stebbing J, et al: An open-label study of tenofovir in HIV-1 and hepatitis B virus co-infected individuals. AIDS 17(1):F7–F10, 2003.

Nunez M, Perez-Olmeda M, Diaz B, et al: Activity of tenofovir on hepatitis B virus replication in HIV-co-infected patients failing or partially responding lamivudine. AIDS 16(17):2352–54, 2002.

Panel on Antiretroviral Guidelines for Adults and Adolescents. Guidelines for the use of antiretroviral agents in HIV-1-infected adults and adolescents. Department of Health and Human Services. December 1, 2009; 1–161. Available at http://www.aidsinfo.nih.gov/ ContentFiles/AdultandAdolescentGL.pdf.

Terrault NA. Treatment of recurrent hepatitis B infection in liver transplant recipients. Liver Transpl 8(suppl 1): S74–81, 2002.

Thromson CA. Prodrug of tenofovir diphosphate approved for combination HIV therapy. Am J Health Syst Pharm 59:18, 2002.

Website: www.viread.com

Tipranavir (Aptivus) TPV

Drug Class: Protease inhibitor

Usual Dose: 500 mg (PO) with ritonavir 200 mg (PO) BID

How Supplied: Oral Capsule, Liquid Filled: 250 mg, Oral Solution: 100 mg/mL

"Usual dose" assumes normal renal/hepatic function. * For renal insufficiency, give usual dose × 1 followed by maintenance dose per CrCl. For dialysis patients, dose the same as for CrCl < 10 mL/min and give supplemental (post-HD/PD dose) immediately after dialysis. CrCl = creatinine clearance; CVVH = continuous veno-venous hemo-filtration; HD/PD = hemodialysis/peritoneal dialysis. See pp. 190–193 for explanations, p. x for abbreviations

Pharmacokinetic Parameters:
Peak serum level: 77–94 mcg/mL
Bioavailability: No data
Excreted unchanged (urine): 44%
Serum half-life (normal/ESRD): 5.5–6 hrs/no data
Plasma protein binding: 99.9%
Volume of distribution (V_d): 7–10 L/kg
Primary Mode of Elimination: Hepatic
Dosage Adjustments*

CrCl 50–80 mL/min	No change
CrCl 10–50 mL/min	No change
CrCl < 10 mL/min	No change
Post-HD dose	No change
Post-PD dose	No change
CVVH dose	No change
Mild hepatic insufficiency	No change
Moderate or severe hepatic insufficiency	Avoid

Drug Interactions: Rifabutin (↑ levels),
clarithromycin (↑ levels), loperamide (↓ levels),
statins (↑ risk of myopathy); abacavir, saquinavir,
tenofovir, zidovudine, amprenavir/RTV,
lopinavir/RTV (↓ levels). Aluminum/magnesium
antacids (↓ absorption 25–30%). Ritonavir (↑
risk of hepatitis). St. John's wort (↓ tipranavir
levels). Keep refrigerated 2–8°C. Metabolized via
CYP 3A4. Maraciroc - dose at 300 mg BID
Adverse Effects: Contraindicated in moderate/
severe hepatic insufficiency. ↑ risk of hepatotoxicity
in HIV patients co-infected with HBV/HCV. Case
reports of intracerebral hemorrhage—use with
caution in patients with coagulopathies.
Allergic Potential: High. Tipranavir is a
sulfonamide; use with caution in patients with
sulfonamide allergies

Safety in Pregnancy: C
Comments: Should be taken with food.
Increased bioavailability when taken with meals.
Must be coadministered with 200 mg ritonavir.
Tipranavir contains a sulfonamide moiety (as do
darunavir and fosamprenavir).
Cerebrospinal Fluid Penetration: No data

REFERENCES:
Barbaro G, Scozzafava A, Mastrolorenzo A, et al.
Highly active antiretroviral therapy: current state
of the art, new agents and their pharmacological
interactions useful for improving therapeutic
outcome. *Curr Pharm Des* 11:1805–43, 2005.

Clotet B. Strategies for overcoming resistance in
HIV-1 infected patients receiving HAART. *AIDS
Rev* 6:123–30, 2004.

Croom KF, Keam SJ. Tipranavir: a ritonavir-boosted
protease inhibitor. *Drugs* 65:1669–79, 2005.

de Mendoza C, Soriano V. Resistance to HIV protease
inhibitors: mechanisms and clinical consequences.
Curr Drug Metab 5:321–8, 2004.

Gulick RM. New antiretroviral drugs. *Clin Microbiol
Infect* 9:186–93, 2003.

Hicks CB, Cahn P, Cooper DA, et al. Durable
efficacy of tipranavir-ritonavir in combination
with an optimised background regimen of
antiretroviral drugs for treatment-experienced
HIV-1-infected patients at 48 weeks in the
Randomized Evaluation of Strategic Intervention
in multi-drug resistant patients with Tipranavir
(RESIST) studies: an analysis of combined data
from two randomized open-label trials. *Lancet*
368:466–75, 2006.

Kandula VR, Khanlou H, Farthing C. Tipranavir: a novel
second-generation nonpeptidic protease inhibitor.
Expert Rev Anti Infect Ther 3:9–21, 2005.

Kashuba AD. Drug-drug interactions and the
pharmacotherapy of HIV infection. *Top HIV Med*
13:64–9, 2005.

Panel on Antiretroviral Guidelines for Adults and
Adolescents. Guidelines for the use of antiretroviral
agents in HIV-1-infected adults and adolescents.
Department of Health and Human Services. December 1,

"Usual dose" assumes normal renal/hepatic function. * For renal insufficiency, give usual dose × 1 followed
by maintenance dose per CrCl. For dialysis patients, dose the same as for CrCl < 10 mL/min and give supplemental (post-HD/PD dose) immediately after dialysis. CrCl = creatinine clearance; CVVH = continuous
veno-venous hemo-filtration; HD/PD = hemodialysis/peritoneal dialysis. See pp. 190–193 for explanations,
p. x for abbreviations

2009; 1–161. Available at http://www.aidsinfo.nih.gov/ ContentFiles/AdultandAdolescentGL.pdf.

Plosker GL, Figgitt DP. Tripanavir. *Drugs* 63:1611–8, 2003.

Turner D, Schapiro JM,Brenner BG, Wainberg MA. The influence of protease inhibitor profiles on selection of HIV therapy in treatment-naïve patients. *Antivir Ther* 9:301–14, 2004.

Yeni P. Tipranavir: a protease inhibitor from a new class with distinct antiviral activity. *J Acquir Immune Defic Syndr* 34 (Suppl 1):S91–4, 2003.

Website: www.aptivus.com

Zidovudine (Retrovir) ZDV

Drug Class: Antiretroviral NRTI (nucleoside reverse transcriptase inhibitor)

Usual Dose: 300 mg (PO) BID (see comments). IV solution 10 mg/mL (dose 1 mg/kg 5–6 x/day)

How Supplied:

Generic—

Oral Capsule: 100 mg

Oral Syrup: 50 mg/5 mL

Oral Tablet: 300 mg

Retrovir—

Intravenous Solution: 10 mg/mL

Oral Capsule: 100 mg

Oral Syrup: 50 mg/5 mL

Oral Tablet: 300 mg

Pharmacokinetic Parameters:

Peak serum level: 1.2 mcg/mL

Bioavailability: 64%

Excreted unchanged (urine): 16%

Serum half-life (normal/ESRD): 1.1/1.4 hrs

Plasma protein binding: < 38%

Volume of distribution (V_d): 1.6 L/kg

Primary Mode of Elimination: Hepatic

Dosage Adjustments*

CrCl 50–80 mL/min	No change
CrCl 10–50 mL/min	No change

CrCl < 10 mL/min	300 mg (PO) QD
HD/PD	100 mg (PO) q6–8h
Post-HD/PD dose	None
CVVH dose	300 mg (PO) QD
Moderate or severe hepatic insufficiency	No information

Drug Interactions: Acetaminophen, atovaquone, fluconazole, methadone, probenecid, valproic acid (↑ zidovudine levels); clarithromycin, nelfinavir, rifampin, rifabutin (↓ zidovudine levels); dapsone, flucytosine, ganciclovir, interferon alpha, bone marrow suppressive/cytotoxic agents (↑ risk of hematologic toxicity); indomethacin (↑ levels of zidovudine toxic metabolite); phenytoin (↑ zidovudine levels, ↑ or ↓ phenytoin levels); ribavirin (↓ zidovudine effect; avoid).

Adverse Effects: Nausea, vomiting, GI upset, diarrhea, malaise, anorexia, leukopenia, severe anemia, macrocytosis, thrombocytopenia, headaches, ↑ SGOT/SGPT, hepatotoxicity, myalgias, myositis, symptomatic myopathy, insomnia, blue/black nail discoloration, asthenia, lactic acidosis with hepatic steatosis (rare, but potentially life-threatening toxicity with use of NRTIs).

Allergic Potential: Low

Safety in Pregnancy: C

Comments: Antagonized by ganciclovir or ribavirin. Also a component of Combivir and Trizivir. Patients on IV therapy should be switched to PO as soon as able to take oral medication. For IV administration, dilute in D5W to a concentration no greater than 4 mg/mL and infuse over 1 hour.

Cerebrospinal Fluid Penetration: 60%

"Usual dose" assumes normal renal/hepatic function. * For renal insufficiency, give usual dose × 1 followed by maintenance dose per CrCl. For dialysis patients, dose the same as for CrCl < 10 mL/min and give supplemental (post-HD/PD dose) immediately after dialysis. CrCl = creatinine clearance; CVVH = continuous veno-venous hemo-filtration; HD/PD = hemodialysis/peritoneal dialysis. See pp. 190–193 for explanations, p. x for abbreviations

REFERENCES:

Barry M, Mulcahy F, Merry C, et al. Pharmacokinetics and potential interactions amongst antiretroviral agents used to treat patients with HIV infection. *Clin Pharmacol* 36:289–304, 1999.

Been-Tiktak AM, Boucher CA, Brun-Vezinet F, et al. Efficacy and safety of combination therapy with delavirdine and zidovudine: a European/Australian phase II trial. *Intern J Antimcrob Agents* 11: 13–21, 1999.

McDowell JA, Lou Y, Symonds WS, et al. Multiple-dose pharmacokinetics and pharmacodynamics of abacavir alone and in combination with zidovudine in human immunodeficiency virus-infected adults. *Antimicrob Agents Chemother* 44:2061–7, 2000.

Montaner JS, Reiss P, Cooper D, et al. A randomized, double-blind trial comparing combinations of nevirapine, didanosine, and zidovudine for HIV-infected patients: The INCAS trial. Italy, the Netherlands, Canada and Australia Study. *J Am Med Assoc* 279:930–7, 1998.

Panel on Antiretroviral Guidelines for Adults and Adolescents. Guidelines for the use of antiretroviral agents in HIV-1-infected adults and adolescents. Department of Health and Human Services. December 1, 2009; 1–161. Available at http://www.aidsinfo.nih.gov/ContentFiles/AdultandAdolescentGL.pdf.

Piscitelli SC, Gallicano KD. Interactions among drugs for HIV and opportunistic infections. *N Engl J Med* 344:984–996, 2001.

Simpson DM. Human immunodeficiency virus-associated dementia: A review of pathogenesis, prophylaxis, and treatment studies of zidovudine therapy. *Clin Infect Dis* 29:19–34, 1999.

"Usual dose" assumes normal renal/hepatic function. * For renal insufficiency, give usual dose × 1 followed by maintenance dose per CrCl. For dialysis patients, dose the same as for CrCl < 10 mL/min and give supplemental (post-HD/PD dose) immediately after dialysis. CrCl = creatinine clearance; CVVH = continuous veno-venous hemo-filtration; HD/PD = hemodialysis/peritoneal dialysis. See pp. 196–199 for explanations, p. ix for abbreviations

Appendix 1†

†   Adapted from: *Top HIV Med.* 2009;17(5):138–145. © 2009, International AIDS Society–USA.

Mutations in the Reverse Transcriptase Gene Associated with Resistance to Reverse Transcriptase Inhibitors

Nucleoside and Nucleotide Analogue Reverse Transcriptase Inhibitors (nRTIs)[a]

Multi-nRTI Resistance: 69 Insertion Complex[b] (affects all nRTIs currently approved by the US FDA)

M41L A62V ▶ 69 Insert K70R L210W T215Y/F K219Q/E

Multi-nRTI Resistance: 151 Complex[c] (affects all nRTIs currently approved by the US FDA except tenofovir)

A62V V75I F77L F116Y Q151M

Multi-RTI Resistance: Thymidine Analogue-Associated Mutations[d,e] (TAMs; affect all nRTIs currently approved by the US FDA)

M41L D67N K70R L210W T215Y/F K219Q/E

Abacavir[f,g] K65R L74V Y115F M184V

Didanosine[g,h] K65R L74V

Mutations in the Reverse Transcriptase Gene Associated with Resistance to Reverse Transcriptase Inhibitors (cont'd)

Nucleoside and Nucleotide Analogue Reverse Transcriptase Inhibitors (nRTIs)[a] (cont'd)

	41 (M)	65 (K)	67 (D)	70 (K)	184 (M)	210 (L)	215 (T)	219 (K)
Emtricitabine		R			V / I			
Lamivudine		R			V / I			
Stavudine[d,e,g,i,j,k]	L	R	N	R		W	Y / F	Q / E
Tenofovir[l]		R		E				
Zidovudine[d,e,i,k]	L		N	R		W	Y / F	Q / E

Nonnucleoside Analogue Reverse Transcriptase Inhibitors (NNRTIs)[a,m]

	100 (L)	101 (K)	103 (K)	106 (V)	108 (V)	181 (Y)	188 (Y)	190 (G)	225 (P)
Efavirenz	I	P	N	M	I	C / I	L	S / A	H

Etravirine[n]

	V 90	A 98	L 100	K 101	V 106	E 138	V 179	Y 181	G 190	M 230
	I	G	I	E	I	A	D	C	S	L
				H			F	I	A	
				P			T	V		

Nevirapine

	L 100	K 101	K 103	V 106	V 108	Y 181	G 188	G 190
	I	P	N	A	I	C	C	A
				M		I	L	
							H	

Mutations in the Protease Gene Associated with Resistance to Protease Inhibitors[o,p,q]

Atazanavir +/– ritonavir[r]

Pos	10	16	20	24	32	33	34	36	46	48	50	53	54	60	62	64	71	73	82	84	85	88	90	93
aa	L	G	K	L	V	L	E	M	M	G	I	F	I	D	I	I	A	G	V	I	I	N	L	L
	F	E	R	I	I	F	Q	L	I	V	L	L	L	E	V	L	V	C	A	V	V	S	M	M
	V		M			V		V	L		V	Y	M			M	I	S	T					
	C		I										A			V	T	T	F					
			T														L	A	I					
			V																					

Darunavir/ritonavir[s]

Pos	11	32	33	47	50	54	74	76	84	89
aa	V	V	L	I	I	I	T	L	I	L
	I	I	F	V	V	M	P	V	V	V
						L				

Fosamprenavir/ritonavir

Pos	10	32	46	47	50	54	73	76	82	84	90
aa	L	V	M	I	I	I	G	L	V	I	L
	F	I	I	V	L	V	S	V	A	V	M
	I		L		V				F		
	R				M				S		
	V								T		

Indinavir/ritonavir[t]

Pos	10	20	24	32	36	46	54	71	73	76	77	82	84	90
aa	L	K	L	V	M	M	I	A	G	L	V	V	I	L
	I	M	I	I	I	I	V	V	S	V	I	A	V	M
	R	R				L		T	A			F		
	V											T		

Lopinavir/ritonavir[u]

Pos	10	20	24	32	33	46	47	50	53	54	63	71	73	76	82	84	90
aa	L	K	L	V	L	M	I	I	F	I	L	A	G	L	V	I	L
	F	M	I	I	F	I	V	V	L	V	P	V	S	V	A	V	M
	I	R				L	A			L		T			F		
	R									A					T		
	V									M					S		
										T							
										S							

Protease Inhibitors (continued)

Nelfinavir[t,v]

Position	10	30	36	46	71	77	82	84	88	90
Wild type	L	**D**	M	M	A	V	V	I	N	L
Mutation	F	N	I	I	V	I	A	V	D	M
	I			L	T		F		S	
							T			
							S			

Saquinavir/ritonavir[t]

Position	10	24	48	54	62	71	73	77	82	84	90
Wild type	L	L	**G**	I	I	A	G	V	V	I	L
Mutation	I	I	V	V	V	V	S	I	A	V	M
				L		T			F		
									T		
									S		

Tipranavir/ritonavir[w]

Position	10	13	20	33	35	36	43	46	47	54	58	69	74	82	83	84	90
Wild type	L	I	K	L	E	M	K	M	I	I	**Q**	H	**T**	**V**	**N**	**I**	L
Mutation	V	V	M	F	G	I	T	L	V	A	E	K	P	L	D	V	M
			R							M				T			
			V							V							

Mutations in the Envelope Gene Associated with Resistance to Entry Inhibitors

Enfuvirtide[x]

Position	36	37	38	39	40	42	43
Wild type	G	I	V	Q	Q	N	N
Mutation	D	V	A	R	H	T	D
	S		M				
			E				

Maraviroc[y]

See User Note

Mutations in the Integrase Gene Associated with Resistance to Integrase Inhibitors

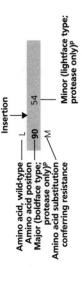

	Y	Q	N
Raltegravir[z]	**143**	**148**	**155**
	R	H	H
	H	K	
	C	R	

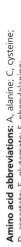

MUTATIONS

Insertion →

— L —

— 90 — **54**

M

Amino acid, wild-type
Amino acid position
Major (boldface type; protease only)[p]
Amino acid substitution conferring resistance

Minor (lightface type; protease only)[p]

Amino acid abbreviations: A, alanine; C, cysteine;
D, aspartate; E, glutamate; F, phenylalanine;
G, glycine; H, histidine; I, isoleucine; K, lysine;
L, leucine; M, methionine; N, asparagine; P, proline;
Q, glutamine; R, arginine; S, serine; T, threonine;
V, valine; W, tryptophan; Y, tyrosine.

USER NOTES

a. Some nucleoside (or nucleotide) analogue reverse transcriptase inhibitor (nRTI) mutations, like T215Y and H208Y,[1] may lead to viral hypersusceptibility to the non-nucleoside analogue reverse transcriptase inhibitors (NNRTIs), including etravirine,[2] in nRTI-treated individuals. The presence of these mutations may improve subsequent virologic response to NNRTI-containing regimens (nevirapine or efavirenz) in NNRTI-naive individuals,[3-7] although no clinical data exist for improved response to etravirine in NNRTI-experienced individuals.

b. The 69 insertion complex consists of a substitution at codon 69 (typically T69S) and an insertion of 2 or more amino acids (S-S, S-A, S-G, or others). The 69 insertion complex is associated with resistance to all nRTIs currently approved by the US FDA when present with 1 or more thymidine analogue–associated mutations (TAMs) at codons 41, 210, or 215.[8] Some other amino acid changes from the wild-type T at codon 69 without the insertion may be associated with broad nRTI resistance.

c. Tenofovir retains activity against the Q151M complex of mutations.[8]

d. Mutations known to be selected by thymidine analogues (M41L, D67N, K70R, L210W, T215Y/F, and K219Q/E, termed TAMs) also confer reduced susceptibility to all approved nRTIs.[9] The degree to which cross-resistance is observed depends on the specific mutations and number of mutations involved.[10-13] Mutations in the C-terminal reverse transcriptase domains, including RNase H, outside of the regions depicted in the figure may prove to be important for HIV-1 drug resistance.[14] The clinical relevance of these in vitro findings remains unclear. Recent analyses showed no clear effect on phenotypic susceptibility to efavirenz or nevirapine in already NNRTI-resistant clinical isolates.[15] Moreover, connection domain mutations were not clearly associated with reduced phenotypic susceptibility or virologic response to etravirine in the DUET trials.[16] Thus, they are not depicted on the figure bars.

e. Although reverse transcriptase changes associated with the E44D and V118I mutations may have an accessory role in increased resistance to nRTIs in the presence of TAMs, their clinical relevance is very limited.[17-19]

f. The M184V mutation alone does not appear to be associated with a reduced virologic response to abacavir in vivo.[20,21] When associated with TAMs, M184V increases abacavir resistance.[20,21]

g. As with tenofovir, the K65R mutation may be selected by didanosine, abacavir, or stavudine (particularly in patients with nonsubtype-B clades) and is associated with decreased viral susceptibility to these drugs.[20,22,23] Data are lacking on the potential negative impact of K65R on clinical response to didanosine.

h. The presence of 3 of the following mutations—M41L, D67N, L210W, T215Y/F, K219Q/E—is associated with resistance to didanosine.[24] The presence of K70R or M184V alone does not decrease virologic response to didanosine.[25]

i. K65R is selected frequently (4%–11%) in patients with nonsubtype-B clades for whom stavudine-containing regimens are failing in the absence of tenofovir.[26,27]

j. The presence of M184V appears to delay or prevent emergence of TAMs.[28] This effect may be overcome by an accumulation of TAMs or other mutations.

k. The T215A/C/D/E/G/H/I/L/N/S/V substitutions are revertant mutations at codon 215 that confer increased risk of virologic failure of zidovudine or stavudine in antiretro-viral-naive patients.[29-31] The T215Y mutant may emerge quickly from 1 of these mutations in the presence of zidovudine or stavudine.[32,33]

l. The presence of K65R is associated with a reduced virologic response to tenofovir.[8] A reduced response also occurs in the presence of 3 or more TAMs inclusive of either M41L or L210W.[8] The presence of TAMs or combined treatment with zidovudine prevents the emergence of K65R in the presence of tenofovir.[34-36]

m. The sequential use of nevirapine and efavirenz (in either order) is not recommended because of cross-resistance between these drugs.[37]

n. Resistance to etravirine has been extensively studied only in the context of coadministration with darunavir/ritonavir. In this context, mutations associated with virologic outcome have been assessed and their relative weights (or magnitudes of impact) assigned. In addition, phenotypic cutoff values have been calculated, and assessment of genotype-phenotype correlations from a large clinical database have determined relative importance of the various mutations. These 2 approaches are in agreement for many, but not all, mutations and weights.[38-40] The single mutations Y181C/I/V, K101P, and L100I reduce but do not preclude clinical utility. The presence of K103N alone does not affect etravirine response.[41] Accumulation of several mutations results in greater reductions in susceptibility and virologic response than do single mutations.[42,43]

o. Often, numerous mutations are necessary to substantially impact virologic response to a ritonavir-boosted protease inhibitor (PI).[44] In some specific circumstances, atazanavir might be used unboosted. In such cases, the mutations that are selected are the same as with ritonavir-boosted atazanavir, but the relative frequency of mutations may differ.

p. Resistance mutations in the protease gene are classified as "major" or "minor."

Major mutations in the protease gene are defined as those selected first in the presence of the drug or those substantially reducing drug susceptibility. These mutations tend to be the primary contact residues for drug binding.

Minor mutations generally emerge later than major mutations and by themselves do not have a substantial effect on phenotype. They may improve replication of viruses containing major mutations. Some minor mutations are present as common polymorphic changes in HIV-1 nonsubtype-B clades.

q. Ritonavir is not listed separately, as it is currently used only at low dose as a pharmacologic booster of other PIs.

r. Many mutations are associated with atazanavir resistance. Their impacts differ, with I50L, I84V, and N88S having the greatest effect. Higher atazanavir levels obtained with ritonavir boosting increase the number of mutations required for loss of activity. The presence of M46I plus L76V might increase susceptibility to atazanavir.[45]

s. HIV-1 RNA response to ritonavir-boosted darunavir correlates with baseline susceptibility and the presence of several specific PI mutations. Reductions in response are associated with increasing numbers of the mutations indicated in the figure bar. The negative impact of the protease mutations I47V, I54M, T74P, and I84V and the positive impact of the protease mutation V82A on virologic response to darunavir/ritonavir were shown in 2 data sets independently.[46,47] Some of these mutations appear to have a greater effect on susceptibility than others (eg, I50V vs V11I). A median darunavir phenotypic fold-change greater than 10 (low clinical cutoff) occurs with 3 or more of the 2007 IAS–USA mutations listed for darunavir[48] and is associated with a diminished virologic response.[49]

t. The mutations depicted on the figure bar cannot be considered comprehensive because little relevant research has been reported in recent years to update the resistance and cross-resistance patterns for this drug.

u. In PI-experienced patients, the accumulation of 6 or more of the mutations indicated on the figure bar is associated with a reduced virologic response to lopinavir/ritonavir.[50,51] The product information states that accumulation of 7 or 8 mutations confers resistance to the drug.[52] However, there is emerging evidence that specific mutations, most notably I47A (and possibly I47V) and V32I, are associated with high-level resistance.[53-55] The addition of L76V to 3 PI resistance–associated mutations substantially increases resistance to lopinavir/ritonavir.[45]

v. In some nonsubtype-B HIV-1, D30N is selected less frequently than are other PI mutations.[56]

w. Clinical correlates of resistance to tipranavir are limited by the paucity of clinical trials and observational studies of the drug. Lists of mutations associated with accumulating resistance have been presented, with some conflicting results. In vitro studies and initial analysis of clinical data show mutations L33F, V82L/T, and I84V as having substantial contributions. Confirmatory studies are pending. A number of mutations (L24I, I50L/V, I54L, and L76V) are associated with decreased resistance in vitro and improved short-term virologic response if 2 or more are present.

x. Resistance to enfuvirtide is associated primarily with mutations in the first heptad repeat (HR1) region of the gp41 envelope gene. However, mutations or polymorphisms in other regions of the envelope (eg, the HR2 region or those yet to be identified) as well as coreceptor usage and density may affect susceptibility to enfuvirtide.[57-59]

y. The activity of CC chemokine receptor 5 (CCR5) antagonists is limited to patients with virus that uses only CCR5 for entry (R5 virus). Viruses that use both CCR5 and CXC chemokine receptor 4 (CXCR4; termed dual/mixed [D/M]) or only CXCR4 (X4 virus) do not respond to treatment with CCR5 antagonists. Virologic failure of these drugs frequently is associated with outgrowth of D/M or X4 virus from a preexisting minority population present at levels below the limit of assay detection. Mutations in HIV-1 gp120 that allow the virus to bind to the drug-bound form of CCR5 have been described in viruses from some patients whose virus remained R5 after virologic failure of a CCR5 antagonist. Most of these mutations are found in the V3 loop, the major determinant of viral tropism. There is as yet no consensus on specific signature mutations for CCR5 antagonist resistance, so they are not depicted in the figure. Some CCR5 antagonist-resistant viruses selected in vitro have shown mutations in gp41 without mutations in V3; the clinical significance of such mutations is not yet known.

z. Raltegravir failure is associated with integrase mutations in at least 3 distinct genetic pathways defined by 2 or more mutations including (1) a signature (major) mutation at Q148H/K/R, N155H, or Y143R/H/C; and (2) 1 or more additional minor mutations. Minor mutations described in the Q148H/K/R pathway include L74M plus E138A, E138K, or G140S. The most common mutational pattern in this pathway is Q148H plus G140S, which also confers the greatest loss of drug susceptibility. Mutations described in the N155H pathway include this major mutation plus either L74M, E92Q, T97A, E92Q plus T97A, Y143H, G163K/R, V151I, or D232N.[60] The Y143R/H/C mutation is uncommon.[61-65]

REFERENCES TO THE USER NOTES

---

1. Clark SA, Shulman NS, Bosch RJ, Mellors JW. Reverse transcriptase mutations 118I, 208Y, and 215Y cause HIV-1 hypersusceptibility to non-nucleoside reverse transcriptase inhibitors. *AIDS.* 2006;20:981–984.

2. Picchio G, Vingerhoets J, Parkin N, Azijn H, de Bethune MP. Nucleoside-associated mutations cause hypersusceptibility to etravirine. [Abstract 23.] *Antivir Ther.* 2008;13 (Suppl 3):A25.

3. Shulman NS, Bosch RJ, Mellors JW, Albrecht MA, Katzenstein DA. Genetic correlates of efavirenz hypersusceptibility. *AIDS.* 2004;18:1781–1785.

4. Demeter LM, DeGruttola V, Lustgarten S, et al. Association of efavirenz hypersusceptibility with virologic response in ACTG 368, a randomized trial of abacavir (ABC).

5. Haubrich RH, Kemper CA, Hellmann NS, et al. The clinical relevance of nonnucleoside reverse transcriptase inhibitor hypersusceptibility: a prospective cohort analysis. *AIDS.* 2002;16:F33–F40.

6. Tozzi V, Zaccarelli M, Narciso P, et al. Mutations in HIV-1 reverse transcriptase potentially associated with hypersusceptibility to non-nucleoside reverse-transcriptase inhibitors: effect on response to efavirenz-based therapy in an urban observational cohort. *J Infect Dis.* 2004;189:1688–1695.

7. Katzenstein DA, Bosch RJ, Hellmann N, et al. Phenotypic susceptibility and virological outcome in

nucleoside-experienced patients receiving three or four antiretroviral drugs. *AIDS*. 2003;17:821–830.

8. Miller MD, Margot N, Lu B, et al. Genotypic and phenotypic predictors of the magnitude of response to tenofovir disoproxil fumarate treatment in antiretroviral-experienced patients. *J Infect Dis*. 2004;189:837–846.

9. Whitcomb JM, Parkin NT, Chappey C, Hellman NS, Petropoulos CJ. Broad nucleoside reverse-transcriptase cross-resistance in human immunodeficiency virus type 1 clinical isolates. *J Infect Dis*. 2003;188:992–1000.

10. Larder BA, Kemp SD. Multiple mutations in HIV-1 reverse transcriptase confer high-level resistance to zidovudine (AZT). *Science*. 1989;246:1155–1158.

11. Kellam P, Boucher CA, Larder BA. Fifth mutation in human immunodeficiency virus type 1 reverse transcriptase contributes to the development of high-level resistance to zido-vudine. *Proc Natl Acad Sci USA*. 1992;89:1934–1938.

12. Calvez V, Costagliola D, Descamps D, et al. Impact of stavudine phenotype and thymidine analogues mutations on viral response to stavudine plus lamivudine in ALTIS 2 ANRS trial. *Antivir Ther*. 2002;7:211–218.

13. Kuritzkes DR, Bassett RL, Hazelwood JD, et al. Rate of thymidine analogue resistance mutation accumulation with zidovudine- or stavudine-based regimens. *JAIDS*. 2004;36:600–603.

14. Yap SH, Sheen CW, Fahey J, et al. N348I in the connection domain of HIV-1 reverse transcriptase confers zidovudine and nevirapine resistance. *PLoS Med*. 2007;4:e335.

15. Paredes R, Tambuyzer L, Pou C, et al. Effect of RT connection domain mutations on efavirenz and nevirapine phenotypic susceptibility in NNRTI-resistant clinical HIV-1 isolates. [Abstract 53.] *Antivir Ther*. 2009;14(Suppl 1):A57.

16. Vingerhoets J, Tambuyzer L, Paredes R, et al. Effect of mutations in the RT connection domain on phenoytpic susceptibility and virologic response to etravirine. [Abstract 33.] *Antivir Ther*. 2009; 14(Suppl 1):A35.

17. Romano L, Venturi G, Bloor S, et al. Broad nucleoside-analogue resistance implications for human immunodeficiency virus type 1 reverse-transcriptase mutations at codons 44 and 118. *J Infect Dis*. 2002;185:898–904.

18. Walter H, Schmidt B, Werwein M, Schwingel E, Korn K. Prediction of abacavir resistance from genotypic data: impact of zidovudine and lamivudine

resistance in vitro and in vivo. *Antimicrob Agents Chemother*. 2002;46:89–94.

19. Mihailidis C, Dunn D, Pillay D, Pozniak A. Effect of isolated V118I mutation in reverse transcriptase on response to first-line antiretroviral therapy. *AIDS*. 2008;22:427–430.

20. Harrigan PR, Stone C, Griffin P, et al. Resistance profile of the human immunodeficiency virus type 1 reverse transcriptase inhibitor abacavir (1592U89) after monotherapy and combination therapy. CNA2001 Investigative Group. *J Infect Dis*. 2000;181:912–920.

21. Lanier ER, Ait-Khaled M, Scott J, et al. Antiviral efficacy of abacavir in antiretroviral therapy-experienced adults harbouring HIV-1 with specific patterns of resistance to nucleoside reverse transcriptase inhibitors. *Antivir Ther*. 2004;9:37–45.

22. Winters MA, Shafer RW, Jellinger RA, Mamtora G, Gingeras T, Merigan TC. Human immunodeficiency virus type 1 reverse transcriptase genotype and drug susceptibility changes in infected individuals receiving dideoxyinosine monotherapy for 1 to 2 years. *Antimicrob Agents Chemother*. 1997;41:757–762.

23. Svarovskaia ES, Margot NA, Bae AS, et al. Low-level K65R mutation in HIV-1 reverse transcriptase of treatment-experienced patients exposed to abacavir or didanosine. *JAIDS*. 2007;46:174–180.

24. Marcelin AG, Flandre P, Pavie J, et al. Clinically relevant genotype interpretation of resistance to didanosine. *Antimicrob Agents Chemother*. 2005;49:1739–1744.

25. Molina JM, Marcelin AG, Pavie J, et al. Didanosine in HIV-1-infected patients experiencing failure of antiretroviral therapy: a randomized placebo-controlled trial. *J Infect Dis*. 2005;191:840–847.

26. Hawkins CA, Chaplin B, Idoko J, et al. Clinical and genotypic findings in HIV-infected patients with the K65R mutation failing first-line antiretroviral therapy in Nigeria. *JAIDS*. 2009;52:228–234.

27. Wallis C, Sanne I, Venter F, Mellors J, Stevens W. Varied patterns of HIV-1 drug resistance on failing first-line antiretroviral therapy in South Africa. *JAIDS*. 2009;Epub ahead of print.

28. Kuritzkes DR, Quinn JB, Benoit SL, et al. Drug resistance and virologic response in NUCA 3001, a randomized trial of lamivudine versus zidovudine versus zidovudine plus lamivudine in previously untreated patients. *AIDS*. 1996;10:975–981.

29. Riva C, Violin M, Cozzi-Lepri A, et al. Transmitted virus with substitutions at position 215 and risk

of virological failure in antiretroviralnaive patients starting highly active antiretroviral therapy. [Abstract 124.] *Antivir Ther.* 2002;7:S103.

30. Chappey C, Wrin T, Deeks S, Petropoulos CJ. Evolution of amino acid 215 in HIV-1 reverse transcriptase in response to intermittent drug selection. [Abstract 32.] *Antivir Ther.* 2003;8:S37.

31. Violin M, Cozzi-Lepri A, Velleca R, et al. Risk of failure in patients with 215 HIV-1 revertants starting their first thymidine analog-containing highly active antiretroviral therapy. *AIDS.* 2004;18:227–235.

32. Garcia-Lerma JG, MacInnes H, Bennett D, Weinstock H, Heneine W. Transmitted human immunodeficiency virus type 1 carrying the D67N or K219Q/E mutation evolves rapidly to zidovudine resistance in vitro and shows a high replicative fitness in the presence of zidovudine. *J Virol.* 2004;78:7545–7552.

33. Lanier ER, Ait-Khaled M, Craig C, Scott J, Vavro C. Effect of baseline 215D/C/S 'revertant' mutations on virological response to lamivudine/zidovudine-containing regimens and emergence of 215Y upon virological failure. [Abstract 146.] *Antivir Ther.* 2002;7:S120.

34. Parikh UM, Zelina S, Sluis-Cremer N, Mellors JW. Molecular mechanisms of bidirectional antagonism between K65R and thymidine analog mutations in HIV-1 reverse transcriptase. *AIDS.* 2007;21:1405–1414.

35. Parikh UM, Barnas DC, Faruki H, Mellors JW. Antagonism between the HIV-1 reverse-transcriptase mutation K65R and thymidine-analogue mutations at the genomic level. *J Infect Dis.* 2006;194:651–660.

36. Von Wyl V, Yerly S, Boni J, et al. Factors associated with the emergence of K65R in patients with HIV-1 infection treated with combination antiretroviral therapy containing tenofovir. *Clin Infect Dis.* 2008;46:1299–1309.

37. Antinori A, Zaccarelli M, Cingolani A, et al. Cross-resistance among nonnucleoside reverse transcriptase inhibitors limits recycling efavirenz after nevirapine failure. *AIDS Res Hum Retroviruses.* 2002;18:835–838.

38. Benhamida J, Chappey C, Coakley E, Parkin NT. HIV-1 genotype algorithms for prediction of etravirine susceptibility: novel mutations and weighting factors identified through correlations to phenotype. [Abstract 130.] *Antivir Ther.* 2008; 13(Suppl 3):A142.

39. Coakley E, Chappey C, Benhamida J, et al. Biological and clinical cut-off analyses for etravirine in the PhenoSense HIV assay. [Abstract 122.] *Antivir Ther.* 2008;13(Suppl 3):A134.

40. Peeters M, Nijs S, Vingerhoets J, et al. Determination of phenotypic clinical cut-offs for etravirine: pooled week 24 results of the DUET-1 and DUET-2 trials. [Abstract 121.] *Antivir Ther.* 2008; 13(Suppl 3):A133.

41. Etravirine [package insert]. Bridgewater, NJ: Tibotec Therapeutics; 2008.

42. Vingerhoets J, Peeters M, Azijn H, et al. An update of the list of NNRTI mutations associated with decreased virological response to etravirine: multivariate analyses on the pooled DUET-1 and DUET-2 clinical trial data. [Abstract 24.] *Antivir Ther.* 2008; 13(Suppl 3):A26.

43. Scherrer AU, Hasse B, von Wyl V, et al. Prevalence of etravirine mutations and impact on response to treatment in routine clinical care: Swiss HIV Cohort Study (SHCS). *HIV Med.* 2009;10:647–656.

44. Hirsch MS, Gunthard HF, Schapiro JM, et al. Antiretroviral drug resistance testing in adult HIV-1 infection: 2008 recommendations of an International AIDS Society–USA panel. *Clin Infect Dis.* 2008;47:266–285.

45. Norton M, Young T, Parkin N, et al. Prevalence, mutational patterns, and phenotypic correlates of the L76V protease mutation in relation to LPV-associated mutations. [Abstract 854.] 15th Conference on Retroviruses and Opportunistic Infections. February 3–6, 2008; Boston, MA.

46. De Meyer S, Descamps D, Van Baelen B, et al. Confirmation of the negative impact of protease mutations I47V, I54M, T74P and I84V and the positive impact of protease mutation V82A on virological response to darunavir/ritonavir. [Abstract 126.] *Antivir Ther.* 2009;14(Suppl 1):A147.

47. Descamps D, Lambert-Niclot S, Marcelin AG, et al. Mutations associated with virological response to darunavir/ritonavir in HIV-1-infected protease inhibitor-experienced patients. *J Antimicrob Chemother.* 2009;63:585–592.

48. Johnson VA, Brun-Vézinet F, Clotet B, et al. Update of the drug resistance mutations in HIV-1: 2007. *Top HIV Med.* 2007;15:119–125.

49. De Meyer S, Dierynck I, Lathouwers E, et al. Phenotypic and genotypic determinants of resistance to darunavir: analysis of data from treatment-experienced patients in POWER 1, 2, 3

and DUET-1 and 2. [Abstract 31.] *Antivir Ther.* 2008;13(Suppl 3):A33.

50. Masquelier B, Breilh D, Neau D, et al. Human immunodeficiency virus type 1 genotypic and pharmacokinetic determinants of the virological response to lopinavir-ritonavir-containing therapy in protease inhibitor-experienced patients. *Antimicrob Agents Chemother.* 2002;46:2926–2932.

51. Kempf DJ, Isaacson JD, King MS, et al. Identification of genotypic changes in human immunodeficiency virus protease that correlate with reduced susceptibility to the protease inhibitor lopinavir among viral isolates from protease inhibitor-experienced patients. *J Virol.* 2001;75:7462–7469.

52. Lopinavir/ritonavir [package insert]. Abbott Park, IL: Abbott Laboratories; 2008.

53. Mo H, King MS, King K, Molla A, Brun S, Kempf DJ. Selection of resistance in protease inhibitor-experienced, human immunodeficiency virus type 1-infected subjects failing lopinavir- and ritonavir-based therapy: mutation patterns and baseline correlates. *J Virol.* 2005;79:3329–3338.

54. Friend J, Parkin N, Liegler T, Martin JN, Deeks SG. Isolated lopinavir resistance after virological rebound of a ritonavir/lopinavir-based regimen. *AIDS.* 2004;18:1965–1966.

55. Kagan RM, Shenderovich M, Heseltine PN, Ramnarayan K. Structural analysis of an HIV-1 protease I47A mutant resistant to the protease inhibitor lopinavir. *Protein Sci.* 2005;14:1870–1878.

56. Gonzalez LMF, Brindeiro RM, Aguiar RS, et al. Impact of nelfinavir resistance mutations on in vitro phenotype, fitness and replication capacity of HIV-1 with subtype B and C proteases. [Abstract 56.] *Antivir Ther.* 2004;9:S65.

57. Reeves JD, Gallo SA, Ahmad N, et al. Sensitivity of HIV-1 to entry inhibitors correlates with envelope/coreceptor affinity, receptor density, and fusion kinetics. *Proc Natl Acad Sci USA.* 2002;99:16249–16254.

58. Reeves JD, Miamidian JL, Biscone MJ, et al. Impact of mutations in the coreceptor binding site on human immunodeficiency virus type 1 fusion, infection, and entry inhibitor sensitivity. *J Virol.* 2004; 78:5476–5485.

59. Xu L, Pozniak A, Wildfire A, et al. Emergence and evolution of enfuvirtide resistance following long-term therapy involves heptad repeat 2 mutations within gp41. *Antimicrob Agents Chemother.* 2005;49:1113–1119.

60. Hazuda DF, Miller MD, Nguyen BY, Zhao J, for the P005 Study Team. Resistance to the HIV-integrase inhibitor raltegravir: analysis of protocol 005, a phase II study in patients with triple-class resistant HIV-1 infection. *Antivir Ther.* 2007;12:S10.

61. Miller MD, Danovich RM, Ke Y, et al. Longitudinal analysis of resistance to the HIV-1 integrase inhibitor raltegravir: results from P005 a phase II study in treatment-experienced patients. [Abstract 6.] *Antivir Ther.* 2008;13:A8.

62. Fransen S, Gupta S, Danovich R, et al. Loss of raltegravir susceptibility in treated patients is conferred by multiple non-overlapping genetic pathways. [Abstract 7.] *Antivir Ther.* 2008;13:A9.

63. Hatano H, Lampiris H, Huang W, et al. Virological and immunological outcomes in a cohort of patients failing integrase inhibitors. [Abstract 10.] *Antivir Ther.* 2008;13:A12.

64. Da Silva D, Pellegrin I, Anies G, et al. Mutational patterns in the HIV-1 integrase related to virological failures on raltegravir-containing regimens. [Abstract 12.] *Antivir Ther.* 2008;13:A14.

65. Ceccherini-Silberstein F, Armenia D, D'Arrigo R, et al. Virological response and resistance in multiexperienced patients treated with raltegravir. [Abstract 18.] *Antivir Ther.* 2008;13:A20.

Adapted from: *Top HIV Med.* 2009;17(5):138–145. © 2009, International AIDS Society–USA.

Appendix 2

SELECTED KEY INTERNET RESOURCES

- AIDSinfo—A Service of the Department of Health and Human Services (www. aidsinfo.nih.gov)
- Chronic Hepatitis C: Current Disease Management (http://digestive.niddk.nih.gov/ ddiseases/pubs/chronichepc/)
- Clinical Care Options (www.clinicaloptions.com/HIV.aspx)
- Comprehensive HIV/AIDS Resource (www.thebody.com)
- Hep C Connection (www.hepc-connection.org)
- HIV Drug Interactions: www.HIV-druginteractions.org
- HIV Hepatitis Resources (www.mpaetc.org/hep)
- HIV and Hepatitis.com (www.hivandhepatitis.com)
- HIV and Observations (blogs.jwatch.org/hiv-id-observations/)
- International AIDS Society—USA (www.iasusa.org)
- Johns Hopkins Hepatitis C and HIV Coinfection Information (www.hopkins-hivguide. org/diagnosis/opportunistic_infections/viral/full_hepatitis_c.html)
- Journal Watch: AIDS Clinical Care (aids-clinical-care.jwatch.org)
- Medscape HIV/AIDS (www.medscape.com/hiv)
- National AIDS Treatment Advocacy Project (www.natap.org)
- National Clinicians' Post-exposure Prophylaxis Hotline (www.ucsf.edu/hivcntr/ Hotlines/PEPline.html)
- National HIV/AIDS Clinicians' Consultation Center (www.nccc.ucsf.edu/)
- National Institute of Allergy and Infectious Diseases (www3.niaid.nih.gov/)
- National Library of Medicine—AIDS Portal (sis.nlm.nih.gov/hiv.html)
- National Library of Medicine—MedlinePlus AIDS page (www.nlm.nih.gov/medlineplus/)

REFERENCE

1. Krakower D, Kwan CK, Yassa DS, Colvin RA. iAIDS: HIV-Related Internet Resources for the Practicing Clinician <http://www.ncbi.nlm.nih.gov/pubmed/20738185>. Clin Infect Dis 2010, Aug 25.

INDEX